JAMA
Guide to Statistics and Methods

Edward H. Livingston, MD
Roger J. Lewis, MD, PhD

Notice

Medicine is an ever-changing science. As new research and clinical experience broaden our knowledge, changes in treatment and drug therapy are required. The authors and the publisher of this work have checked with sources believed to be reliable in their efforts to provide information that is complete and generally in accord with the standards accepted at the time of publication. However, in view of the possibility of human error or changes in medical sciences, neither the authors nor the publisher nor any other party who has been involved in the preparation or publication of this work warrants that the information contained herein is in every respect accurate or complete, and they disclaim all responsibility for any errors or omissions or for the results obtained from use of the information contained in this work. Readers are encouraged to confirm the information contained herein with other sources. For example and in particular, readers are advised to check the product information sheet included in the package of each drug they plan to administer to be certain that the information contained in this work is accurate and that changes have not been made in the recommended dose or in the contraindications for administration. This recommendation is of particular importance in connection with new or infrequently used drugs.

JAMA Guide to Statistics and Methods

Editors

Edward H. Livingston, MD
Roger J. Lewis, MD, PhD

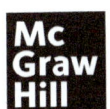

New York   Chicago   San Francisco   Athens
London   Madrid   Mexico City   Milan
New Delhi   Singapore   Sydney   Toronto

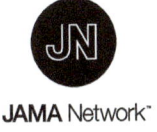

JAMA Network

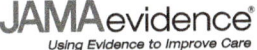

Using Evidence to Improve Care

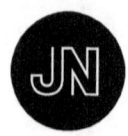

JAMA Network™

JAMA Guide to Statistics and Methods
Copyright © 2020 American Medical Association. All rights reserved. Published by McGraw-Hill Education. Except as permitted under the United States Copyright Act of 1976, no part of this publication may be reproduced or distributed in any form or by any means, or stored in a data base or retrieval system, without the prior written permission of the publisher.

JAMAevidence® is a registered trademark of the American Medical Association.

1 2 3 4 5 6 7 8 9   LCR   24 23 22 21 20 19

ISBN: 978-1-260-45532-8
MHID: 1-260-45532-7

JAMA Network Journals:
Editor in Chief: Howard Bauchner, MD
Executive Managing Editor: Annette Flanagin, RN, MA
Deputy Editor, Clinical Reviews and Education: Edward H. Livingston, MD
Assistant Editor: Kate Pezalla, MA
Cover Illustrator: Andy Rekito, MS

McGraw-Hill Professional:
This book was set in Minion Pro, Regular, 10/12 pt, by MPS Limited.
The editors were Susan Barnes and Rhiannon Wong.
The production supervisor was Richard Ruzycka.
Project management was provided by Jyoti Shaw and Poonam Bisht, MPS Limited.

This book is printed on acid-free paper.

Library of Congress Cataloging-in-Publication Data

Names: Livingston, Edward H., editor., Lewis, Roger J., editors. | JAMA Network, issuing body.
Title: JAMA guide to statistics and methods / [edited by] Edward H. Livingston, Roger J. Lewis.
Description: New York : McGraw-Hill Education, [2020] | Includes
 bibliographical references and index. | Summary: "A new, accessible guide to explanations about statistical analytic approaches and methods used in medical research from the experts at JAMA"— Provided by publisher.
Identifiers: LCCN 2019022195 | ISBN 9781260455328 (alk. paper) | ISBN 1260455327 (alk. paper) | ISBN 9781260455335 (ebook)
Subjects: MESH: Statistics as Topic | Biomedical Research
Classification: LCC R853.S7 | NLM WA 950 | DDC 610.72/7—dc23
LC record available at https://lccn.loc.gov/2019022195

McGraw-Hill Education books are available at special quantity discounts to use as premiums and sales promotions or for use in corporate training programs. To contact a representative, please visit the Contact Us pages at www.mhprofessional.com.

CONTENTS

Organizational Structure of This Book — xxiv
  Interventional Studies
    Trial Strategy and Design
    Enrollment, Allocation of Treatment, and Ethics
    Measurement Outcome and Analysis and Interpretation of Results
    Application of Results
  Observational Studies
    Study Strategy and Design
    Assessment of Risk Factors and Exposures
    Measurement Outcome and Analysis and Interpretation of Results
    Application of Results
  Practical Guide to Data Sets

Foreword — xxvii
Preface — xxxi
Editors and Contributors — xxxiii

INTERVENTIONAL STUDIES
Trial Strategy and Design

Noninferiority Trials: Is a New Treatment Almost as Effective as Another? — 1

Use of the Method
  Why Are Noninferiority Trials Conducted?
  What Are the Limitations of Noninferiority Trials?
  Why Was a Noninferiority Trial Conducted in This Case?
  How Should the Results Be Interpreted?
Caveats to Consider When Looking at a Noninferiority Trial

Dose-Finding Trials: Optimizing Phase 2 Data in the Drug Development Process 9

Use of the Method
    Why Are Dose-Response Models Used?
    What Are the Limitations of Dose-Response Modeling?
    Why Did the Authors Use Dose-Response Modeling in This Particular Study?
    How Should the Dose-Response Findings Be Interpreted in This Particular Study?
Caveats to Consider When Looking at Results Based on a Dose-Response Model

Pragmatic Trials: Practical Answers to "Real World" Questions 17

Use of the Method
    Why Are Pragmatic Trials Conducted?
    Description of the Method
What Are the Limitations of Pragmatic Trials?
Why Was a Pragmatic Trial Conducted in This Case?
How Should the Results Be Interpreted?

Cluster Randomized Trials: Evaluating Treatments Applied to Groups 25

Use of the Method
    Why Is Cluster Randomization Used?
    What Are Limitations of Cluster Randomization?
    Why Did the Authors Use Cluster Randomization in This Particular Study?
    How Should Cluster Randomization Findings Be Interpreted in This Particular Study?
Caveats to Consider When Looking at a Cluster Randomized Trial

The Stepped-Wedge Clinical Trial: Evaluation by Rolling Deployment   33

Use of the Method
   Why Is a Stepped-Wedge Clinical Trial Design Used?
   Description of the Stepped-Wedge Clinical Trial Design
Limitations of the Stepped-Wedge Design
How Was the Stepped-Wedge Design Used?
How Should a Stepped-Wedge Clinical Trial Be Interpreted?

Sample Size Calculation for a Hypothesis Test   41

Use of the Method
   Why Is Power Analysis Used?
   What Are the Limitations of Power Analysis?
   Why Did the Authors Use Power Analysis in This Particular Study?
   How Should This Method's Findings Be Interpreted in This Particular Study?
Caveats to Consider When Looking at Results Based on Power Analysis

Minimal Clinically Important Difference: Defining What Really Matters to Patients   49

Use of the Method
   Why Is the MCID Used?
   What Are the Limitations of MCID Derivation Methods?
   Why Did the Authors Use MCID in This Particular Study?
   How Should MCID Findings Be Interpreted in This Particular Study?
Caveats to Consider When Looking at Results Based on MCIDs

Enrollment, Allocation of Treatment, and Ethics

Randomization in Clinical Trials: Permuted Blocks and Stratification — 57

Explanation of the Concept
    What Are Permuted Blocks and Stratified Randomization?
    Why Are Permuted Blocks and Stratified Randomization Important?
Limitations of Permuted Block Randomization and Stratified Randomization
    How Were These Approaches to Randomization Used?
    How Does the Approach to Randomization Affect the Trial's Interpretation?

Equipoise in Research: Integrating Ethics and Science in Human Research — 65

What Is Equipoise?
Why Is Equipoise Important?
What Are the Limitations of Equipoise?
How Is Equipoise Applied in This Case?
How Does Equipoise Influence the Interpretation of the Study?

Measurement Outcomes and Analysis and Interpretation of Results

Time-to-Event Analysis — 73

Use of the Method
    Why Is Time-to-Event Analysis Used?
    What Are the Limitations of the Proportional Hazards Model?
    How Should Time-to-Event Findings Be Interpreted in This Particular Study?
Caveats to Consider When Looking at Results from a Time-to-Event Analysis

The "Utility" in Composite Outcome Measures: Measuring What Is Important to Patients   81

Why Are Composite End Points Used in Clinical Studies?

Limitations of Composite End Points
How Were Composite End Points Used in This Study?

How Does the Use of a Composite End Point Affect the Interpretation of This Study?

Missing Data: How to Best Account for What Is Not Known   89

Use of the Method
    Why Are These Methods Used?
    What Are the Limitations of These Methods?
    Why Did the Authors Use This Method in This Particular Study?
    How Should This Method's Findings Be Interpreted in This Particular Study?

Caveats to Consider When Looking at the Results in This Study Based on This Method

The Intention-to-Treat Principle: How to Assess the True Effect of Choosing a Medical Treatment   97

Use of the Method
    Why Is ITT Analysis Used?
    What Are the Limitations of ITT Analysis?
    Why Did the Authors Use ITT Analysis in This Particular Study?

Caveats to Consider When Looking at Results Based on ITT Analysis

Analyzing Repeated Measurements Using Mixed Models   105

Use of the Method

    Why Are Mixed Models Used for Repeated Measures Data?

    What Are the Limitations of Mixed Models?

    Why Did the Authors Use Mixed Models in This Particular Study?

Caveats to Consider When Looking at Results From Mixed Models

Logistic Regression: Relating Patient Characteristics to Outcomes   113

Use of the Method

    Why Is Logistic Regression Used?

    Description of the Method

    What Are the Limitations of Logistic Regression?

    Why Did the Authors Use Logistic Regression in This Study?

    How Should the Results of Logistic Regression Be Interpreted in This Particular Study?

Caveats to Consider When Assessing the Results of a Logistic Regression Analysis

Logistic Regression Diagnostics: Understanding How Well a Model Predicts Outcomes   121

Use of the Method

    Why Are Logistic Regression Model Diagnostics Used?

    Description of the Method

    What Are the Limitations of Logistic Regression Diagnostics?

    Why Did the Authors Use Logistic Regression Diagnostics in This Particular Study?

    How Should the Results of Logistic Regression Diagnostics Be Interpreted in This Particular Study?

Caveats to Consider When Assessing the Results of Logistic Regression Diagnostics

Number Needed to Treat: Conveying the Likelihood of a Therapeutic Effect   129

Explanation of the Concept
    What Is the NNT?
    Why Is the NNT Important?
Limitations and Alternatives to the NNT
    How Was the Concept of NNT Applied in This Particular Study?
    How Should the NNT Be Interpreted in the Study by Zhao et al?

Multiple Comparison Procedures   137

Use of the Method
    Why Are Multiple Comparison Procedures Used?
    What Are the Limitations of Multiple Comparison Procedures?
    Why Did the Authors Use Multiple Comparison Procedures in This Particular Study?
    How Should This Method's Findings Be Interpreted in This Particular Study?
Caveats to Consider When Looking at Multiple Comparison Procedures
    To Adjust or Not
    Confirmatory vs Exploratory
    FWER vs FDR
    Definition of Family

Gatekeeping Strategies for Avoiding False-Positive Results in Clinical Trials With Many Comparisons   145

Use of the Method
    Why Is Serial Gatekeeping Used?
    Description of the Method
What Are the Limitations of Gatekeeping Strategies?
How Was Gatekeeping Used in This Case?
How Should the Results Be Interpreted?

Multiple Imputation: A Flexible Tool for Handling Missing Data　　153

Use of the Method
    Why Is Multiple Imputation Used?
    What Are the Limitations of Multiple Imputation?
    Why Did the Authors Use Multiple Imputation in This Particular Study?
    How Should Multiple Imputation Findings Be Interpreted in This Particular Study?
Caveats to Consider When Looking at Results Based on Multiple Imputation

Interpretation of Clinical Trials That Stopped Early　　161

Use of the Method
    Why Is Early Stopping Used?
    What Are the Limitations of Early Stopping?
    Why Did the Authors Use Early Stopping in This Study?
    How Should Early Stopping Be Interpreted in This Particular Study?
Caveats to Consider When Looking at a Trial That Stopped Early

Bayesian Analysis: Using Prior Information to Interpret the Results of Clinical Trials　　169

Prior Information
    What Is Prior Information?
    Why Is Prior Information Important?
Limitations of Prior Information
How Was Prior Information Used?
How Should the Trial Results Be Interpreted in Light of the Prior Information?

Application of Results

Decision Curve Analysis 175

Use of the Method
    Why Is DCA Used?
    What Are the Limitations of the DCA Method?
    Why Did the Authors Use DCA in This Particular Study?
    How Should DCA Findings Be Interpreted in This Particular Study?
Caveats to Consider When Looking at Results Based on DCA

Methods for Evaluating Changes in Health Care Policy— The Difference-in-Differences Approach 183

Use of the Method
    Why Was the Difference-in-Differences Method Used?
    What Are the Limitations of the Difference-in-Differences Method?
    Why Did the Authors Use the Difference-in-Differences Method?
    How Should the Findings Be Interpreted?
Caveats to Consider When Assessing the Results of a Difference-in-Differences Analysis

OBSERVATIONAL STUDIES
Study Strategy and Design

Case-Control Studies: Using "Real-world" Evidence to Assess Association 191

Explanation of the Method
    What Are Case-Control and Nested Case-Control Studies?
    Why Are Case-Control Studies Used?
Limitations of Case-Control Studies
How Was the Method Applied in This Case?
How Does the Case-Control Design Affect the Interpretation of the Study?

Meta-analyses Can Be Credible and Useful: A New Standard — 199

Overview
The Existing Evidence
Improvements
Conclusions

Mendelian Randomization — 207

Use of the Method
    Why Is Mendelian Randomization Used?
    What Are the Limitations of Mendelian Randomization?
    How Did the Authors Use Mendelian Randomization?
Caveats to Consider When Evaluating Mendelian Randomization Studies

Using the E-Value to Assess the Potential Effect of Unmeasured Confounding in Observational Studies — 215

Why Is the E-Value Used?
What Are the Limitations of the E-Value?
Why Did the Authors Use the E-Value in This Particular Study?
How Should the E-Value Findings Be Interpreted in This Particular Study?
Caveats to Consider When Looking at Results Based on the E-Value

Assessment of Risk Factors and Exposures

Confounding by Indication in Clinical Research — 223

Addressing Confounding in Clinical Research
Use of Methods to Control Confounding

CONTENTS **xv**

What Are the Limitations of Methods to Control for Confounding?
How Should the Results Be Interpreted?
Caveats to Consider When Interpreting an Analysis Intended to Adjust for Confounding by Indication

Mediation Analysis 231

Use of the Method
    Why Is Mediation Analysis Used?
    Description of Mediation Analysis
    What Are the Limitations of Mediation Analysis?
    Why Did the Authors Use Mediation Analysis?
Caveats to Consider When Assessing the Results of Mediation Analysis

Measurement Outcome and Analysis and Interpretation of Results

Odds Ratios—Current Best Practice and Use 239

Why Report Odds Ratios From Logistic Regression?
What Are the Limitations of Odds Ratios?
How Did the Authors Use Odds Ratios?
How Should the Findings Be Interpreted?
What Caveats Should the Reader Consider?

Marginal Effects—Quantifying the Effect of Changes in Risk Factors in Logistic Regression Models 247

Use of Marginal Effects
    Why Are Marginal Effects Used?
    What Are Marginal Effects?

What Are the Limitations of Marginal Effects?

How Should the Marginal Effects Be Interpreted in Cummings et al?

Adjusting for Covariates: A Source of False Findings in Published Research Studies   255

Treatment Effects in Multicenter Randomized Clinical Trials   261

Estimating Treatment Effects in Multicenter Clinical Trials

   Why Are Differences Between Centers Considered When Estimating Treatment Effects?

   How Are Center Effects Incorporated into Estimates of Treatment Effects?

Limitations of Estimates of Treatment Effects from Multicenter Clinical Trials

How Were the Multicenter Data Analyzed in the Study by Dodick et al?

How Should the Results From This Study Be Interpreted?

The Propensity Score   269

Use of the Method

   Why Were Propensity Methods Used?

   What Are the Limitations of Propensity Score Methods?

   Why Did the Authors Use Propensity Methods?

   How Should the Findings Be Interpreted?

What Caveats Should the Reader Consider When Assessing the Results of Propensity Analyses?

Using Free-Response Receiver Operating Characteristic Curves to Assess the Accuracy of Machine Diagnosis of Cancer 277

Why Are FROC Curves Used?
How Are FROC Curves Constructed?
What Are the Limitations of FROC Curves?
How Should the FROC Curves Be Interpreted in This Study?
Caveats to Consider When Looking at FROC Curves

Random-Effects Meta-analysis: Summarizing Evidence With Caveats 285

Why Is Random-Effects Meta-analysis Used?
Description of Random-Effects Meta-analysis
Why Did the Authors Use Random-Effects Meta-analysis?
What Are Limitations of a Random-Effects Meta-analysis?
Caveats to Consider When Assessing the Results of a Random-Effects Meta-analysis
How Should the Results of a Random-Effects Meta-analysis Be Interpreted in This Particular Study?

Bayesian Hierarchical Models 293

Why Is a BHM Used?
What Are the Limitations of BHMs?
How Were BHMs Used in This Case?
How Should BHMs Be Interpreted?

Application of Results

Evaluating Discrimination of Risk Prediction Models: The C Statistic 301

Use of the Method
    Why Are C Statistics Used?
    What Are the Limitations of the C Statistic?
    Why Did the Authors Use C Statistics in Their Study?
    How Should the Findings Be Interpreted?
Caveats to Consider When Using C Statistics to Assess Predictive Model Performance

Overview of Cost-effectiveness Analysis 309

The Use of Cost-effectiveness Analysis
Description of Cost-effectiveness Analysis
Limitation in the Use of Cost-effectiveness Analysis
How Was the Cost-effectiveness Analysis Performed in This Study?
How Should the Cost-effectiveness Analysis Be Interpreted in This Study?

Choosing a Time Horizon in Cost and Cost-effectiveness Analyses 317

The Use of Time Horizon in a Cost-effectiveness Analysis
Limitations Regarding Selection of Time Horizons
How Was Time Horizon Defined and Used in the Study?
How Does the Time Horizon Selected by Wittenborn et al Affect the
    Interpretation of the Study?

On Deep Learning for Medical Image Analysis 325

Opening the Deep Learning Black Box
What Are the Limitations of Deep Learning Methods?

PRACTICAL GUIDE TO DATA SETS

A Checklist to Elevate the Science of Surgical Database Research   333

Tips for Analyzing Large Data Sets From the *JAMA Surgery* Statistical Editors   341

Study Population Considerations
Methodological and Sample Size Considerations
Data Elements and Presentation
Analytic and Statistical Considerations
Conclusions

Practical Guide to Surgical Data Sets: Healthcare Cost and Utilization Project National Inpatient Sample (NIS)   349

Introduction to the Healthcare Cost and Utilization Project
Strengths of Administrative Data
Limitations of Administrative Data and the HCUP Databases
    Administrative Data Limitations
    NIS Limitations
Critical Methodologic Considerations
Unique Capabilities of HCUP

Practical Guide to Surgical Data Sets: Surveillance, Epidemiology, and End Results (SEER) Database   359

Introduction
Data Considerations
    Data Sources

Time Trend Data
Cancer Data
Treatment Data
Statistical Considerations
Conclusions

Practical Guide to Surgical Data Sets: Medicare Claims Data — 367

Introduction
Pros and Cons of Medicare Data
Potential Avenues of Research
    Comparative Effectiveness Research
    Health Policy Evaluation
    Understanding Variation
Where to Find More Information

Practical Guide to Surgical Data Sets: Military Health System Tricare Encounter Data — 375

Introduction
Use of the Data
    Salient and Unique Features of the Data Set
    How Are Data Compiled?
    What Are Common Outcomes That Can Be Studied?
    What Are the Limitations With This Data Set?
Statistical Considerations
Where to Find More Information

Practical Guide to Surgical Data Sets: Veterans Affairs Surgical Quality Improvement Program (VASQIP) 383

Advent of the Veterans Affairs Surgical Quality Improvement Program
Data Considerations
- Patients
- Procedure
- Hospital
- Outcomes

Utility and Unique Features of VASQIP
Statistical Considerations
Conclusions

Practical Guide to Surgical Data Sets: National Surgical Quality Improvement Program (NSQIP) and Pediatric NSQIP 391

Introduction
Data Elements and Considerations
- Access and Logistics
- Variables and Outcomes
- Statistical Methodology
- Limitations

Conclusions

Practical Guide to Surgical Data Sets: Metabolic and Bariatric Surgery Accreditation and Quality Program (MBSAQIP) 399

Introduction
Data Considerations for the MBSAQIP Participant Use File

Deidentification of Patients, Facilities, and Clinicians
MBSAQIP PUF Content
Outcomes
Statistical Considerations
MBSAQIP PUF Advantages and Limitations
Conclusions

Practical Guide to Surgical Data Sets: National Cancer Database (NCDB)   407

Introduction
Data Element Considerations
    Hospital Variables
    Tumor Characteristics
    Treatment Variables
    Outcomes
Analytic and Statistical Considerations
Conclusions

Practical Guide to Surgical Data Sets: National Trauma Data Bank (NTDB)   415

Introduction
Data Compilation and Structure
Methods
Limitations
Recommended Reading
Conclusions

Practical Guide to Surgical Data Sets: Society for Vascular Surgery Vascular Quality Initiative (SVS VQI)   423

Features of the Data Set
Statistical Considerations
Conclusions

Practical Guide to Surgical Data Sets: Society of Thoracic Surgeons (STS) National Database   431

Introduction
Data Element Considerations
   Adult Cardiac Surgery Database (ACSD)
   Congenital Heart Surgery Database
   General Thoracic Surgery Database
   Data Source
   Outcomes and Other Key Measures
   Accessing Data
   Statistical Considerations
   Limitations
Conclusions

Glossary	439
Index	467

ORGANIZATIONAL STRUCTURE OF THIS BOOK

Interventional Studies	Trial Strategy and Design	Enrollment, Allocation of Treatment, and Ethics
	• Noninferiority Trials • Dose-Finding Trials • Pragmatic Trials • Cluster Randomized Trials • The Stepped-Wedge Clinical Trial • Sample Size Calculation for a Hypothesis Test • Minimal Clinically Important Difference	• Randomization in Clinical Trials • Equipoise in Research
Observational Studies	Study Strategy and Design	Assessment of Risk Factors and Exposures
	• Case-Control Studies • Meta-analyses Can Be Credible and Useful • Mendelian Randomization • Using the E-Value to Assess the Potential Effect of Unmeasured Confounding in Observational Studies	• Confounding by Indication in Clinical Research • Mediation Analysis
Practical Guide to Data Sets	• 13 Articles	

Measurement Outcome and Analysis and Interpretation of Results

- Time-to-Event Analysis
- The "Utility" in Composite Outcome Measures
- Missing Data
- The Intention-to-Treat Principle
- Analyzing Repeated Measurements Using Mixed Models
- Logistic Regression
- Logistic Regression Diagnostics
- Number Needed to Treat
- Multiple Comparison Procedures
- Gatekeeping Strategies for Avoiding False-Positive Results in Clinical Trials With Many Comparisons
- Multiple Imputation
- Interpretation of Clinical Trials That Stopped Early
- Bayesian Analysis

Application of Results

- Decision Curve Analysis
- Methods for Evaluating Changes in Health Care Policy—The Difference-in-Differences Approach

Measurement Outcome and Analysis and Interpretation of Results

- Odds Ratios—Current Best Practice and Use
- Marginal Effects—Quantifying the Effect of Changes in Risk Factors in Logistic Regression Models
- Adjusting for Covariates
- Treatment Effects in Multicenter Randomized Clinical Trials
- The Propensity Score
- Using Free-Response Receiver Operating Characteristic Curves to Assess the Accuracy of Machine Diagnosis of Cancer
- Random-Effects Meta-analysis
- Bayesian Hierarchical Models

Application of Results

- Evaluating Discrimination of Risk Prediction Models
- Overview of Cost-effectiveness Analysis
- Choosing a Time Horizon in Cost and Cost-effectiveness Analysis
- On Deep Learning for Medical Image Analysis

FOREWORD

The evidence-based medicine (EBM) movement—perhaps officially launched in 1991 with the first article in the medical literature that used the term,[1,2] but with antecedents that go back considerably further—advocates that systematic summaries of the highest quality relevant evidence should inform our clinical care.[3-5] With this premise, clinicians should have some understanding of what constitutes more vs less trustworthy evidence. The widespread acceptance of the principle, and the corollary regarding physician familiarity with evidentiary standards, has resulted in a major change in medical education. Requirements exist throughout North America, and in many other countries, that both undergraduate and postgraduate medical training include attention to skills of accurately interpreting the medical literature.

As EBM was being launched, *JAMA* became a champion for the development and dissemination of the new approach to clinical practice.[4-6] *JAMA*'s *Users' Guides to the Medical Literature* provided the core educational materials for EBM, and became established as required reading for frontline clinicians, and medical educators, in understanding the literature and using the literature to inform clinical practice. The series has provided the core material for all subsequent EBM educational resources.

Although the Users' Guides have played a key role in EBM education they have, as any resource will, limitations that require complementary material. The Users' Guides all have a broad scope, addressing how clinicians should read primary articles and systematic reviews informing choice of therapy, evaluating claims of harm, establishing prognosis, evaluating diagnostic tests, and so on. *JAMA*, again wisely and with the initiative to innovation, recognized the limitation: the articles do not focus on specific methodologic and statistical issues that clinicians would ideally understand when using the medical literature to guide their care.

This is particularly relevant because the statistical and methodologic world has not stood still. Clinicians may not be familiar with research methods introduced after they completed training. Recognizing the unmet clinician needs, *JAMA* introduced its Guide to Statistics and Methods series to provide a more granular and specific discussion regarding statistics and research methodology. The series has proved very successful, with over 55 publications to date.

The articles address a number of crucial themes in understanding the research literature. Within the broad category of interventional studies, issues addressed have included trial strategy and design; enrollment, allocation of treatment, and ethics; measurement of outcomes, analyses, and interpretation of results; and application of results. Issues relevant to observational studies have included study strategy and design; assessment of risk factors and exposure; measurement of outcomes, analyses, and interpretation of results; and application of results. Another group of 13 articles within the series offer practical guides to surgical data sets.

These guides on statistical and methodologic issues are highly relevant to clinicians. First, they address statistical and analytic approaches and methods used in research reported in *JAMA* and JAMA Network journal articles. These research articles use the particular statistical tests or methodologic approaches under discussion, and thus provide—a key to any EBM educational material—relevant examples. In addition, the articles address concepts that clinicians will repeatedly see in the medical literature.

Another great merit of the *JAMA* Guide to Statistics and Methods series is its accessibility. The articles are written in plain English, using language practicing clinicians can easily understand, avoiding complex mathematics or the use of arcane technical language, and presenting material graphically whenever possible. Linking the methods articles to published research reports further enhances accessibility and usefulness of the statistical and methodologic concepts discussed.

Although I am a methodologist, as with any scientist, the scope of my expertise is limited, and I am vulnerable to ignorance in areas that have developed and expanded after I received my training. Thus, I have a number of articles in the series among my favorites: those in which my understanding was limited, and in which I needed lucid explanations to gain a grasp of new concepts. For example, neural networks have been around since the 1980s, but have only gained popularity since the increasing sophistication that has accompanied advances in machine learning, and in particular in application to medical imaging. An article addressing convolutional neural networks applied to medical imaging opened the black box, providing a clear and compelling explanation of the fundamental principles underlying the method. The article also links to a very helpful video.

Although I have been involved in primary interventional studies, they have almost exclusively been randomized trials. As a clinical epidemiologist, I am also familiar with standard observational cohort and case-control studies, but much less so with less common and more complex observational study designs such as stepped-wedge clinical trials. The design made feasible a study of a quality improvement intervention to reduce complications after myocardial infarction that could not have succeeded within a conventional randomized trial. The article in this series on stepped-wedge clinical trial design clearly explains the advantages and limitations of this approach. As a methodologist, I was gratified to learn that although a naïve analysis suggested a benefit, the sophisticated analysis that was possible because of the stepped-wedge design showed a different result. While the intervention was ongoing, clinical care was improving independently, and the optimal adjusted analysis demonstrated that it was this secular improvement, rather than the intervention, that improved outcomes.

Now, *JAMA* has wisely and helpfully collected the articles in the series into a single book, which has also been incorporated into JAMAevidence online.[7] Clinicians interested in deepening their understanding of the articles that guide their clinical practice will find the collection a highly accessible and extremely informative source of information.

Gordon Guyatt, MD, MSc
McMaster University

References

1. Department of Clinical Epidemiology & Biostatistics, McMaster University. How to read clinical journals, I: why to read them and how to start reading them critically. *Can Med Assoc J*. 1981;124(5):555-558.
2. Evidence-Based Medicine Working Group. Evidence-based medicine: a new approach to teaching the practice of medicine. *JAMA*. 1992;268(17):2420-2425.
3. Guyatt G. Evidence-based medicine. *ACP J Club (Ann Intern Med)*. 1991;114 (suppl 2):A-16.
4. Evidence-based medicine—an oral history website. http://ebm.jamanetwork.com. Accessed August 17, 2014.
5. Smith R, Rennie D. Evidence-based medicine—an oral history. *JAMA*. 2014;311(4):365-367.
6. Guyatt GH, Rennie D. Users' Guides to the Medical Literature. *JAMA*. 1993;270(17):2096-2097.
7. JAMAevidence website. https://jamaevidence.mhmedical.com/. Accessed April 4, 2019.

PREFACE

The quantity and diversity of scientific publications are vast and rapidly expanding. Yet, the quality of the underlying methodology is highly variable and many studies have poor study design or analysis. While editors at traditional journals invest substantial efforts to help ensure published studies are performed and interpreted correctly, readers of those journals will be better equipped to apply study results to their individual clinical practice if they appreciate the strengths and weaknesses of the underlying research methodology. With the increasing popularity of preprint servers, clinicians will read scientific reports prior to rigorous peer review, which requires the ability to independently evaluate the design, analysis, and interpretation of clinical studies. Now, more than ever, clinicians must have sufficient understanding of study methodology to judge if what they are reading is likely to be valid and applicable to the patients they treat.

Statistics is generally not a very popular course in medical school; thus, many clinicians do not have a firm understanding of traditional study design and statistical analysis. Many medical statistics courses emphasize mathematics along with myriad assumptions and rules that do not resonate with clinicians who pursued medical school because of their love of biologic science and interest in helping others, rather than an interest in mathematics. Further, there are many new statistical methods that are increasingly important in clinical research that clinicians may have never seen before.

The *JAMA Guide to Statistics and Methods* was created to help clinicians overcome these challenges. Research methods are described in plain English without reliance on equations and without any assumption that the reader understands the field of statistics. We distinguish between statistics and methods: statistics are mathematical approaches to describing collections of data and associated uncertainty, whereas methods refer to how a study was designed or some other aspect of how a study was organized and conducted. Each article explains how a statistical or methodologic concept, or the results of a statistical analysis, should be applied or interpreted in an example research article published in *JAMA* or JAMA Network journals, along with the limitations associated with the data and the methodology used to evaluate them. The intent of these guides is to enable clinicians to better understand research findings so that they can competently assess if study results are reliable enough to adopt them into clinical practice.

This book is organized into major sections: Interventional Studies and Observational Studies. Each of these has 4 subsections. For Interventional Studies these subsections are (1) Trial Strategy and Design, (2) Enrollment, Allocation of Treatment, and Ethics, (3) Measurement of Outcomes, Analyses, and Interpretation of Results, and (4) Application of Results. The subsections for Observational Studies are similar: (1) Study Strategy and Design, (2) Assessment of Risk Factors and Exposures, (3) Measurement of Outcomes, Analyses, and Interpretation of Results, and (4) Application of Results. A third section provides guides for interpreting studies of large surgical data sets to enable clinicians to better understand these types of studies.

We thank the contributors to this series who represent leaders in clinical research, methods, and statistics. They are listed on the following pages.

The *JAMA Guide to Statistics and Methods* is not meant to be a comprehensive overview of all possible methodology used in medical research. Rather, by basing topics on recently published articles, methods emphasized are those commonly in use. For clinicians negotiating the ever-expanding medical literature, these topics will be the ones that they are likely to see and must understand to determine the relevancy of research findings to their clinical practice.

Edward H. Livingston, MD
Roger J. Lewis, MD, PhD

EDITOR AND CONTRIBUTORS

EDITOR

Roger J. Lewis, MD, PhD is Chair of the Department of Emergency Medicine at Harbor-UCLA Medical Center, Professor and Vice Chair in the Department of Emergency Medicine at the David Geffen School of Medicine at UCLA, and the Senior Medical Scientist at Berry Consultants, LLC. Dr Lewis is a member of the National Academy of Medicine of the National Academies and a Fellow of both the Society for Clinical Trials and the American Statistical Association.

CONTRIBUTORS

David B. Allison, PhD
Office of Energetics and Nutrition Obesity Research Center
Department of Biostatistics
School of Public Health
University of Alabama at Birmingham
Birmingham, Alabama

David Arterburn, MD
Kaiser Permanente Washington Health Research Institute
Department of Medicine
University of Washington, Seattle
Seattle, Washington

Anirban Basu, PhD
The Comparative Health Outcomes, Policy, and Economics (CHOICE) Institute
Departments of Pharmacy, Health, Services and Economics
University of Washington, Seattle
Seattle, Washington

Karl Y. Bilimoria, MD, MS
Surgical Outcomes and Quality Improvement Center
Department of Surgery and Center for Healthcare Studies
Feinberg School of Medicine
Northwestern University
Chicago, Illinois

Kristine Broglio, MS
Berry Consultants, LLC
Austin, Texas

Jing Cao, PhD
Department of Statistical Science
Southern Methodist University
Dallas, Texas

Lawrence Carin, PhD
Duke University
Durham, North Carolina

Danny Chu, MD
Department of Cardiothoracic
 Surgery
University of Pittsburgh School
 of Medicine
Pittsburgh, Pennsylvania

Jason T. Connor, PhD
Berry Consultants, LLC
Austin, Texas
University of Central Florida
 College of Medicine
Orlando, Florida

Ralph B. D'Agostino Sr, PhD
Department of Mathematics and
 Statistics
Boston University
Boston, Massachusetts

Sapan S. Desai, MD, PhD, MBA
Performance Improvement
Department of Vascular Surgery
Northwest Community
 Hospital
Arlington Heights, Illinois

Michelle A. Detry, PhD
Berry Consultants, LLC
Austin, Texas

Justin B. Dimick, MD, MPH
The Center for Healthcare
 Outcomes and Policy
Institute for Healthcare Policy
 and Innovation
Department of Surgery
University of Michigan School of
 Medicine,
Department of Health Policy &
 Management
University of Michigan School of
 Public Health
Ann Arbor, Michigan
Surgical Innovation Editor,
 JAMA Surgery

Kemi M. Doll, MD, MSCR
Division of Gynecologic
 Oncology
Department of Obstetrics and
 Gynecology
University of Washington,
 Seattle
Seattle Cancer Care Alliance
Seattle, Washington

Bryan E. Dowd, PhD
Division of Health Policy and
 Management
School of Public Health
University of Minnesota,
 Minneapolis
Minneapolis, Minnesota

Susan S. Ellenberg, PhD
Department of Biostatistics, Epidemiology, and Informatics
Perelman School of Medicine
University of Pennsylvania
Philadelphia, Pennsylvania

Connor A. Emdin, DPhil
Center for Genomic Medicine
Massachusetts General Hospital
Harvard Medical School
Boston, Massachusetts,
Cardiovascular Disease Initiative
Broad Institute
Cambridge, Massachusetts

Farhood Farjah, MD, MPH
Department of Surgery
University of Washington
Seattle, Washington

Mark Fitzgerald, PhD
Berry Consultants, LLC
Austin, Texas

Amir A. Ghaferi, MD, MS
Department of Surgery
University of Michigan School of Medicine
Institute for Healthcare Policy and Innovation
Ann Arbor, Michigan

Steven N. Goodman, MD, PhD
Department of Health Research and Policy
Meta-research Innovation Center at Stanford
Department of Medicine
Stanford University School of Medicine
Palo Alto, California

Adil H. Haider, MD, MPH
Department of Surgery
Brigham and Women's Hospital
Center for Surgery and Public Health
Harvard Medical School
Boston, Massachusetts
Deputy Editor, *JAMA Surgery*

Sebastien Haneuse, PhD
Department of Biostatistics
Harvard T.H. Chan School of Public Health
Boston, Massachusetts

Zain G. Hashmi, MBBS
Center for Surgery and Public Health
Harvard Medical School and Harvard School of Public Health
Department of Surgery
Brigham & Women's Hospital
Boston, Massachusetts
Department of Surgery
Sinai Hospital of Baltimore
Baltimore, Maryland

Jason S. Haukoos, MD, MSc
Department of Emergency Medicine
University of Colorado School of Medicine
Denver, Colorado

Elliott R. Haut, MD, PhD
Department of Surgery
Johns Hopkins University School of Medicine
Department of Health Policy and Management
Johns Hopkins Bloomberg School of Public Health
Baltimore, Maryland

Robert D. Herbert, PhD
Neuroscience Research Australia (NeuRA)
School of Medical Sciences
Faculty of Medicine
University of New South Wales
Sydney, New South Wales, Australia

Terry Hyslop, PhD
Department of Biostatistics and Bioinformatics
Duke University
Durham, North Carolina
Statistical Editor, *JAMA Surgery*

John P. A. Ioannidis, MD, DSc
Departments of Medicine and Health Research and Policy
Meta-Research Innovation Center at Stanford
Stanford University School of Medicine
Palo Alto, California

Telba Z. Irony, PhD
Office of Biostatistics and Epidemiology
Center for Biologics Evaluation and Research
US Food and Drug Administration
Silver Spring, Maryland

Kamal M. F. Itani, MD
Veterans Affairs Boston Healthcare System
Boston University
Harvard Medical School
Boston, Massachusetts

Amy H. Kaji, MD, PhD
Department of Emergency Medicine
Harbor-UCLA Medical Center
David Geffen School of Medicine at UCLA
Torrance, California,
Los Angeles Biomedical Research Institute
Los Angeles, California
Statistical Editor, *JAMA Surgery*

Sekar Kathiresan, MD
Center for Genomic Medicine
Massachusetts General Hospital
Harvard Medical School
Boston, Massachusetts
Cardiovascular Disease Initiative
Broad Institute
Cambridge, Massachusetts

Amit V. Khera, MD
Center for Genomic Medicine
Massachusetts General Hospital
Harvard Medical School
Boston, Massachusetts,
Cardiovascular Disease
　Initiative
Broad Institute
Cambridge, Massachusetts

Melina R. Kibbe, MD
Department of Surgery
University of North Carolina at
　Chapel Hill
Chapel Hill, North Carolina
Editor, *JAMA Surgery*

Helena Chmura Kraemer, PhD
Department of Psychiatry and
　Behavioral Sciences
Stanford University (Emerita)
Palo Alto, California
Statistical Editor, *JAMA Psychiatry*

**Demetrios N. Kyriacou,
MD, PhD**
Departments of Emergency
　Medicine and Preventive
　Medicine
Northwestern University
　Feinberg School of Medicine
Chicago, Illinois
Senior Editor, *JAMA*

Hopin Lee, PhD
Centre for Statistics in Medicine
Nuffield Department of
　Orthopaedics
Rheumatology and
　Musculoskeletal Sciences
University of Oxford
Oxford, United Kingdom
School of Medicine and Public
　Health
University of Newcastle
Newcastel, New South Wales,
　Australia

Roger J. Lewis, MD, PhD
Department of Emergency
　Medicine
Harbor-UCLA Medical Center
Department of Emergency
　Medicine
David Geffen School of Medicine
　at UCLA
Torrance, California,
Los Angeles Biomedical Research
　Institute
Los Angeles, California,
Berry Consultants, LLC
Austin, Texas

Peng Li, PhD
Office of Energetics and
　Nutrition Obesity Research
　Center
Department of Biostatistics
School of Public Health
University of Alabama at
　Birmingham
Birmingham, Alabama

Alex John London, PhD
Department of Philosophy
Carnegie Mellon University
Pittsburgh, Pennsylvania

Yan Ma, PhD
Department of Epidemiology
 and Biostatistics
Milken Institute School of Public
 Health
The George Washington
 University
Washington, District of
 Columbia

Matthew L. Maciejewski, PhD
Center for Health Services
 Research in Primary Care
Durham Veterans Affairs
 Medical Center
Durham Center of Innovation
 to Accelerate Discovery and
 Practice Transformation
 (ADAPT)
Durham Veterans Affairs Health
 Care System
Department of Population
 Health Sciences
Division of General Internal
 Medicine
Department of Medicine
Duke University School of
 Medicine
Durham, North Carolina

**Nader N. Massarweh,
MD, MPH**
Veterans Affairs Health
 Services Research &
 Development
Center for Innovations in
 Quality, Effectiveness and
 Safety
Division of Surgical Oncology
Michael E. DeBakey Department
 of Surgery
Baylor College of Medicine
Houston, Texas

James H. McAuley, PhD
Neuroscience Research Australia
 (NeuRA)
School of Medical Sciences
Faculty of Medicine
University of New South Wales
Sydney New South Wales,
 Australia

Anna E. McGlothlin, PhD
Berry Consultants, LLC
Austin, Texas

Ryan P. Merkow, MD, MS
Surgical Outcomes and Quality
 Improvement Center
Department of Surgery and
 Center for Healthcare Studies
Feinberg School of Medicine
Northwestern University
Chicago, Illinois

William J. Meurer, MD, MS
Department of Emergency
 Medicine
Department of Neurology
University of Michigan,
 Ann Arbor
Ann Arbor, Michigan

Chaya S. Moskowitz, PhD
Department of Epidemiology
 and Biostatistics
Memorial Sloan Kettering
 Cancer Center
New York, New York

Avery B. Nathens, MD, MPH, PhD
Division of Surgery
Sunnybrook Health Sciences Center
University of Toronto
Toronto, Ontario, Canada
American College of Surgeons
Chicago, Illinois

Craig D. Newgard, MD, MPH
Center for Policy and Research in Emergency Medicine
Department of Emergency Medicine
Oregon Health and Science University
Portland, Oregon

Edward C. Norton, PhD
Department of Health Management and Policy
Department of Economics
University of Michigan, Ann Arbor
Ann Arbor, Michigan,
National Bureau of Economic Research
Cambridge, Massachusetts

Timothy M. Pawlik, MD, MPH, PhD
Department of Surgery
Wexner Medical Center
Ohio State University
Columbus, Ohio
Deputy Editor, *JAMA Surgery*

Michael J. Pencina, PhD
Duke Clinical Research Institute
Department of Biostatistics and Bioinformatics
Duke University
Durham, North Carolina

Melanie Quintana, PhD
Berry Consultants, LLC
Austin, Texas

Alfred W. Rademaker, PhD
Department of Preventive Medicine
Feinberg School of Medicine
Northwestern University
Chicago, Illinois
Statistical Editor, *JAMA Surgery*

Mehul V. Raval, MD, MS
Division of Pediatric Surgery
Department of Surgery
Emory University School of Medicine
Children's Healthcare of Atlanta
Atlanta, Georgia

Andrew M. Ryan, PhD
The Center for Healthcare Outcomes and Policy
Institute for Healthcare Policy and Innovation
Department of Health Policy & Management
School of Public Health
University of Michigan, Ann Arbor
Ann Arbor, Michigan

Gillian D. Sanders, PhD
Department of Population Health Sciences
Duke University School of Medicine
Duke Clinical Research Institute
Duke-Margolis Center for Health Policy
Duke University
Durham, North Carolina

Jeffrey L. Saver, MD
Department of Neurology
Ronald Reagan–UCLA Medical Center
David Geffen School of Medicine
University of California
Los Angeles, California

Benjamin R. Saville, PhD
Berry Consultants, LLC
Austin, Texas
Department of Biostatistics
Vanderbilt University School of Medicine
Nashville, Tennessee

Andrew J. Schoenfeld, MD, MSc
Center for Surgery and Public Health
Department of Orthopaedic Surgery
Brigham and Women's Hospital
Harvard Medical School
Boston, Massachusetts

Stephen J. Senn, PhD
Luxembourg Institute of Health
Strassen, Luxembourg
Medical Statistics Group
ScHARR
The University of Sheffield
Sheffield, United Kingdom

Stylianos Serghiou, MD
Department of Health Research and Policy
Stanford University School of Medicine
Meta-research Innovation Center at Stanford
Palo Alto, California

Julie A. Sosa, MD
Department of Surgery
Department of Medicine
Duke University Medical Center
Duke Cancer Institute
Duke Clinical Research Institute
Durham, North Carolina

Harold C. Sox, MD
Patient-Centered Outcomes Research Institute
Washington, DC
Geisel School of Medicine at Dartmouth
Hanover, New Hampshire

Lynne Stokes, PhD
Department of Statistical Science
Southern Methodist University
Dallas, Texas

Elizabeth A. Stuart, PhD
Departments of Mental Health, Biostatistics, and Health Policy and Management

Bloomberg School of Public
   Health
Johns Hopkins University
Baltimore, Maryland

Jonah J. Stulberg, MD, PhD, MPH
Division of Gastrointestinal
   Surgery
Department of Surgery
Surgical Outcomes and Quality
   Improvement Center
Northwestern University
Feinberg School of Medicine
Chicago, Illinois

Dana A. Telem, MD, MPH
Department of Surgery
Center for Healthcare Outcomes
   and Policy
University of Michigan,
   Ann Arbor
Ann Arbor, Michigan

Juliana Tolles, MD, MHS
Department of Emergency
   Medicine
Harbor-UCLA Medical Center
Los Angeles Biomedical Research
   Institute
Torrance, California,
David Geffen School of Medicine
   at UCLA
Los Angeles, California

Gilbert R. Upchurch Jr, MD
Division of Vascular Surgery
University of Virginia,
   Charlottesville
Charlottesville, Virginia

Tyler J. VanderWeele, PhD
Department of Biostatistics
Department of Epidemiology
Harvard T.H. Chan School of
   Public Health
Boston, Massachusetts

Kert Viele, PhD
Berry Consultants, LLC
Austin, Texas

Kabir Yadav, MDCM, MS, MSHS
Department of Emergency Medicine
Harbor-UCLA Medical Center
Los Angeles Biomedical Research
   Institute
Torrance, California

Song Zhang, PhD
Department of Clinical
   Sciences
UT Southwestern Medical
   Center at Dallas
Dallas, Texas

Noninferiority Trials: Is a New Treatment Almost as Effective as Another?

Amy H. Kaji, MD, PhD, and
Roger J. Lewis, MD, PhD

IN THIS CHAPTER

Use of the Method

Why Are Noninferiority Trials Conducted?

What Are the Limitations of Noninferiority Trials?

Why Was a Noninferiority Trial Conducted in This Case?

How Should the Results Be Interpreted?

Caveats to Consider When Looking at a Noninferiority Trial

This JAMA Guide to Statistics and Methods describes the reasons for conducting a noninferiority trial and how to analyze and interpret the results from a trial that did.

Sometimes the goal of comparing a new treatment with a standard treatment is not to find an approach that is more effective but to find a therapy that has other advantages, such as lower cost, fewer adverse effects, or greater convenience with at least similar efficacy to the standard treatment. With other advantages, a treatment that is almost as effective as a standard treatment might be preferred in practice or for some patients. The purpose of a noninferiority trial is to rigorously evaluate a new treatment against an accepted and effective treatment with the goal of demonstrating that it is at least almost as good (ie, not inferior).

In an example published in *JAMA*, Salminen et al described the results of a multicenter noninferiority trial of 530 adults with computed tomography–confirmed acute appendicitis who were randomized either to early appendectomy (the standard treatment) or to antibiotic therapy alone (a potentially less burdensome experimental treatment).[1]

USE OF THE METHOD

Why Are Noninferiority Trials Conducted?

In a traditional clinical trial, a new treatment is compared with a standard treatment or placebo with the goal of demonstrating that the new treatment has greater efficacy. The null hypothesis for such a trial is that the 2 treatments have the same effect. Rejection of this hypothesis, implying that the effects are different, is signaled by a statistically significant *P* value or, alternatively, by a 2-tailed confidence interval that excludes no effect. While the new treatment could be either superior or inferior, the typical trial aims to demonstrate superiority of the new treatment and is known as a superiority trial. Since a superiority trial is capable of identifying both harmful and beneficial effects of a new therapy vs a control (ie, a current therapy), a 2-tailed 95% CI can be used to indicate the upper and lower limits of the difference in treatment effect that are consistent with the observed data. The null hypothesis is rejected, indicating that the new therapy differs from the control, if the confidence interval does not include the result that indicates absence of effect (eg, a risk ratio of 1 or a risk difference of 0).[2] This is equivalent to a statistically significant P value.

Although superiority or inferiority of a new treatment can be demonstrated by a superiority trial, it would generally be incorrect to conclude that the absence of a significant difference in a superiority trial demonstrates that the therapies have similar effects; absence of evidence of a difference is not reliable evidence that there is no difference. An active-controlled noninferiority trial is needed to determine whether a new intervention, which offers other advantages such as decreased toxicity or cost, does not have lesser efficacy than an established treatment.[3-6] Noninferiority trials use known effective treatments as controls because there is little to be gained by demonstrating that a new therapy is not inferior to a sham or placebo treatment.

The objective of a noninferiority trial is to demonstrate that the intervention being evaluated achieves the efficacy of the established therapy within a predetermined acceptable noninferiority margin (Figure 1). The magnitude of this margin depends on what would be a clinically important difference, the expected event rates, and, possibly, regulatory requirements. Other determinants of the noninferiority margin include the known effect of the standard treatment vs placebo; the severity of the disease; toxicity, inconvenience, or cost of the standard treatment; and the primary end point. A smaller noninferiority margin is likely appropriate if the disease under investigation is severe or if the primary end point is death.[3-6]

The sample size required to reliably demonstrate noninferiority depends on both the choice of the noninferiority margin and the assumed true relative effects of the compared

FIGURE 1

Two Different Possible Results of a Noninferiority Trial, Summarized by 1-Tailed Confidence Intervals for the Relative Efficacy of the New and Active-Control Treatments

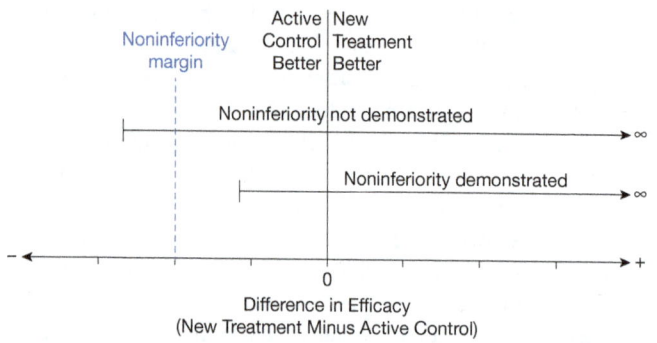

In the top example, the lower limit of the confidence interval lies to the left of the noninferiority margin, demonstrating that the results are consistent with greater inferiority (worse efficacy) than allowed by the noninferiority margin. Thus, the new treatment may be inferior and noninferiority is not demonstrated. In the lower example, the lower limit of the confidence interval lies to the right of the noninferiority margin, demonstrating noninferiority of the new treatment relative to the active-control treatment. The overall result of the trial is defined by the lower limit of the 1-sided confidence interval rather than by the point estimate for the treatment effect, so point estimates are not shown.

treatments.[3-6] An active-controlled noninferiority trial often requires a larger sample size than a superiority trial because the noninferiority margins used in noninferiority studies are generally smaller than the differences sought in superiority trials. Just as important is the assumed effect of the experimental treatment relative to the active-control treatment. The assumed effect may be that the experimental treatment is worse than the control but by a smaller amount than the noninferiority margin, that the 2 treatments are equivalent, or even that the experimental treatment is more effective. These 3 options will result in larger, intermediate, and smaller required sample sizes, respectively, to achieve the same trial power—the chance of demonstrating noninferiority—because they assume progressively better efficacy of the experimental treatment.

Because a noninferiority trial only aims to demonstrate noninferiority and does not aim to distinguish noninferiority from superiority, it is analyzed using a 1-sided confidence interval (Figure 1) or hypothesis test. Typically, a 1-sided 95% or 97.5% CI ($-L$ to ∞; negative values represent inferiority of the experimental treatment) is constructed for the difference between the 2 treatments, and the lower limit, $-L$, is compared with the noninferiority margin. Noninferiority is demonstrated if the lower confidence limit lies above or to the right of the noninferiority margin.[3-6]

What Are the Limitations of Noninferiority Trials?

A negative noninferiority trial does not in general demonstrate inferiority of the experimental treatment, just as a negative superiority trial does not demonstrate equivalence of 2 treatments.

A noninferiority trial is similar to an equivalence trial in that the objective of both is to demonstrate that the intervention matches the action of the established therapy within a prespecified margin. However, the objective of a noninferiority trial is only to demonstrate that the experimental treatment is not substantially worse than the standard treatment, whereas that of an equivalence trial is to demonstrate that the experimental treatment is neither worse than nor better than the standard treatment.[3]

Why Was a Noninferiority Trial Conducted in This Case?

Ever since McBurney demonstrated reduced morbidity from pelvic infections with appendectomy, the standard treatment for acute appendicitis has been surgery, which requires general anesthesia, incurs increased cost, and is associated with postoperative complications, such as wound infections and adhesions. Thus, a less invasive approach with similar efficacy might be preferred by many patients and physicians. Three randomized trials summarized in a recent Cochrane analysis demonstrated equipoise as to whether appendicitis can successfully be treated with antibiotics alone rather than surgery.[7] Because appendectomy is viewed as the standard treatment, it was considered the active control with which the less invasive experimental antibiotic treatment was to be compared.

To design the clinical trial, Salminen et al[1] assumed a surgical treatment success rate of 99% and prespecified a noninferiority margin of −24% based on clinical considerations. This is equivalent to saying that if the rate of treatment success with antibiotics alone could be shown to be no worse than 24% worse than the rate with surgery, then the antibiotic-only strategy would be clinically noninferior. As this study demonstrates, the selection of the noninferiority margin is often subjective rather than based on specific criteria.

How Should the Results Be Interpreted?

The results demonstrated that all but 1 of 273 patients randomized to the surgery group underwent successful appendectomy, resulting in a treatment efficacy of 99.6%. In the antibiotic treatment group, 186 of 256 patients available for follow-up had treatment successes, for a success rate of 72.7%; 70 of the 256 patients underwent surgical intervention within 1 year of initial presentation. Thus, the point estimate for the difference in success rate with the antibiotic-only strategy was −27.0% and the associated 1-tailed 95% CI would range from −31.6% to infinity. Because that interval includes efficacy values worse than the noninferiority margin of −24%, noninferiority cannot be demonstrated.

CAVEATS TO CONSIDER WHEN LOOKING AT A NONINFERIORITY TRIAL

Noninferiority active-controlled trials often require a larger sample size than placebo-controlled trials, in part because the chosen noninferiority margins are often small. The required sample size for a noninferiority trial is highly dependent on the noninferiority margin and the assumed effect of the new treatment; this assumed effect must be clearly stated and realistic.

The primary analysis for a superiority trial should be based on the intention-to-treat (ITT) principle because it is generally conservative in the setting of imperfect adherence to treatment. However, analyzing a noninferiority trial by ITT could make an inferior treatment appear to be noninferior if poor patient adherence resulted in both treatments being similarly ineffective. Thus, when analyzing a noninferiority trial, both ITT and per-protocol analyses should be conducted. The results are most meaningful when both approaches demonstrate noninferiority.

A noninferiority trial does not distinguish between a new treatment that is noninferior and one that is truly superior and cannot demonstrate equivalence.

Acknowledgment

The following disclosures were reported at the time this original article was first published in *JAMA*.

Conflict of Interest Disclosures: None reported.

References

1. Salminen P, Paajanen H, Rautio T, et al. Antibiotic therapy vs appendectomy for treatment of uncomplicated acute appendicitis: the APPAC randomized clinical trial. *JAMA*. 2015;313(23):2340-2348. doi:10.1001/jama.2015.6154.

2. Young KD, Lewis RJ. What is confidence? I: the use and interpretation of confidence intervals. *Ann Emerg Med*. 1997;30(3):307-310. Medline:9287892

3. Kaji AH, Lewis RJ. Are we looking for superiority, equivalence, or noninferiority? *Ann Emerg Med*. 2010;55(5):408-411. Medline:20172627

4. Mulla SM, Scott IA, Jackevicius CA, et al. How to use a non-inferiority trial: Users' Guides to the Medical Literature. *JAMA*. 2012;308:2605-2611. Medline:23268519

5. Tamayo-Sarver JH, Albert JM, Tamayo-Sarver M, Cydulka RK. Advanced statistics: how to determine whether your intervention is different, at least as effective as, or equivalent. *Acad Emerg Med*. 2005;12(6):536-542. Medline:15930406

6. Piaggio G, Elbourne DR, Altman DG, Pocock SJ, Evans SJW; CONSORT Group. Reporting of noninferiority and equivalence randomized trials: an extension of the CONSORT statement. *JAMA*. 2006;295(10):1152-1160. Medline:16522836

7. Wilms IM, de Hoog DE, de Visser DC, Janzing HM. Appendectomy vs antibiotic treatment for acute appendicitis. *Cochrane Database Syst Rev*. 2011;(11):CD008359. Medline:22071846

Dose-Finding Trials: Optimizing Phase 2 Data in the Drug Development Process

Kert Viele, PhD, and Jason T. Connor, PhD

IN THIS CHAPTER

Use of the Method

Why Are Dose-Response Models Used?

What Are the Limitations of Dose-Response Modeling?

Why Did the Authors Use Dose-Response Modeling in This Particular Study?

How Should the Dose-Response Findings Be Interpreted in This Particular Study?

Caveats to Consider When Looking at Results Based on a Dose-Response Model

This JAMA Guide to Statistics and Methods discusses the use of dose-response models in phase 2 studies for identifying promising doses to use in further development of a new drug.

Clinical trials in drug development are commonly divided into 3 categories or phases. The first phase aims to find the range of doses of potential clinical use, usually by identifying the maximum tolerated dose. The second phase aims to find doses that demonstrate promising efficacy with acceptable safety. The third phase aims to confirm the benefit previously found in the second phase using clinically meaningful end points and to demonstrate safety more definitively.

Dose-finding trials—studies conducted to identify the most promising doses or doses to use in later studies—are a key part of the second phase and are intended to answer the dual questions of whether future development is warranted and what dose or doses should be used. If too high a dose is chosen, adverse effects in later confirmatory phase 3 trials may threaten the development program. If too low a dose is chosen, the treatment effect may be too small to yield a positive confirmatory trial and gain approval from a regulatory agency. A well-designed dose-finding trial is able to establish the optimal dose of a medication and facilitate the decision to proceed with a phase 3 trial.

Selection of a dose for further testing requires an understanding of the relationships between dose and both efficacy and safety. These relationships can be assessed by comparing the data from each dose group with placebo, or with the other doses, in a series of pairwise comparisons. This approach is prone to both false-negative and false-positive results because of the large number of statistical comparisons and the relatively small number of patients receiving each dose. These risks can be mitigated by combining data from patients receiving multiple active doses into a single treatment group for comparison with placebo ("pooling"), but only if it is possible to reliably predict which doses are likely to be effective.

In general, dose-response relationships are best examined through dose-response models that make flexible, justifiable assumptions about the potential dose-response relationships and allow the integration of information from all doses used in the trial. This can reduce the risk of both false-negative and false-positive results; incorporating all data into the estimates of efficacy and safety for each dose produces more accurate estimates than evaluating the response to each dose separately.

In an example published in *JAMA*, Gheorghiade et al[1] reported the results of the SOCRATES-REDUCED trial, a randomized placebo-controlled dose-finding clinical trial investigating 4 different target doses of vericiguat for patients with worsening chronic heart failure, with the primary outcome being a reduction in log-transformed level of N-terminal pro-B-type natriuretic peptide. The primary approach to analyzing the dose response, combining the data from patients allocated to the 3 highest target doses (pooling) for comparison with placebo, yielded a negative result ($P = .15$), but a different dose-response model based on linear regression, used in an exploratory secondary analysis, yielded a positive result ($P = .02$).

USE OF THE METHOD

Why Are Dose-Response Models Used?

A dose-response model assumes a general relationship between dose and efficacy or dose and the rates of adverse effects.[2] Ideally, this allows data from patients receiving all doses of the drug to contribute to the estimated dose-response curve, maximizing the statistical power of the study and reducing the uncertainty in the estimates of the effects of each dose. When a sufficiently flexible general relationship is used, the dose-response model correctly identifies doses of low or high efficacy (avoiding the assumption of similar efficacy across doses, as is implied with pooling) while smoothing out spurious highs and lows (avoiding problems that occur when each dose is analyzed separately). A model can produce estimates and confidence intervals for the effect of every dose and often even for drug doses not included in the trial.

Dose-response modeling is first used to determine whether a treatment effect appears to exist and, if so, to estimate dose-specific effects to help optimize subsequent phase 3 trial design. Unlike a confirmatory trial in which a regulatory agency makes a binary decision (eg, to approve or not approve a drug), phase 2 trials are used to inform the next stage of drug development. Therefore, estimation of the magnitude of treatment effects is more important than testing hypotheses regarding treatment effects. Phase 2 dose-finding studies can also be used to predict the likelihood of later phase 3 success through calculation of predictive probabilities.[3]

The assumptions in the dose-response model can be rigid or flexible to match preexisting knowledge of the clinical setting. When accurate, such assumptions can increase the power of a trial design by incorporating known clinical information. When inaccurate, these assumptions compromise the statistical properties of the trial and the interpretability of the results. For example, in the SOCRATES-REDUCED trial, the primary analysis consisted of pooling data from the 3 highest-dose regimens.[1] This approach is most effective when the efficacious region of the dose range can be predicted reliably. The exploratory secondary analysis in the SOCRATES-REDUCED trial was based on a linear regression model. This approach is most effective when a linear dose-response relationship is likely to exist over the range of doses evaluated in the trial.

A common dose-response model is the E_{max} model,[4] which assumes an S-shaped curve for the dose response (eg, a monotonically increasing curve that is flat for low doses, increases for the middle dose range, and then flattens out again for high doses). The model is flexible in that the height of the plateau, the dose location of the increase in efficacy, and the rate of increase may all be informed by the data. Alternatives to the E_{max} model include smoothing models such as a normal dynamic linear model.[5] These models take the raw data and produce a smooth curve that eliminates random highs and lows but maintains the general shape. Normal dynamic linear models are particularly useful for dose responses that may be "inverted U" shaped and may be applicable when the dose response is for an outcome that combines safety and efficacy (low doses may not be efficacious, high doses may be unsafe, resulting in an inverted U shape, with the optimal dose in the middle).

What Are the Limitations of Dose-Response Modeling?

All dose-response models require assumptions regarding the potential shapes of the dose-response curve, although sometimes (eg, with pooling) the assumptions are only implied. When assumptions are incorrect, inferences from the model may be invalid. In the SOCRATES-REDUCED trial, the implied assumption of the primary analysis of similar efficacy among the 3 highest doses was not supported by the data. Similarly, the linear model used in the exploratory secondary analysis assumed that the increase in benefit from one dose to the next was the same between every successive pair of doses. This also does not appear to be strictly consistent with the data obtained in the trial.

Why Did the Authors Use Dose-Response Modeling in This Particular Study?

The authors used dose-response modeling to maximize the power of the primary analysis hypothesis test. If the 3 highest doses had all been similarly effective, pooling of data from these doses would result in higher sample sizes in the treatment group of the primary "treatment vs placebo" hypothesis test and higher power to detect an effect. In the exploratory secondary analysis using the linear dose-response model, the authors used a model that allowed the higher doses to be significantly more efficacious than the lower doses.

How Should the Dose-Response Findings Be Interpreted in This Particular Study?

Figure 2 in the report by Gheorghiade et al[1] shows the key dose-response relationship and suggests that the 10-mg target dose is the most or possibly only effective dose. However, the primary analysis was null, and the protocol called for the statistical secondary analysis only if the primary analysis were significant at $P < .05$. Therefore, although the 10-mg dose appears to be the most promising for investigation in a phase 3 trial, the dose-ranging findings must be considered very tentative. There remains uncertainty regarding how best to estimate the effect of the 10-mg dose. The primary analysis did not evaluate the effect of the 10-mg dose alone, and separate analyses for each dose would be prone to high variation and false-positive results due to multiple comparisons. The exploratory linear model produced an estimated effect for the 10-mg dose under an assumption of linearity. This analysis and its results were considered only exploratory.

CAVEATS TO CONSIDER WHEN LOOKING AT RESULTS BASED ON A DOSE-RESPONSE MODEL

It is often useful to inspect a plot of the dose-response model-based estimates against all data observed in the trial. This allows visual confirmation that the chosen dose-response model captures the general shape of the observed data.

Acknowledgment

The following disclosures were reported at the time this original article was first published in *JAMA*.

Conflict of Interest Disclosures: None reported.

References

1. Gheorghiade M, Greene SJ, Butler J, et al. Effect of vericiguat, a soluble guanylate cyclase stimulator, on natriuretic peptide levels in patients with worsening chronic heart failure and reduced ejection fraction: the SOCRATES-REDUCED randomized trial. *JAMA*. 2015;314(21):2251-2262. doi:10.1001/jama.2015.15734. Medline:26547357
2. Bretz F, Hsu J, Pinheiro J, Liu Y. Dose finding: a challenge in statistics. *Biom J*. 2008;50(4):480-504. Medline:18663758
3. Saville BR, Connor JT, Ayers GD, Alvarez J. The utility of Bayesian predictive probabilities for interim monitoring of clinical trials. *Clin Trials*. 2014;11(4):485-493. Medline:24872363
4. Dragalin V, Hsuan F, Padmanabhan SK. Adaptive designs for dose-finding studies based on sigmoid Emax model. *J Biopharm Stat*. 2007;17(6):1051-1070. Medline:18027216
5. Krams M, Lees KR, Hacke W, Grieve AP, Orgogozo JM, Ford GA; ASTIN Study Investigators. Acute Stroke Therapy by Inhibition of Neutrophils (ASTIN): an adaptive dose-response study of UK-279,276 in acute ischemic stroke. *Stroke*. 2003;34(11):2543-2548. Medline:14563972

Pragmatic Trials: Practical Answers to "Real World" Questions

Harold C. Sox, MD, and
Roger J. Lewis, MD, PhD

IN THIS CHAPTER

Use of the Method

Why Are Pragmatic Trials Conducted?

Description of the Method

What Are the Limitations of Pragmatic Trials?

Why Was a Pragmatic Trial Conducted in This Case?

How Should the Results Be Interpreted?

This JAMA Guide to Statistics and Methods compares pragmatic randomized controlled trials, which focus on important challenges that patients, physicians, and policy makers face in day-to-day life with explanatory trials that seek to test a hypothesis.

The concept of a "pragmatic" clinical trial was first proposed nearly 50 years ago as a study design philosophy that emphasizes answering questions of most interest to decision makers.[1] Decision makers, whether patients, physicians, or policy makers, need to know what they can expect from the available diagnostic or therapeutic options when applied in day-to-day clinical practice. This focus on addressing real-world effectiveness questions influences choices about trial design, patient population, interventions, outcomes, and analysis. Gottenberg et al[2] reported the results of a trial designed to answer the question "If a biologic agent for rheumatoid arthritis is no longer effective for an individual patient, should the clinician recommend another drug with the same mechanism of action or switch to a biologic with a different mechanism of action?" Because the authors included some pragmatic elements in the trial design, this study illustrates the issues that clinicians should consider in deciding whether a trial result is likely to apply to their patients.

USE OF THE METHOD

Why Are Pragmatic Trials Conducted?

Pragmatic trials are intended to help typical clinicians and typical patients make difficult decisions in typical clinical care settings by maximizing the chance that the trial results will apply to patients who are usually seen in practice (external validity). The most important feature of a pragmatic trial is that patients, clinicians, clinical practices, and clinical settings are selected to maximize the applicability of the results to usual practice. Trial procedures and requirements must not inconvenience patients with substantial data collection and should impose a minimum of constraints on usual practice by allowing a choice of medication (within the constraints imposed by the purpose of the study) and dosage, providing the freedom to add cointerventions, and doing nothing to maximize adherence to the study protocol.

The pragmatic trial strategy contrasts with that used for an explanatory trial, the goal of which is to test a hypothesis that the intervention causes a clinical outcome. Explanatory trials seek to maximize the probability that the intervention—and not some other factor—causes the study outcome (internal validity). Explanatory trials seek to give the intervention the best possible chance to succeed by using experts to deliver it, delivering the intervention to patients who are most likely to respond, and administering the intervention in settings that provide expert after-care. Explanatory trials try to prevent any extraneous factors from influencing clinical outcomes, so they exclude patients who might have poor adherence and may intervene to maximize patient and clinician adherence to the study protocol. Explanatory trials are structured to avoid downstream events that could affect study outcomes. If these events occur at different rates in the different study groups, the effect attributed to the intervention may be larger or smaller than its true effect. To avoid this problem, explanatory trials may choose a relatively short follow-up period. Explanatory trials pursue internal validity at the cost of external validity, whereas pragmatic trials place a premium on external validity while maintaining as much internal validity as possible.

Description of the Method

According to Tunis et al,[3] "the characteristic features of [pragmatic clinical trials] are that they (1) select clinically relevant alternative interventions to compare, (2) include a diverse population of study participants, (3) recruit participants from heterogeneous practice settings, and (4) collect data on a broad range of health outcomes." Eligible patients may be defined by presumptive diagnoses, rather than confirmed ones, because treatments are often initiated when the diagnosis is uncertain.[3] Pragmatic trials may compare classes of drugs and allow the physician to choose which drug in the class to use, the dose, and any cointerventions, a freedom that mimics usual practice. Furthermore, the outcome measures are more likely to be patient-reported, global, subjective, and patient-centered (eg, self-reported quality-of-life measures), rather than the more disease-centered end points commonly used in explanatory trials (eg, the results of laboratory tests or imaging procedures).

Both approaches to study design must deal with the cost of clinical trials. Explanatory trials control costs by keeping the trial period as short as possible, consistent with the investigators' ability to enroll enough patients to answer the study question. These trials preferentially recruit patients who will experience the study end point and not leave the study early because of disinterest or death from causes other than the target condition. Investigators in explanatory trials prefer to enroll participants with a high probability of experiencing an outcome in the near term. In contrast, pragmatic trials may control costs by leveraging existing data sources, eg, using disease registries to identify potential participants and using data in electronic health records to identify study outcomes.

Although these concepts sharpen the contrasts between pragmatic and explanatory trials for pedagogical reasons, in reality, many trials have features of both designs, in part to find a reasonable balance between internal validity and external validity.[4,5]

WHAT ARE THE LIMITATIONS OF PRAGMATIC TRIALS?

The main limitation of a pragmatic trial is a direct consequence of choosing to conduct a lean study that puts few demands on patients and clinicians. Data collection may be sparse, and there are few clinical variables with which to identify subgroups of patients who respond particularly well to one of the interventions. The use of the electronic health record as a source of data may save money, but it typically means inconsistent data collection and missing data. Relying on typical clinicians rather than experts in caring for patients with the target condition may lead to increased variability in practice and associated documentation of clinical findings. The variation caused by these shortcomings may reduce statistical precision and the capability of answering the research question unequivocally.

WHY WAS A PRAGMATIC TRIAL CONDUCTED IN THIS CASE?

While Gottenberg et al[2] cite the pragmatism of their study as its main strength, the authors do not explain their study design decisions. However, they imply a pragmatic motivation when they state that the study confirms the superiority of a drug from a different class in a setting that "corresponds to the therapeutic question clinicians face in daily practice." The investigators note that their main limitation of the study was the inability to blind the participants to the identity of the drug they received. Blinding is especially important when the principal study outcomes are those reported by the patient, who may be influenced by knowing the intervention that they received.

HOW SHOULD THE RESULTS BE INTERPRETED?

The study by Gottenberg et al[2] shows that, from the perspective of a population of patients, changing from one class of drugs to another improves the outcomes of care by rheumatologists in a rheumatology subspecialty clinic. This result has limited external validity. It probably applies to other rheumatology clinics, but its application to other settings is unknown. The main pragmatic feature of the study—allowing the rheumatologist to choose from several drugs within a class—implies that the main result applies strictly to the class of drugs rather than to any individual agent. It does not, for example, show that the improvement is the same regardless of which within-class drug the clinician determines. The trial was also pragmatic in that clinicians were aware of the primary treatment and were free to choose cointerventions that would complement it, as would occur in clinical practice.

Several features of this study were not pragmatic, and others raise internal validity concerns. The researchers recruited participants from rheumatology specialty clinics. Although the article does not specify the clinicians who managed the patient's rheumatoid arthritis during the study, the clinicians were presumably rheumatologists in the participating practices. Even though the results apply to patients in a specialty clinic, whether they apply to patients managed by primary care physicians, with or without expert consultation, is unknown. The authors also did not specify the intensity of follow-up; was it typical of rheumatoid arthritis patients receiving biologic agents or did the study protocol specify more intensive follow-up? The primary outcome measure was a score based on the erythrocyte sedimentation rate and a count of involved joints. The article does not identify the person who assessed the primary outcome. Assigning this task to the managing physician would be consistent with a pragmatic design, but it would also raise concerns about biased outcome assessment because the person measuring the outcome would know the treatment assignment.

The terms "explanatory" and "pragmatic" mark the ends of a spectrum of study designs. Typically, as noted by Thorpe and co-authors of the PRECIS (Pragmatic-Explanatory Continuum Indicator Summary) article,[5] some features of a study are pragmatic and others are explanatory, as the study by Gottenberg et al illustrates and as would be expected because internal validity and external validity are typically achieved at the cost of one another. Whether the authors label their study as pragmatic or explanatory, readers should pay close attention to the study characteristics that maximize its applicability to their patients and their practice style.

Acknowledgment

The following disclosures were reported at the time this original article was first published in *JAMA*.

Conflict of Interest Disclosures: None reported.

Disclaimer: Dr Sox is an employee of the Patient-Centered Outcomes Research Institute (PCORI). This article does not represent the policies of PCORI.

References

1. Schwartz D, Lellouch J. Explanatory and pragmatic attitudes in therapeutical trials. *J Chronic Dis*. 1967;20(8):637-648. Medline:4860352
2. Gottenberg J-E, Brocq O, Perdriger A, et al. Non–TNF-targeted biologic vs a second anti-TNF drug to treat rheumatoid arthritis in patients with insufficient response to a first anti-TNF drug. *JAMA*. 2016;316(11):1172-1180. doi:10.1001/jama.2016.13512
3. Tunis SR, Stryer DB, Clancy CM. Practical clinical trials: increasing the value of clinical research for decision making in clinical and health policy. *JAMA*. 2003;290(12):1624-1632. Medline:14506122
4. Zwarenstein M, Treweek S, Gagnier JJ, et al. CONSORT group; Pragmatic Trials in Healthcare (Practihc) group. Improving the reporting of pragmatic trials: an extension of the CONSORT statement. *BMJ*. 2008;337:a2390. doi:10.1136/bmj.a2390. Medline:19001484
5. Thorpe KE, Zwarenstein M, Oxman AD, et al. A Pragmatic-Explanatory Continuum Indicator Summary (PRECIS): a tool to help trial designers. *J Clin Epidemiol*. 2009;62(5):464-475. Medline:19348971

Cluster Randomized Trials: Evaluating Treatments Applied to Groups

William J. Meurer, MD, MS, and
Roger J. Lewis, MD, PhD

IN THIS CHAPTER

Use of the Method

Why Is Cluster Randomization Used?

What Are Limitations of Cluster Randomization?

Why Did the Authors Use Cluster Randomization in This Particular Study?

How Should Cluster Randomization Findings Be Interpreted in This Particular Study?

Caveats to Consider When Looking at a Cluster Randomized Trial

This JAMA Guide to Statistics and Methods describes the reasons for using cluster randomization in a clinical trial and how to analyze and interpret the results from a trial that did.

Sometimes a new treatment is best introduced to an entire group of patients rather than to individual patients. Examples include when the new approach requires procedures be followed by multiple members of a health care team or when the new technique is applied to the environment of care (eg, a method for cleaning a hospital room before it is known which patient will be assigned the room). This avoids confusion that could occur if all caregivers had to keep track of which patients were being treated the old way and which were being treated the new way.

One approach to evaluate the efficacy of such treatments—treatments for which the application typically involves changes at the level of the health care practice, hospital unit, or even health care system—is to conduct a cluster randomized trial. In a cluster randomized trial, study participants are randomized in groups or clusters so that all members within a single group are assigned to either the experimental intervention or the control.[1,2] This contrasts with the more familiar randomized clinical trial (RCT) in which randomization occurs at the level of the individual participant, and the treatment assigned to one study participant is essentially independent of the treatment assigned to any other. In a cluster randomized trial, the cluster is the unit randomized, whereas in a traditional RCT, the individual study participant is randomized. In both types of trials, however, the outcomes of interest are recorded for each participant individually.

Although there are both theoretical and pragmatic reasons for using cluster randomization in a clinical trial, doing so introduces a fundamental challenge to those analyzing and interpreting the results of the trial: study participants from the same cluster (eg, patients treated within the same medical practice or hospital unit) tend to be more similar to each other than participants from different clusters.[2] This nearly universal fact violates a common assumption of most statistical tests, namely, that individual observations are independent of each other. To obtain valid results, a cluster randomized trial must be analyzed using statistical methods that account for the greater similarity between individual participants from the same cluster compared with those from different clusters.[2-4]

In a *JAMA* article, Curley et al[5] reported the results of the RESTORE trial, a cluster randomized clinical trial evaluating a nurse-implemented, goal-directed sedation protocol for children with acute respiratory failure receiving mechanical ventilation in the intensive care setting, comparing this approach with usual care. The trial evaluated the primary hypothesis that the intervention group—patients treated in intensive care units (ICUs) using the goal-directed sedation protocol—would have a shorter duration of mechanical ventilation. Thirty-one pediatric ICUs, the "clusters," were randomized to either implement the goal-directed sedation protocol or continue their usual care practices.

USE OF THE METHOD

Why Is Cluster Randomization Used?

Cluster randomization should be used when it would be impractical or impossible to assign and correctly deliver the experimental and control treatments to individual study participants.[1,2] Typical situations include the study of interventions that must be implemented by multiple team members, that affect workflow, or that alter the structure of care delivery. As in the RESTORE trial, interventions that involve training multidisciplinary health care teams are practically difficult to conduct using individual-level randomization, as health care practitioners cannot easily unlearn a new way of taking care of patients.

Cluster randomization is often used to reduce the mixing or contamination of treatments in the 2 groups of the trial, as might occur if patients in the control group start to be treated using some of the approaches included in the experimental treatment group, perhaps because the practitioners become habituated to the experimental approach or perceive it to be superior.[1,2] For example, consider an injury prevention trial testing the effect of offering bicycle helmets to students in a classroom on the incidence of subsequent head injury. If a conventional RCT were conducted and half of the students in each classroom received helmets, it is likely that some of the other half of students would inform their parents about the ongoing intervention and many of these children might also begin to use bicycle helmets. Contamination is a form of crossover between treatment groups and will generally reduce the observed treatment effect using the usual intent-to-treat analysis.[6] Cluster randomization may also be used to reduce potential selection bias. Physicians choosing individual patients from their practice to consent for randomization may tend to enroll patients with specific characteristics (eg, lesser or greater illness severity), reducing the external validity of the trial. Assignment of the treatment group at the practice level, with the application of the assigned treatment to all patients treated within the practice, may minimize this problem.

Using a cluster randomized design also can offer practical advantages. For example, if 2 or more treatments are considered to be within the standard of care, and depending on the risks associated with treatment, streamlined consent procedures or even integration of general and research consents may be used to reduce barriers to participation and ensure a truly representative patient population is enrolled in the trial.[1,7]

What Are Limitations of Cluster Randomization?

Any time data are clustered, the statistical analysis must use techniques that account for the likeness of cluster members.[2,3] Extensions of the more-familiar regression models that are appropriate for the analysis of clustered data include generalized estimating equations (as used in the RESTORE trial), mixed linear models, and hierarchical models. While the proper use of these approaches is complex, the informed reader should be alert to statements that the analysis method was selected to account for the similarity or correlations of data within each cluster. The intracluster correlation coefficient (ICC) quantifies the likeness within clusters and ranges from 0 to 1, although it is frequently in the 0.02 to 0.1 range.[4] A value of 0 means each member of the cluster is not more like the other members, with respect to the measured characteristic, than they are to the population at large, so each additional individual contributes the same amount of new information. In contrast, a value of 1 means that each member of the cluster is exactly the same as the others in the cluster, so any participants beyond the first contribute no additional information at all. A larger ICC, representing greater similarity of results within clusters, will decrease the effective sample size of the trial, reducing the precision of estimates of treatment effects and the power of the trial.[2] If the ICC is high, the effective sample size will be closer to the number of groups, and if the ICC is low, the effective sample size will be closer to the total number of individuals in the trial.

It is often impossible to maintain blinding of treatment assignment in a cluster randomized trial, both because of the nature of treatments and because of the number of patients in a given location all receiving the same treatment. It is well known that trials evaluating nonblinded interventions have a greater risk of bias.

Why Did the Authors Use Cluster Randomization in This Particular Study?

The RESTORE trial investigators used cluster randomization because they were introducing a nurse-implemented, goal-directed sedation protocol that required a change in behavior among multiple caregivers within each ICU. A major component of the experimental intervention was educating the critical care personnel regarding the perceived benefits and risks of sedation agents and use patterns relative to others. Had individual-level randomization been used to allocate patients, it is highly likely that the patients randomized to standard care would have received care that was somewhere between the prior standard and the new protocol, because all ICU caregivers would have been informed about the scientific and pharmacological basis for the goal-directed sedation protocol.

How Should Cluster Randomization Findings Be Interpreted in This Particular Study?

As in any clinical trial, randomization may or may not work effectively to create similar groups of patients. In the RESTORE trial, some differences between the intervention groups were observed that might partially explain the negative primary outcome. Specifically, the intervention group had a greater proportion of younger children—a group that is more difficult to sedate.[8] The RESTORE trial investigators used randomization in blocks to ensure balance of pediatric ICU sizes between groups; methods exist to balance groups in cluster trials on multiple factors simultaneously.[9] Although the RESTORE trial yielded a negative primary outcome, the authors noted some promising secondary outcomes related to clinicians' perception of patient comfort. However, these assessments were unblinded and thus may be subject to bias.

CAVEATS TO CONSIDER WHEN LOOKING AT A CLUSTER RANDOMIZED TRIAL

When evaluating a cluster randomized trial, the first consideration is whether the use of clustering was well justified. Would it have been possible to use individual-level randomization and maintain fidelity in treatment allocation and administration? What would be the likelihood of contamination? Cluster randomization cannot minimize baseline differences between 2 treatment groups as efficiently as individual-level randomization. The design must be justified for scientific or logistical reasons to accept this trade-off.[10]

Second, the usual sources of bias should be considered, such as patient knowledge of treatment assignment and unblinded assessments of outcome. Although not specific to cluster randomized trials, these sources of bias tend to be more problematic.

Third, it is important to consider whether the intracluster correlation was appropriately accounted for in the design, analysis, and interpretation of the trial.[1,10] During the design, the likely ICC should be considered to ensure the planned sample size is adequate. The analysis should be based on statistical methods that account for clustering, such as generalized estimating equations.

Finally, the interpretation should consider the extent with which the 2 treatment groups contained an adequate number, size, and similarity of clusters and whether any clusters were lost to follow-up.

Acknowledgment

The following disclosures were reported at the time this original article was first published in *JAMA*.

Conflict of Interest Disclosures: None reported.

References

1. Campbell MK, Elbourne DR, Altman DG; CONSORT group. CONSORT statement: extension to cluster randomised trials. *BMJ*. 2004;328(7441):702-708. Medline:15031246
2. Wears RL. Advanced statistics: statistical methods for analyzing cluster and cluster-randomized data. *Acad Emerg Med*. 2002;9(4):330-341. Medline:11927463
3. Dawid AP. Conditional independence in statistical theory. *J R Stat Soc Series B*. 1979;41:1-31.

4. Killip S, Mahfoud Z, Pearce K. What is an intracluster correlation coefficient? *Ann Fam Med*. 2004;2(3):204-208. Medline:15209195

5. Curley MA, Wypij D, Watson RS, et al. Protocolized sedation vs usual care in pediatric patients mechanically ventilated for acute respiratory failure. *JAMA*. 2015;313(4):379-389. Medline:25602358

6. Detry MA, Lewis RJ. The intention-to-treat principle. *JAMA*. 2014;312(1): 85-86. Medline:25058221

7. Huang SS, Septimus E, Kleinman K, et al. Targeted versus universal decolonization to prevent ICU infection. *N Engl J Med*. 2013;368(24):2255-2265. Medline:23718152

8. Anand KJ, Willson DF, Berger J, et al. Tolerance and withdrawal from prolonged opioid use in critically ill children. *Pediatrics*. 2010;125(5):e1208-e1225. Medline:20403936

9. Scott PA, Meurer WJ, Frederiksen SM, et al. A multilevel intervention to increase community hospital use of alteplase for acute stroke (INSTINCT). *Lancet Neurol*. 2013;12(2):139-148. Medline:23260188

10. Ivers NM, Taljaard M, Dixon S, et al. Impact of CONSORT extension for cluster randomised trials on quality of reporting and study methodology. *BMJ*. 2011;343:d5886. Medline:21948873

The Stepped-Wedge Clinical Trial: Evaluation by Rolling Deployment

Susan S. Ellenberg, PhD

IN THIS CHAPTER

Use of the Method
Why Is a Stepped-Wedge Clinical Trial Design Used?
Description of the Stepped-Wedge Clinical Trial Design
Limitations of the Stepped-Wedge Design
How Was the Stepped-Wedge Design Used?
How Should a Stepped-Wedge Clinical Trial Be Interpreted?

This JAMA Guide to Statistics and Methods discusses the stepped-wedge approach to cluster randomized clinical trial design, in which clusters are randomized to the order in which they receive the experimental regimen.

Cluster randomized trials are studies in which groups of individuals, for example those associated with specific clinics, families, or geographical areas, are randomized between an experimental intervention and a control.[1] A stepped-wedge design is a type of cluster design in which the clusters are randomized to the order in which they receive the experimental regimen. All clusters begin the study with the control intervention, and by the end of the trial (assuming no unexpected and unacceptable safety issues arise), all clusters are receiving the experimental regimen.

USE OF THE METHOD

Why Is a Stepped-Wedge Clinical Trial Design Used?

Cluster randomized trials have been performed for many decades, even centuries,[2] but the statistical underpinnings of such designs have been worked out only relatively recently.[3,4] The primary motivation for a cluster design is to study treatments that can be delivered only in a group setting (eg, an educational approach in a classroom setting) or to avoid contamination in the delivery of each regimen (eg, a behavioral intervention that could be delivered individually but in settings in which those randomized to different approaches are in close contact with each other and might learn about and then adopt the alternative regimen).[1] Clusters are typically identified prospectively and randomized to receive the experimental or control intervention. However, there are exceptions, such as the ring vaccination trial conducted during the 2014-2015 Ebola epidemic, in which clusters were defined around newly identified cases.[5]

If a cluster randomized trial is deemed necessary or desirable in a specific setting, but resource limitations permit only a gradual implementation of the experimental regimen, a stepped-wedge design may be considered as the fairest way to determine which clusters receive the experimental regimen earlier and which later. Stepped-wedge designs have benefits similar to those of crossover trials because outcomes within a cluster may be compared between the time intervals in which a cluster received the control and the experimental interventions. This controls for the unique characteristics of the cluster when making the treatment comparison. One attractive aspect of stepped-wedge designs is that all participants in all clusters ultimately receive the experimental regimen, thereby ensuring that all participants have an opportunity to potentially benefit from the intervention. This can be advantageous when strong beliefs exist regarding the efficacy of a treatment regimen. When limited resources preclude making the treatment regimen widely available from the start, the use of randomization to determine which clusters get early access to the treatment regimen may appeal to participants' sense of fairness.

Description of the Stepped-Wedge Clinical Trial Design

Important considerations in designing a stepped-wedge trial include the number of clusters, the number of "steps" (time points at which the changeovers from control to intervention occur), the duration of treatment at each step, and the balance of prognostic characteristics across the clusters receiving the intervention at each step. The required sample size (total number of participants) to achieve a given level of power decreases as the numbers of clusters and steps increase. Maximum power for a given number of clusters is achieved when each cluster has its own step, but more typically multiple clusters are randomized to change at the same time to limit trial duration.[6] The risk of bias decreases as the number of clusters increases, as more clusters improve the likelihood of achieving similar prognoses across clusters, and as the trial duration decreases, reducing the effect of temporal trends.

LIMITATIONS OF THE STEPPED-WEDGE DESIGN

As with cluster randomized designs generally, stepped-wedge designs require larger sample sizes, often much larger, than would be required for randomized trials in which individual study participants are randomized to receive the experimental or control intervention. Efficiency is reduced because of the need to account for the similarities among participants within a given cluster; ie, the extent to which individuals within a cluster are more alike than they are similar to the study population as a whole. Consequently, each individual in a cluster provides less information about the study findings than would occur if the randomization had been by individual. For example, suppose the outcome of a trial was 1-year survival, and in 1 cluster the prognosis of participants was so good that every participant in the cluster was certain to survive at least 1 year. Then the information from that cluster is the same whether there are 100 participants or only 1 participant. When participants are randomized individually, the factors that influence outcomes are balanced within each participating site, and in an analysis appropriately stratified by site, the comparisons will not be affected by site differences in prognosis. Even though randomization of clusters is intended to balance prognosis, such balance cannot be ensured with a small number of clusters (eg, 10-20), which is common in many cluster randomized trials. The randomization can be stratified according to characteristics that are considered to relate to prognosis (eg, mean socioeconomic status of cluster participants), but this is often difficult to do precisely. Unless the number of clusters is quite large, stratification by more than 1 or 2 variables is not feasible.

Another limitation of the stepped-wedge design is the potential for confounding by temporal trends. When changes in clinical care are occurring over a short time, comparisons of outcomes between earlier and later periods may be influenced by background changes that affect the outcome of interest irrespective of the intervention being tested. Another time-dependent phenomenon that can influence stepped-wedge trials is the effect of accumulating experience with the intervention. If more experience enhances the likelihood that the intervention will be successful, participants in clusters randomized earlier in the trial will more likely benefit. Time dependency concerns must be balanced against the advantage that the before-after comparison within clusters balances the unknown as well as the known characteristics of cluster participants. To address the time dependency, the time factor must be accounted for in the analysis.

HOW WAS THE STEPPED-WEDGE DESIGN USED?

Huffman and colleagues[7] reported results of the QUIK trial, an investigation of a quality improvement intervention intended to reduce complications following myocardial infarction. A stepped-wedge design was used rather than a standard cluster randomized design because this approach allowed all the participating hospitals to receive the experimental intervention during the course of the study and also had the advantage of controlling for potential differences in study participant characteristics by comparing outcomes within a cluster during different periods.[8] The authors did not pursue an individually randomized design, which also would have controlled for both cluster characteristics and temporal trends. Individual randomization for quality improvement interventions would probably not be feasible within individual participating hospitals because the intervention would be difficult to isolate to individual patients. Sixty-three hospitals were included in the study and were randomized in groups of 12 or 13 that would initiate the intervention at 1 of 4 randomization points. The duration of each of the 4 steps was 4 months. After adjusting for within-hospital clustering and temporal trends, the prognostic characteristics of the trial participants in the 2 treatment groups were similar.

HOW SHOULD A STEPPED-WEDGE CLINICAL TRIAL BE INTERPRETED?

Huffman et al did not find a significant benefit of the quality improvement intervention. Although unadjusted analyses did suggest benefit, appropriate statistical analysis adjusting for time trends markedly attenuated the benefit. In this case, it is possible that the quality of care was improving while the study was progressing independent of the study intervention, highlighting the importance of accounting for time trends (clearly shown in Figures 2A and 2B in the article[7]) when analyzing the results of stepped-wedge trials.

Concerns have been raised about the difficulties in obtaining informed consent from patients in stepped-wedge trials.[9] Obtaining individual informed consent is often difficult in cluster randomized trials because individuals receiving treatment in a particular cluster may not be able to avoid exposure to the intervention assigned to that cluster. In the QUIK trial, consent was not obtained from patients who received the assigned intervention but it was obtained for 30-day follow-up. The investigators noted that this requirement may have introduced selection bias because of refusals by some participants.

Stepped-wedge clinical trials offer a way to evaluate an intervention in a system in which the ultimate goal is to implement the intervention at all sites yet retain the ability to objectively evaluate the intervention's efficacy.

Acknowledgment

The following disclosures were reported at the time this original article was first published in *JAMA*.
Conflict of Interest Disclosures: None reported.

References

1. Meurer WJ, Lewis RJ. Cluster randomized trials: evaluating treatments applied to groups. *JAMA*. 2015;313(20):2068-2069. Medline:26010636
2. Moberg J, Kramer M. A brief history of the cluster randomised trial design. *J R Soc Med*. 2015;108(5):192-198. Medline:26022551
3. Cornfield J. Randomization by group: a formal analysis. *Am J Epidemiol*. 1978;108(2):100-102. Medline:707470
4. Donner A, Birkett N, Buck C. Randomization by cluster: sample size requirements and analysis. *Am J Epidemiol*. 1981;114(6):906-914. Medline:7315838
5. Henao-Restrepo AM, Camacho A, Longini IM, et al. Efficacy and effectiveness of an rVSV-vectored vaccine in preventing Ebola virus disease: final results from the Guinea ring vaccination, open-label, cluster-randomised trial (Ebola Ça Suffit!). *Lancet*. 2017;389(10068):505-518. Medline:28017403
6. Baio G, Copas A, Ambler G, Hargreaves J, Beard E, Omar RZ. Sample size calculation for a stepped wedge trial. *Trials*. 2015;16:354. Medline:26282553
7. Huffman MD, Mohanan PP, Devarajan R, et al. Effect of a quality improvement intervention on clinical outcomes in patients in India with acute myocardial infarction: the ACS QUIK randomized clinical trial. *JAMA*. 2018;319(6):567-578. doi:10.1001/jama.2017.21906.
8. Huffman MD, Mohanan PP, Devarajan R, et al. Acute coronary syndrome quality improvement in Kerala (ACS QUIK): rationale and design for a cluster-randomized stepped-wedge trial. *Am Heart J*. 2017;185:154-160. Medline:28267469
9. Taljaard M, Hemming K, Shah L, Giraudeau B, Grimshaw JM, Weijer C. Inadequacy of ethical conduct and reporting of stepped wedge cluster randomized trials: results from a systematic review. *Clin Trials*. 2017;14(4):333-341. Medline:28393537

Sample Size Calculation for a Hypothesis Test

Lynne Stokes, PhD

IN THIS CHAPTER

Use of the Method

Why Is Power Analysis Used?

What Are the Limitations of Power Analysis?

Why Did the Authors Use Power Analysis in This Particular Study?

How Should This Method's Findings Be Interpreted in This Particular Study?

Caveats to Consider When Looking at Results Based on Power Analysis

This JAMA Guide to Statistics and Methods explains the importance of considering sample size when interpreting study results, how the power analysis can help calculate the appropriate sample size, and the potential pitfalls of this approach.

Koegelenberg et al[1] reported the results of a randomized clinical trial (RCT) that investigated whether treatment with a nicotine patch in addition to varenicline produced higher rates of smoking abstinence than varenicline alone. The primary results were positive; that is, patients receiving the combination therapy were more likely to achieve continuous abstinence at 12 weeks than patients receiving varenicline alone. The absolute difference in the abstinence rate was estimated to be approximately 14%, which was statistically significant at level $\alpha = .05$.

These findings differed from the results reported in 2 previous studies[2,3] of the same question, which detected no difference in treatments. What explains this difference? One explanation offered by the authors is that the previous studies "…may have been inadequately powered," which means the sample size in those studies may have been too small to identify a difference between the treatments tested.

USE OF THE METHOD

Why Is Power Analysis Used?

The sample size in a research investigation should be large enough that differences occurring by chance are rare but should not be larger than necessary, to avoid waste of resources and to prevent exposure of research participants to risk associated with the interventions. With any study, but especially if the study sample size is very small, any difference in observed rates can happen by chance and thus cannot be considered statistically significant.

In developing the methods for a study, investigators conduct a power analysis to calculate sample size. The power of a hypothesis test is the probability of obtaining a statistically significant result when there is a true difference in treatments. For example, suppose, as Koegelenberg et al[1] did, that the smoking abstinence rate were 45% for varenicline alone and 14% larger, or 59%, for the combination regimen. Power is the probability that, under these conditions, the trial would detect a difference in rates large enough to be statistically significant at a certain level α (ie, α is the probability of a type I error, which occurs by rejecting a null hypothesis that is actually true).

Power can also be thought of as the probability of the complement of a type II error. If we accept a 20% type II error for a difference in rates of size d, we are saying that there is a 20% chance that we do not detect the difference between groups when the difference in their rates is d. The complement of this, $0.8 = 1 - 0.2$, or the statistical power, means that when a difference of d exists, there is an 80% chance that our statistical test will detect it.

Figure 2 illustrates the relationship between sample size and power for the test described. The top light blue line shows the power for the parameter settings above (baseline rate of 45% and minimum detectable difference, or MDD, of 14%), when significance level α is set to .05. For this scenario, the authors' target sample size of 398 (199 in each group) will produce a power of 80%. All these values (45%, 14%, .05, 80%) must be selected at the planning stage of the study to carry out this calculation. The significance level and power are "rule-of-thumb" choices and are typically not based on the specifics of the study. If the researcher wants to reduce the probability of making a type I error ($\alpha = .05$) or to increase the probability of detecting the specified difference (power = 80%), then these values can be changed. Either change will require a larger sample size.

Selecting the baseline rate and MDD requires the expertise of the researcher. The baseline rate is typically available from the literature, because this rate is often based on a therapy that has

FIGURE 2

Power for Detecting Difference and Sample Size

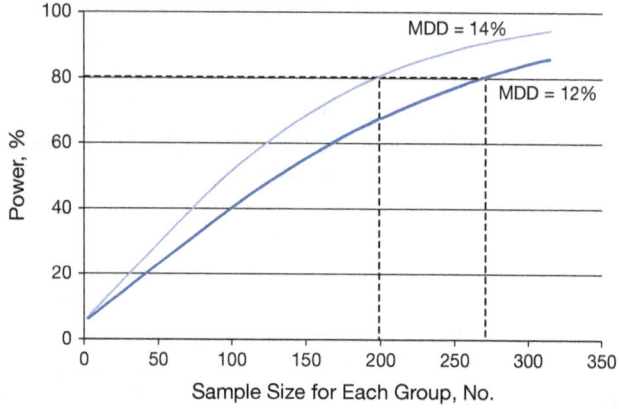

For a baseline rate of 45% and a minimum detectable difference (MDD) of 14%, the target sample size of 398 (199 in each group) will produce a power of 80% when α is set to .05. When the MDD is 12%, the resulting sample size is 542 (2 × 271) to achieve a power of 80%.

been studied. The MDD choice is more subjective. It should be a clinically meaningful rate difference, or a scientifically important rate difference, or both, that is also feasible to detect. For example, if the combination therapy of varenicline and nicotine patch increased abstinence by 0.1%, this difference would not be of practical benefit, would require an extremely large sample size, and would thus be too small a setting for the MDD. If the MDD were specified as 50%, the new therapy would have to be 95% effective (45% + 50%) before there would be a high chance of detecting any difference, so would be too large for the MDD. The authors based their choice of MDD = 14% on a compromise between their judgment of a clinically important difference, 12%, and the scientifically meaningful value of 16%. The 16% rate was the observed difference in a study that compared varenicline alone and together with nicotine gum.[4] Thus, the ability to confirm a difference that is slightly smaller for a related treatment was considered scientifically important.

What Are the Limitations of Power Analysis?

Calculation of sample size requires predictions of baseline rates and MDD, which may not be readily available, before the study begins. The sample size is especially sensitive to the MDD. This is illustrated by the blue line in Figure 2, which shows the sample size needed in this study if the MDD were set to 12%. The resulting sample size is 542 (2×271) to achieve a power of 80%.

This method of conducting a power analysis might also produce the incorrect sample size if the data analysis conducted differs from that planned. For example, if abstinence were affected by other covariates, such as age, and the groups were unbalanced on this variable, other analyses might be used, such as logistic regression models accounting for covariate differences. The sample size that would be appropriate for one analysis may be too large or small to achieve the same power with another analytic procedure.

Why Did the Authors Use Power Analysis in This Particular Study?

The number of research participants available for any study is limited by resources. However, the authors were aware that previous studies comparing these treatments had found no significant difference in abstinence rates. This can occur even if a difference exists if the sample size is too small. The authors wanted to ensure that their sample size was adequate to detect even a small but clinically important difference, so they carefully evaluated sample size.

How Should This Method's Findings Be Interpreted in This Particular Study?

A power analysis can help with the interpretation of study findings when statistically significant effects are not found. However, because the findings in the study by Koegelenberg et al[1] were statistically significant, interpretation of a lack of significance was unnecessary. If no statistically significant difference in abstinence rates had been found, the authors could have noted that, "The study was sufficiently powered to have a high chance of detecting a difference of 14% in abstinence rates. Thus, any undetected difference is likely to be of little clinical benefit."

CAVEATS TO CONSIDER WHEN LOOKING AT RESULTS BASED ON POWER ANALYSIS

Sample size calculation based on any power analysis requires input from the researcher prior to the study. Some of these are assumptions and predictions of fact (such as the baseline rate), which may be incorrect. Others reflect the clinical judgment of the researcher (eg, MDD), with which the reader may disagree. If a statistically significant effect is not found, the reader should assess whether either of these is a concern.

The reader should also not interpret a lack of significance for an outcome other than the one on which the power analysis was based as confirmation that no difference exists, because the analysis is specific to the parameter settings. For example, no significant difference was found in this study for most adverse events rates, although the power analysis does not apply to these rates. Thus, the sample size may not be adequate to interpret that finding to confirm that no meaningful difference in these outcomes exists.

Acknowledgment

The following disclosures were reported at the time this original article was first published in *JAMA*.

Conflict of Interest Disclosures: None reported.

References

1. Koegelenberg CFN, Noor F, Bateman ED, et al. Efficacy of varenicline combined with nicotine replacement therapy vs varenicline alone for smoking cessation: a randomized clinical trial. *JAMA*. 2014;312:155-161. doi:10.1001/jama.2014.7195.
2. Hajek P, Smith KM, Dhanji AR, McRobbie H. Is a combination of varenicline and nicotine patch more effective in helping smokers quit than varenicline alone? A randomised controlled trial. *BMC Med*. 2013;11:140. Medline:23718718
3. Ebbert JO, Burke MV, Hays JT, Hurt RD. Combination treatment with varenicline and nicotine replacement therapy. *Nicotine Tob Res*. 2009;11(5):572-576. Medline:19351781
4. Besada NA, Guerrero AC, Fernandez MI, Ulibarri MM, Jiménez-Ruiz CA. Clinical experience from a smokers clinic combining varenicline and nicotine gum. *Eur Respir J*. 2010;36(suppl 54):462s.

JAMAevidence
Using Evidence to Improve Care

Minimal Clinically Important Difference: Defining What Really Matters to Patients

Anna E. McGlothlin, PhD, and
Roger J. Lewis, MD, PhD

IN THIS CHAPTER

Use of the Method

Why Is the MCID Used?

What Are the Limitations of MCID Derivation Methods?

Why Did the Authors Use MCID in This Particular Study?

How Should MCID Findings Be Interpreted in This Particular Study?

Caveats to Consider When Looking at Results Based on MCIDs

This JAMA Guide to Statistics and Methods explains minimal clinically important difference, a concept in which clinicians define the smallest benefit of value to patients to help determine whether a therapy improves a subjective outcome enough from the perspective of the patient.

When assessing the clinical utility of therapies intended to improve subjective outcomes, the amount of improvement that is important to patients must be determined.[1] The smallest benefit of value to patients is called the minimal clinically important difference (MCID). The MCID is a patient-centered concept, capturing both the magnitude of the improvement and also the value patients place on the change. Using patient-centered MCIDs is important for studies involving patient-reported outcomes,[2] for which the clinical importance of a given change may not be obvious to clinicians selecting treatments. The MCID defines the smallest amount an outcome must change to be meaningful to patients.[1]

For example, Hinman et al[3] reported findings from a clinical trial evaluating whether acupuncture (needle, laser, and sham laser) improved pain or overall functional outcomes compared with no acupuncture among patients with chronic knee pain. Pain was measured on a numerical rating scale and functional status by the Western Ontario and McMaster Universities Osteoarthritis Index (WOMAC) score. The MCIDs for both end points were based on prior experience with these scoring systems. The MCID for pain was determined using an expert consensus, or Delphi approach,[4] while the MCID for function was determined using an "anchor" approach, based on patients' qualitative assessments of their own responses to treatment.[5]

USE OF THE METHOD

Why Is the MCID Used?

The appropriate clinical interpretation of changes on a numerical scale must consider not only statistical significance, but also whether the observed change is meaningful to patients. Identical changes on a numerical scale may have different clinical importance in different patient populations (eg, different ages, disease severity, injury type). Furthermore, statistical significance is linked to the sample size. Given a large enough sample, statistical significance between groups may occur with very small differences that are clinically meaningless.[6]

When determining how many patients to enroll in a study, the calculation usually reflects the intention to reliably find a clinically important effect of a treatment, such as the MCID. The smaller the treatment effect sought, the larger the required number of study participants.[7]

The MCID can be calculated using consensus, anchor, and distribution-based methods. Consensus (also known as Delphi) methods convene an expert panel to provide independent assessments of what constitutes a clinically relevant change. The assessments are then revised after the panel members review each other's assessments. This process is repeated until a consensus is reached regarding a numerical value for the MCID. The MCID for the pain assessment scale used in Hinman et al[3] was determined by the Delphi method using a panel of 6 rheumatology experts.[4]

Anchor-based methods determine the MCID by associating the change in the numerical scale for an outcome to some other subjective and independent assessment of improvement. For example, patients may be asked if they felt "about the same," "a little bit better," or "quite a bit better" after receiving treatment. These categorical responses are then related to the numerical measurement scale used in the study, "anchoring" the numerical outcome scale to the qualitative, categorical assessment that is presumably more meaningful to patients. The MCID for the WOMAC measure of functional status in the study by Hinman et al[3] was based on the 75th percentile of the WOMAC score; 75% of patients categorizing themselves as having experienced benefit (the anchor) had an improvement equal to or larger than the derived MCID using this definition.[5]

Distribution-based methods for defining the MCID involve neither expert opinion nor patient assessments. These methods rely on the statistical properties of the distribution of outcome scores, particularly how widely the scores vary between patients. These methods determine what magnitude of change is required to show that the change in an outcome measure in response to an intervention is more than would be expected from chance alone. Because distribution-based methods are not derived from individual patients, they probably should not be used to determine an MCID.[6]

What Are the Limitations of MCID Derivation Methods?

Consensus methods use clinical and domain experts, rather than patients, to define the MCID. In many settings, expert opinion may not be a valid and reliable way to determine what is important to patients.

Anchor-based methods are limited by the choice of anchor, which is a subjective assessment. For example, when an anchor is based on asking a patient whether he or she improved after receiving treatment, the response may be susceptible to recall bias. A patient's current status tends to influence recollection of the past. The anchor's validity and reliability are crucial for determination of a valid MCID.

Anchor-based methods may be influenced by the statistical distribution of scores within each category of the anchor. If the data are highly skewed, such as occurs with length-of-stay information because of the occasional outlying patient with a complicated clinical course, the derivation of the MCID may be affected by the outliers. Furthermore, anchor methods often rely on an MCID estimate derived from only a subset of patients (those within a particular category of the anchor). Not accounting for information from patients outside of this group may result in erroneous MCID estimates if the characteristics of the excluded patients differ from those who were included.

Because distribution-based methods are based on purely statistical reasoning, they can only identify a minimal detectable effect: that is, an effect that is unlikely to be attributable to random measurement error. The lack of an anchor that links the numeric scores to an assessment of what is important to patients causes distribution-based methods to fall short of identifying important, clinically meaningful outcomes for patients. In fact, the term MCID is sometimes replaced by "minimal detectable change" when the difference is calculated by distribution-based methods.[6] Distribution-based methods are not recommended as a first-line means for determining MCID.

Ideally, determination of the MCID should consider different thresholds in different subsets of the population. For example, patients with substantial amounts of pain at baseline might require greater pain reduction to perceive treatment benefit compared with those patients who have little baseline pain.

Why Did the Authors Use MCID in This Particular Study?

Hinman et al[3] specified an MCID for each end point to establish an appropriate sample size for their study and to facilitate clinically meaningful interpretation of the final outcome data. The number of patients enrolled was selected to provide sufficient power (ie, probability) for detecting a change in outcomes resulting from the intervention that was at least as large as the MCID for each end point.

How Should MCID Findings Be Interpreted in This Particular Study?

The actual treatment effects observed in the study of Hinman et al[3] were quite modest, ranging from an improvement of 0.9 to 1.2 units in pain, relative to an MCID of 1.8 units, and an improvement of 4.4 to 5.1 units in function, relative to an MCID of 6 WOMAC units. Although there were statistically significant differences between groups, the clinical importance of these differences is uncertain.[3]

CAVEATS TO CONSIDER WHEN LOOKING AT RESULTS BASED ON MCIDS

In the study by Hinman et al,[3] the observed effect is smaller than the predefined MCID, yet the differences between groups still achieved statistical significance. This phenomenon is not uncommon and occurred in another recently published study in *JAMA* on the effect of vagal nerve stimulation for obesity treatment.[8] This occurs because the study sample size is selected to achieve a high probability of detecting a benefit equal to the MCID, resulting in a substantial chance of demonstrating statistical significance even when the effect of an intervention is smaller than the MCID.

In the study by Hinman et al,[3] acupuncture therapies were compared with control groups by measuring difference in mean changes in pain and function scores. An alternative experimental design would be based on a "responder analysis," namely, comparing the proportion of patients within each therapy who experienced a change greater than the MCID. This type of data presentation could be more informative because it focuses on patients who experience an improvement at least as large as the MCID.[2] This approach is useful when the data are highly skewed by outliers in such a way that the calculated mean value may be above the MCID even when most patients do not have an effect greater than the MCID.

A fundamental aspect of MCIDs that is often ignored is the need to consider potential improvements from an intervention in relation to costs and complications. When selecting an MCID for a clinical trial, defining a meaningful improvement from the patient's perspective ideally involves considering all aspects of clinical care, both favorable and unfavorable.

Acknowledgment

The following disclosures were reported at the time this original article was first published in *JAMA*.
Conflict of Interest Disclosures: None reported.

References

1. Jaeschke R, Singer J, Guyatt GH. Measurement of health status: ascertaining the minimal clinically important difference. *Control Clin Trials*. 1989;10(4):407-415. Medline:2691207
2. Guidance for industry: patient-reported outcome measures: use in medical product development to support labeling claims. Food and Drug Administration. http://www.fda.gov/downloads/Drugs/Guidances/UCM193282.pdf. Accessed August 27, 2014.
3. Hinman RS, McCrory P, Pirotta M, et al. Acupuncture for chronic knee pain: a randomized clinical trial. *JAMA*. 2014;312(13):1313-1322. doi:10.1001/jama.2014.12660
4. Bellamy N, Carette S, Ford PM, et al. Osteoarthritis antirheumatic drug trials: III, setting the delta for clinical trials: results of a consensus development (Delphi) exercise. *J Rheumatol*. 1992;19(3):451-457. Medline:1578462
5. Tubach F, Ravaud P, Baron G, et al. Evaluation of clinically relevant changes in patient reported outcomes in knee and hip osteoarthritis: the minimal clinically important improvement. *Ann Rheum Dis*. 2005;64(1):29-33. Medline:15208174
6. Turner D, Schünemann HJ, Griffith LE, et al. The minimal detectable change cannot reliably replace the minimal important difference. *J Clin Epidemiol*. 2010;63(1):28-36. Medline:19800198
7. Livingston EH, Elliot A, Hynan L, Cao J. Effect size estimation: a necessary component of statistical analysis. *Arch Surg*. 2009;144(8):706-712. Medline:19687373
8. Ikramuddin S, Blackstone RP, Brancatisano A, et al. Effect of reversible intermittent intra-abdominal vagal nerve blockade on morbid obesity: the ReCharge randomized clinical trial. *JAMA*. 2014;312(9):915-922. Medline:25182100

Randomization in Clinical Trials: Permuted Blocks and Stratification

Kristine Broglio, MS

IN THIS CHAPTER

Explanation of the Concept

What Are Permuted Blocks and Stratified Randomization?

Why Are Permuted Blocks and Stratified Randomization Important?

Limitations of Permuted Block Randomization and Stratified Randomization

How Were These Approaches to Randomization Used?

How Does the Approach to Randomization Affect the Trial's Interpretation?

This JAMA Guide to Statistics and Methods explains the rationale for permuted block randomization and for stratifying randomization in clinical trials.

The most compelling way to establish that an intervention definitively causes a clinical outcome is to randomly allocate patients into treatment groups. Randomization helps to ensure that a certain proportion of patients receive each treatment and that the treatment groups being compared are similar in both measured and unmeasured patient characteristics.[1,2] Simple or unrestricted, equal randomization of patients between 2 treatment groups is equivalent to tossing a fair coin for each patient assignment.[2,3] As the sample size increases, the 2 groups will become more perfectly balanced. However, this balance is not guaranteed when there are relatively few patients enrolled in a trial. In the coin toss scenario, obtaining several consecutive heads, for example, is more likely than typically perceived.[1,4] If a long series of assignments to 1 group occurred when randomizing patients in a clinical trial, imbalances between the groups would occur.

Imbalances between groups can be minimized in small sample–size studies by restricting the randomization procedure. Restricted randomization means that simple randomization is applied within defined groups of patients. Two articles published in *JAMA* used restrictions on the randomization procedure: Bilecen et al[5] used permuted block randomization, a restricted randomization method used to help ensure the balance of the number of patients assigned to each treatment group.[3] Kim et al[6] used a stratified randomization scheme together with permuted block randomization. Stratified randomization is a restricted randomization method used to balance one or a few prespecified prognostic characteristics between treatment groups.[1]

EXPLANATION OF THE CONCEPT

What Are Permuted Blocks and Stratified Randomization?

The permuted block technique randomizes patients between groups within a set of study participants, called a block. Treatment assignments within blocks are determined so that they are random in order but that the desired allocation proportions are achieved exactly within each block. In a 2-group trial with equal allocation and a block size of 6, 3 patients in each block would be assigned to the control and 3 to the treatment and the ordering of those 6 assignments would be random. For example, with treatment labels A and B, possible blocks might be: ABBABA, BABBAA, and AABABB. As each block is filled, the trial is guaranteed to have the desired allocation to each group.

Stratified randomization requires identification of key prognostic characteristics that are measurable at the time of randomization and are considered to be strongly associated with the primary outcome. The categories of the prognostic characteristics define the strata and the total number of strata for randomization is the product of the number of categories across the selected prognostic characteristics.[1,7] Randomization is then performed separately within each stratum.[7] For example, if randomization were stratified by sex (men vs women) and age (<40, 40-59, ≥60 years), there would be a total of 6 strata. Randomization within each stratum could be a simple randomization or could be a permuted block randomization.

Why Are Permuted Blocks and Stratified Randomization Important?

The most efficient allocation of patients for maximizing statistical power is often equal allocation into groups. Power to detect a treatment effect is increased as the standard error of the treatment-effect estimate is decreased. In a 2-group setting, allocating more patients to 1 group would reduce the standard error for that 1 group but doing so would decrease the sample size and increase the standard error in the other group. The standard error of the treatment effect or the difference between the groups is therefore minimized with equal allocation.[8] Permuted block randomization avoids such imbalances.[2] This is an important consideration for trials with planned interim analyses because interim analyses may be conducted using small sample sizes resulting in a greater chance of having large imbalances in the allocation of patients between groups.[1,4,7]

Stratified randomization ensures balance between treatment groups for the selected, measurable prognostic characteristics used to define the strata. Because stratified randomization essentially produces a randomized trial within each stratum, stratification can be used when different patient populations are being enrolled or if it is important to analyze results within the subgroups defined by the stratifying characteristics.[3,7] For example, when there are concerns that an intervention is influenced by patient sex, stratification might occur by sex. Because patients are randomly allocated both in the male and female groups, the effect of the intervention can be tested for the entire population and—assuming sufficient sample size—separately in men and women.

LIMITATIONS OF PERMUTED BLOCK RANDOMIZATION AND STRATIFIED RANDOMIZATION

The main limitation of permuted block randomization is the potential for bias if treatment assignments become known or predictable.[1,9] For example, with a block size of 4, if an investigator knew the first 3 assignments in the block, the investigator also would know with certainty the assignment for the next patient enrolled. The use of reasonably large block sizes, random block sizes, and strong blinding procedures such as double-blind treatment assignments and identical-appearing placebos are strategies used to prevent this.

In stratified randomization, the number of strata should be fairly limited, such as 3 or 4, but even fewer strata should be used in trials enrolling relatively few research participants.[7,10] There is no particular statistical disadvantage to stratification, but strata do result in more complex randomization procedures.[3] In some settings, stratified randomization may not be possible because it is simply not feasible to determine a patient's prognostic characteristics before getting a treatment assignment, such as in an emergency setting. An alternative to stratification is to prespecify a statistical adjustment for the key characteristics in the primary analysis that are thought to influence outcomes and may not be completely balanced between groups by the randomization procedure. Another alternative to stratification is minimization.[7] Minimization considers the current balance of the key prognostic characteristics between treatment groups and if an imbalance exists, assigns future patients as necessary to rebalance the groups.[7] For example, if the experimental group had a smaller proportion of women than did the control group and the next patient to be randomized is a woman, a minimization procedure might assign that patient to the experimental group. Minimization can be more complex than stratification, but is effective and can accommodate more factors than stratification.[7]

How Were These Approaches to Randomization Used?

Bilecen et al[5] reported a single-center randomized clinical trial comparing a fibrinogen concentrate with placebo in reducing intraoperative bleeding during high-risk cardiac surgery, with a total sample size of 120 patients. In this study, patients were randomized according to a permuted block randomization scheme with a block size of 4. With this randomization scheme, the entire randomization list can be generated before a single patient is enrolled. Random treatment assignments are generated in groups of 4, by randomly selecting 2 of the assignments to be to the control group and then allowing the remaining 2 assignments to be to the treatment group. As each patient is randomized into the trial, the patient receives the next sequential assignment on the randomization list. The study by Bilecen et al had an equal number of patients randomized into the 2 treatment groups. The block sizes were small, so randomization was performed centrally and blinding procedures were in place to minimize the ability of the investigators to predict the randomization sequence.

Kim et al[6] performed a multicenter clinical trial assessing the hemoglobin response at 12 weeks among patients undergoing radical gastrectomy after administration of ferric carboxymaltose or placebo. A total of 454 patients were randomized using both stratification and permuted blocks with random block sizes. Randomization was stratified at each site based on the clinical stage of gastric cancer. For this randomization scheme, a randomization list can be generated prior to the start of the trial as well, but 1 randomization list must be generated for each site and clinical stage strata. A sequence of block sizes is randomly generated where allowable block sizes were 2, 4, or 6 in this study. Within each block, half of the assignments are randomly selected to be to the control group and remaining assignments are allowed to be to the treatment group. As each patient is randomized into the trial, the patient receives the next sequential assignment on the randomization list specific to his/her site and clinical cancer stage. The use of a random block size ensures that the next randomization assignment cannot be guessed. Because this was a multicenter trial with 7 sites, randomization within each site ensures that a site discontinuing participation in the trial or enrolling poorly would not affect the overall balance of the treatment groups.[2,7] Stratifying by clinical cancer stage ensures that the control and intervention groups are balanced on this 1 important prognostic characteristic.

The treatment groups were nearly equal in size and were balanced for cancer stage. While Kim et al did not report the primary efficacy results by cancer stage subgroups, it would have been appropriate to do so.

How Does the Approach to Randomization Affect the Trial's Interpretation?

In a clinical trial, the ultimate goal of the randomization procedure is to create similar treatment groups that allow an unbiased comparison. Restricted randomization procedures such as stratified randomization and permuted block randomization create balance between important prognostic characteristics and are useful when conducting randomized trials enrolling relatively few patients.[3] In the cases of the trials by Bilecen et al and by Kim et al, the restricted randomization procedures minimized the risk of biased study results by ensuring balanced treatment groups.

Acknowledgment

The following disclosures were reported at the time this original article was first published in *JAMA*.

Conflict of Interest Disclosures: None reported.

References

1. Pocock SJ. Allocation of patients to treatment in clinical trials. *Biometrics*. 1979;35(1):183-197. Medline:497334
2. Lachin JM. Statistical properties of randomization in clinical trials. *Control Clin Trials*. 1988;9(4):289-311. Medline:3060315
3. Lachin JM, Matts JP, Wei LJ. Randomization in clinical trials: conclusions and recommendations. *Control Clin Trials*. 1988;9(4):365-374. Medline:3203526
4. Zelen M. The randomization and stratification of patients to clinical trials. *J Chronic Dis*. 1974;27(7-8):365-375. Medline:4612056
5. Bilecen S, de Groot JAH, Kalkman CJ, et al. Effect of fibrinogen concentrate on intraoperative blood loss among patients with intraoperative bleeding during high-risk cardiac surgery: a randomized clinical trial. *JAMA*. 2017; 317(7):738-747. Medline:28241354

6. Kim Y-W, Bae J-M, Park Y-K, et al. FAIRY Study Group. Effect of intravenous ferric carboxymaltose on hemoglobin response among patients with acute isovolemic anemia following gastrectomy: the FAIRY Randomized Clinical Trial. *JAMA*. 2017;317(20):2097-2104. Medline:28535237

7. Kernan WN, Viscoli CM, Makuch RW, Brass LM, Horwitz RI. Stratified randomization for clinical trials. *J Clin Epidemiol*. 1999;52(1):19-26. Medline:9973070

8. Hey SP, Kimmelman J. The questionable use of unequal allocation in confirmatory trials. *Neurology*. 2014;82(1):77-79. Medline:24306005

9. Matts JP, Lachin JM. Properties of permuted-block randomization in clinical trials. *Control Clin Trials*. 1988;9(4):327-344. Medline:3203524

10. Therneau TM. How many stratification factors are "too many" to use in a randomization plan? *Control Clin Trials*. 1993;14(2):98-108. Medline:8500309

Equipoise in Research: Integrating Ethics and Science in Human Research

Alex John London, PhD

IN THIS CHAPTER

What Is Equipoise?

Why Is Equipoise Important?

What Are the Limitations of Equipoise?

How Is Equipoise Applied in This Case?

How Does Equipoise Influence the Interpretation of the Study?

This JAMA Guide to Statistics and Methods reviews the concept of equipoise, which allows for randomization of interventions while also respecting the rights of human subjects in clinical research.

The principle of equipoise states that, when there is uncertainty or conflicting expert opinion about the relative merits of diagnostic, prevention, or treatment options, allocating interventions to individuals in a manner that allows the generation of new knowledge (eg, randomization) is ethically permissible.[1,2] The principle of equipoise reconciles 2 potentially conflicting ethical imperatives: to ensure that research involving human participants generates scientifically sound and clinically relevant information while demonstrating proper respect and concern for the rights and interests of study participants.[1]

Lascarrou et al[3] reported the results of a randomized trial designed to investigate whether the "routine use of the video laryngoscope for orotracheal intubation of patients in the ICU increased the frequency of successful first-pass intubation compared with use of the Macintosh direct laryngoscope." Intubation in the intensive care unit (ICU) is associated with the potential for serious adverse events, and video laryngoscopy in the ICU has gained support from some clinicians who believe it to be superior to direct laryngoscopy. Such practitioners may therefore regard it as unethical to randomize study participants to direct laryngoscopy because they consider it to be an inferior intervention. But requiring uncertainty of individual clinicians to conduct a clinical trial gives too much ethical weight to personal judgment, hindering valuable research without providing benefit to patients. Therefore, it is important to understand the role of conflicting expert medical judgment in establishing equipoise and how this principle applies to the trial conducted by Lascarrou et al.[3]

WHAT IS EQUIPOISE?

Two features of medical research pose special challenges for the goal of ensuring respect and concern for the rights and interests of participants. First, to generate reliable information, research often involves design features that alter the way participants are treated. For example, randomization and blinding are commonly used to reduce selection bias and treatment bias.[4] Controlling how interventions are allocated and what researchers and participants know about who is receiving which interventions helps to more clearly distinguish the effects of the intervention from confounding effects. But randomization severs the link between what a participant receives and the recommendation of a treating clinician with an ethical duty to provide the best possible care for the individual person. In the study by Lascarrou et al,[3] patients were randomized to undergo intubation with the video laryngoscope or the direct laryngoscope, independent of the preference of the treating physician.

Second, medical research involves exposing people to interventions whose risks and potential therapeutic, prophylactic, or diagnostic merits may be unknown, unclear, or the subject of disagreement within the medical community. In the present case, some clinicians may maintain that video laryngoscopy is the superior strategy for orotracheal intubation in the ICU, others may disagree, while others judge that there is not sufficient evidence to warrant a strong commitment for or against this approach.

The principle of equipoise states that if there is uncertainty or conflicting expert opinion about the relative therapeutic, prophylactic, or diagnostic merits of a set of interventions, then it is permissible to allocate a participant to receive an intervention from this set, so long as there is not consensus that an alternative intervention would better advance that participant's interests.[1,2,5-7]

In the present case, there is equipoise between video and direct laryngoscopy because experts disagree about their relative clinical merits. These disagreements are reflected in variations in clinical practices. If it is ethically permissible for patients to receive care from expert clinicians in good professional standing with differing medical opinions about what constitutes optimal treatment, then it ordinarily cannot be wrong to permit participants to be randomized to those same treatment alternatives.[5] Although randomization removes the link between what a participant receives and the recommendation of a particular clinician, the presence of equipoise ensures that each participant receives an intervention that would be recommended or utilized by at least a reasonable minority of informed expert clinicians.[1,5,6] Equipoise thus ensures that randomization is consistent with respect for participant interests because it guarantees that no participant receives care known to be inferior to any available alternative.

WHY IS EQUIPOISE IMPORTANT?

Ensuring equipoise helps researchers and institutional review boards (IRBs) fulfill 3 ethical obligations. First, to "disturb" equipoise studies must be designed to generate information that resolves uncertainty or reduces divergence in opinion among qualified medical experts. Such studies are likely to have both social and scientific values. Second, any risks to which participants are exposed must be reasonable in light of the value of the information a study is likely to produce.[5,6] IRBs must make this determination before participants are enrolled.

Third is the obligation to show respect for potential participants as autonomous decision makers. Explaining during the informed consent process the nature of the uncertainty or conflict in medical judgment that a study is designed to resolve allows each individual to decide whether to participate by understanding the relevant uncertainties, their effects on that person's own interests, and how their resolution will contribute to improving the state of medical care.

WHAT ARE THE LIMITATIONS OF EQUIPOISE?

Since its introduction, the concept of equipoise has received numerous formulations, creating the potential for confusion and misunderstanding[2,7] and spurring criticism and debate. One criticism holds that the version of equipoise described here is too permissive because it allows randomization even when individual clinicians are not uncertain about how best to treat a patient.[8] The trial conducted by Lascarrou et al[3] represents a case in which some clinicians have strong preferences for one modality of treatment over others. Requiring individual clinician uncertainty entrenches unwarranted variation in patient care by preventing participants from being offered the choice of participating in a study in which they might be allocated to interventions that would be recommended or utilized by other medical experts. If it is ethically acceptable for patients to receive care from informed, expert clinicians who favor different interventions, then it ordinarily cannot be unethical to allow patients to be randomized to the alternatives that such clinicians recommend. Legitimate disagreement among informed experts signifies that the clinical community lacks a basis for judging that patients are better off with one modality over the other.

An interpretation of equipoise that requires uncertainty on the part of the individual clinician is not ethically justified because it prevents studies that are likely to improve the quality of patient care without the credible expectation that this restriction will improve patient outcomes.

Another criticism is that equipoise is unlikely ever to exist, or to persist for long.[9] This objection applies most directly to the view that equipoise only exists if the individual clinician believes that the interventions offered in a trial are of exactly equal expected value.[10] On this view, equipoise would often disappear even though different experts retain conflicting medical recommendations. It therefore appears poorly suited to the goals of promoting the production of valuable information and protecting the interests of study participants.

HOW IS EQUIPOISE APPLIED IN THIS CASE?

Lascarrou et al[3] did not explicitly discuss equipoise in their study. However, the consent process approved by the ethics committee reflects the judgment that the interventions in the trial "were considered components of standard care" and patients who lacked decisional capacity could be enrolled even if no surrogate decision maker was present.

Ensuring that a study begins in and is designed to disturb a state of equipoise provides credible assurance to participants and other stakeholders that patients in medical distress can be enrolled in a study that will help improve patient care in emergency settings without concern that their health interests will be knowingly compromised in the process.

HOW DOES EQUIPOISE INFLUENCE THE INTERPRETATION OF THE STUDY?

In the past, strongly held beliefs about the effectiveness of treatments ranging from bloodletting to menopausal hormone therapy have proven to be false. Intubation in the ICU is associated with the potential for serious adverse events. Because video laryngoscopy is increasingly championed as the superior method for orotracheal intubation in the ICU, careful study of its relative merits and risks in comparison to conventional direct laryngoscopy addresses a question of clinical importance. The findings of Lascarrou et al[3] suggest that perceived merits of video laryngoscopy do not translate into superior clinical outcomes and may be associated with higher rates of life-threatening complications. This result underscores the importance of conducting clinical research before novel interventions become widely incorporated into clinical practice, even if those interventions appear to offer clear advantages over existing alternatives.

Acknowledgment

The following disclosures were reported at the time this original article was first published in *JAMA*.

Conflict of Interest Disclosures: None reported.

References

1. Freedman B. Equipoise and the ethics of clinical research. *N Engl J Med*. 1987;317(3):141-145. Medline:3600702
2. London AJ. Clinical equipoise: foundational requirement or fundamental error? In: Steinbock B, ed. *The Oxford Handbook of Bioethics*. Oxford, UK: Oxford University Press; 2007:571-595.
3. Lascarrou JB, Boisrame-Helms J, Bailly A, et al. Clinical Research in Intensive Care and Sepsis (CRICS) Group. Video laryngoscopy vs direct laryngoscopy on successful first-pass orotracheal intubation among ICU patients: a randomized clinical trial. *JAMA*. 2017;317(5):483-493. doi:10.1001/jama.2016.20603
4. Guyatt G, Rennie D, Meade MO, Cook DJ. *Users' Guides to the Medical Literature: A Manual for Evidence-Based Clinical Practice*. 3rd ed. New York, NY: McGraw-Hill; 2015.
5. London AJ. Reasonable risks in clinical research: a critique and a proposal for the Integrative Approach. *Stat Med*. 2006;25(17):2869-2885. Medline:16810711
6. Miller PB, Weijer C. Rehabilitating equipoise. *Kennedy Inst Ethics J*. 2003;13(2):93-118. Medline:14569997
7. van der Graaf R, van Delden JJ. Equipoise should be amended, not abandoned. *Clin Trials*. 2011;8(4):408-416. Medline:21746767
8. Hellman D. Evidence, belief, and action: the failure of equipoise to resolve the ethical tension in the randomized clinical trial. *J Law Med Ethics*. 2002;30(3):375-380. Medline:12497697
9. Sackett DL. Equipoise, a term whose time (if it ever came) has surely gone. *CMAJ*. 2000;163(7):835-836. Medline:11033713
10. Lilford RJ, Jackson J. Equipoise and the ethics of randomization. *J R Soc Med*. 1995;88(10):552-559. Medline:8537943

Time-to-Event Analysis

Juliana Tolles, MD, MHS, and
Roger J. Lewis, MD, PhD

IN THIS CHAPTER

Use of the Method

Why Is Time-to-Event Analysis Used?

What Are the Limitations of the Proportional Hazards Model?

How Should Time-to-Event Findings Be Interpreted in This Particular Study?

Caveats to Consider When Looking at Results from a Time-to-Event Analysis

This JAMA Guide to Statistics and Methods discusses the use of time-to-event analysis to evaluate the risk of an adverse outcome from a medical treatment.

Time-to-event analysis, also called survival analysis, was used in the study by Nissen et al[1] to compare the risk of major adverse cardiovascular events (MACE) in a noninferiority trial of a combination of naltrexone and bupropion vs placebo for overweight or obese patients with cardiovascular risk factors. The authors used a type of time-to-event analysis called Cox proportional hazards modeling to compare the risk of MACE in the 2 groups, concluding that the use of naltrexone-bupropion increased the risk of MACE per unit time by no more than a factor of 2.

USE OF THE METHOD

Why Is Time-to-Event Analysis Used?

One way to evaluate how a medical treatment affects patients' risk of an adverse outcome is to analyze the time intervals between the initiation of treatment and the occurrence of such events. That information can be used to calculate the hazard for each treatment group in a clinical trial. The hazard is the probability that the adverse event will occur in a defined time interval. For example, Nissen et al[1] could measure the number of patients who experience MACE while taking naltrexone-bupropion during week 8 of the study and calculate the risk that an individual patient will experience MACE during week 8, assuming that the patient has not had MACE before week 8. This concept of a discrete hazard rate can be extended to a hazard function, which is generally a continuous curve that describes how the hazard changes over time. The hazard function shows the risk at each point in time and is expressed as a rate or number of events per unit of time.[2]

Calculating the hazard function using time-to-event observations is challenging because the event of interest is usually not observed in all patients. Thus, the time to the event occurrence for some patients is invisible—or censored—and there is no way to know if the event will occur in the near future, the distant future, or never. Censoring may occur because the patient is lost to follow-up or did not experience the event of interest before the end of the study period. In the study by Nissen et al,[1] only 243 patients experienced MACE before the termination of the study, resulting in 8662 censored observations, meaning there were 8662 patients for whom it is not known when they experienced MACE, if ever. Common nonparametric statistical tests, such as the Wilcoxon rank sum test, could be used to compare the time intervals seen in the 2 groups if the analysis was limited to only the 243 patients who had observed events; however, when censored data are excluded from analysis, the information contained in the experience of the other 8662 patients is lost. While it is unknown when in the future, if ever, these patients will experience an event, the knowledge that these patients did not experience MACE during their participation in the trial is informative. The information contained in censored observations varies: patients whose data are censored early, such as a patient who is lost to follow-up in the first weeks of a study, contribute less information than those who are observed for a long time before censoring. However, all observations provide some information, and to avoid bias, methods of analysis that can accommodate censoring are used for time-to-event studies.

Kaplan-Meier plots and the Cox proportional hazards model are examples of methods for analyzing time-to-event data that account for censored observations. A Kaplan-Meier curve plots the fraction of "surviving" patients (those who have not experienced an event) against time for each treatment group. The height of the Kaplan-Meier curve at the end of each time interval is determined by taking the fraction or proportion of patients who remained event-free at the end of the prior time interval and multiplying that proportion by the fraction of patients who survive the current time interval without experiencing an event. The value of the Kaplan-Meier curve at the end of the current time interval then becomes the starting value for the next time interval. This iterative and cumulative multiplication process begins with the first time interval and continues in a stepwise manner along the Kaplan-Meier curve; the Kaplan-Meier curve is thus sometimes called the "product limit estimate" of the survival curve. Censoring is properly taken into account because only patients still being followed up at the beginning of each time interval are considered in determining the fraction "surviving" at the end of that time interval.[3] Figures 2A and 2B in the article by Nissen et al[1] plot the cumulative incidence of MACE in each group vs time, an "upside-down" version of Kaplan-Meier, which provides similar information.

While a Kaplan-Meier plot elegantly represents differences between different groups' survival curves over time, it gives little indication of their statistical significance. The statistical significance of observed differences can be tested with a log-rank test.[3] This test, however, does not account for confounding variables, such as differences in patient demographics between groups.

The Cox proportional hazards model both addresses the problem of censoring and allows adjustment for multiple prognostic independent variables, or confounders such as age and sex. The model assumes a "baseline" hazard function exists for individuals whose independent predictor variables are all equal to their reference value. The baseline hazard function is not explicitly defined but is allowed to take any shape. The output of a Cox proportional hazards model is a hazard ratio for each independent predictor variable, which defines how much the hazard is multiplied for each unit change in the variable of interest as compared with the baseline hazard function. Hazard ratios can be calculated for all independent variables, both confounders and intervention variables.

What Are the Limitations of the Proportional Hazards Model?

The Cox proportional hazards model relies on 2 important assumptions. The first is that data censoring is independent of outcome of interest. If the placebo patients in the trial by Nissen et al[1] were both less likely to experience MACE and less likely to follow up with trial investigators because they did not experience weight loss, the probability of censoring and the risk of MACE would be correlated, threatening the validity of the analysis. The second assumption is that the hazard functions, representing the risk of an event over time, are proportional to each other for all patient groups. In other words, the hazard functions all have the same shape and differ only in overall magnitude; the effect of each independent predictor or confounder is on the overall magnitude of the hazard function. In this trial, it is reasonable to assume that the baseline hazard function for MACE in patients taking placebo looks like a line with a positive slope: age likely increases the hazard of a cardiovascular event. The assumption of proportional hazards means that the hazard function of MACE in patients taking naltrexone-bupropion is assumed to be the baseline hazard multiplied by an unknown, constant value. This assumption would be violated if, for example, patients taking the drug experience an early increase in risk of MACE after initiating treatment as a result of adverse effects but then experience decreased risk over the long-term as they lose weight. In that scenario, the treatment group hazard function would be shaped like a peak with a long tail and would not be proportional to the baseline hazard function.

How Should Time-to-Event Findings Be Interpreted in This Particular Study?

The trial was designed as a noninferiority study and statistically powered to assess the null hypothesis that the hazard ratio of naltrexone-bupropion to placebo for MACE is greater than 2.0 at the 25% interim analysis point. Using a Cox proportional hazard model with randomized treatment as a predictor, the estimated hazard ratio was 0.59 (95% CI, 0.39-0.90). It can therefore be concluded that the hazard ratio of MACE associated with the active treatment was less than 2.0. Although it might be tempting to conclude that the hazard ratio is smaller (eg, less than 1.0), the hypothesis testing structure of the noninferiority trial only allowed a rigorous conclusion to be drawn about the hypothesis that the hazard ratio was less than 2.0.

CAVEATS TO CONSIDER WHEN LOOKING AT RESULTS FROM A TIME-TO-EVENT ANALYSIS

Nissen et al[1] used a Cox proportional hazards model to estimate the hazard ratio associated with naltrexone-bupropion compared with placebo for MACE in overweight or obese patients with cardiovascular risk factors. This trial likely meets the assumptions of the Cox proportional hazards model: the censoring is likely to be independent of hazard, and the hazard functions for all groups are likely to be roughly proportional. Readers should interpret with caution any time-to-event analysis in which the probability of being lost to follow-up or the duration of observation is likely to be correlated with the risk of experiencing an event. Readers should also be cautious in accepting Cox proportional hazards models in which the hazard function of a treatment group is unlikely to be proportional to the baseline hazard. If 2 survival curves cross at any point, such as seen in the far right of Figure 2B in the article by Nissen et al,[1] this might suggest that the hazard ratio between the 2 groups has reversed and the proportionality assumption has been violated (Figure 3). There are also several diagnostic tests that researchers can use to verify the proportionality assumption, including using Kaplan-Meier curves, testing

FIGURE 3

Time to MACE in the Final End-of-Study Analysis

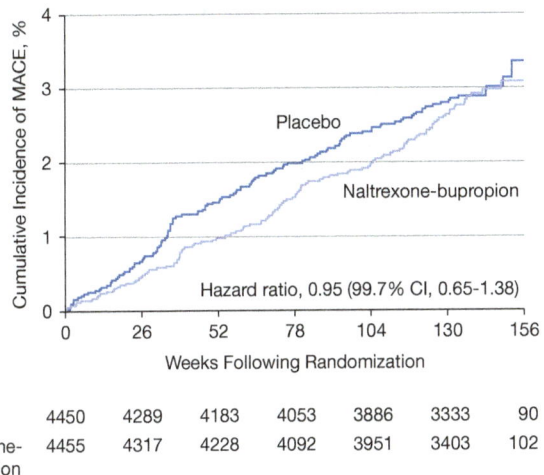

The survival curves cross in this figure from Nissen et al,[1] suggesting that the proportionality assumption may have been violated. MACE indicates major adverse cardiovascular events.

the significance of time-dependent covariates, and plotting Schoenfeld residuals.[4] Selection of an appropriate verification method depends on the types of covariates used in the Cox proportional hazards model.

Acknowledgment

The following disclosures were reported at the time this original article was first published in *JAMA*.

Conflict of Interest Disclosures: None reported.

References

1. Nissen SE, Wolski KE, Prcela L, et al. Effect of naltrexone-bupropion on major adverse cardiovascular events in overweight and obese patients with cardiovascular risk factors: a randomized clinical trial. *JAMA*. 2016;315(10): 990-1004. doi:10.1001/jama.2016.1558.
2. Lee ET. *Statistical Methods for Survival Analysis*. 2nd ed. New York, NY: John Wiley & Sons; 1992.
3. Young KD, Menegazzi JJ, Lewis RJ. Statistical methodology: IX, Survival analysis. *Acad Emerg Med*. 1999;6(3):244-249. Medline:10192678
4. Hess KR. Graphical methods for assessing violations of the proportional hazards assumption in Cox regression. *Stat Med*. 1995;14(15):1707-1723. Medline:7481205

The "Utility" in Composite Outcome Measures: Measuring What Is Important to Patients

Telba Z. Irony, PhD

IN THIS CHAPTER

Why Are Composite End Points Used in Clinical Studies?

Limitations of Composite End Points

How Were Composite End Points Used in This Study?

How Does the Use of a Composite End Point Affect the Interpretation of This Study?

This JAMA Guide to Statistics and Methods reviews the use of composite outcome measures in clinical trials and discusses how their use should influence interpretations of trial results.

There are many harmful manifestations of atherosclerotic cardiovascular disease (ASCVD). Because all of these manifestations are undesirable, combining the most important ones into a single study outcome measure can simplify efforts to measure the overall effect of the disease on health outcomes. For example, ASCVD can result in myocardial infarction (MI), stroke, or death. Each of these is to be avoided, and how well an intervention reduces the risk of any of these occurring can be measured by combining all of these clinical outcomes into a single composite end point. A composite end point is an outcome that is defined as occurring if 1 or more of the components occur. For ASCVD, one of the most common composites is called major adverse cardiovascular events (MACE). Because a composite outcome occurs more frequently than its individual components, composites can reduce the number of study participants required to achieve the desired power of a study, making it easier and less expensive to conduct a clinical trial.

A study by Kavousi et al[1] demonstrates the benefits and limitations of composite outcomes. This study assessed the utility of coronary artery calcification (CAC) testing for estimating the probability of incident ASCVD in low-risk women using a composite end point that included nonfatal MI, coronary heart disease (CHD) death, and stroke. Overall, the authors found that CAC "was associated with an increased risk of ASCVD and modest improvement in prognostic accuracy compared with traditional risk factors."[1]

WHY ARE COMPOSITE END POINTS USED IN CLINICAL STUDIES?

Composite end points may be used in a clinical trial (or in observational studies) if the target disease has several clinically important consequences and the study is intended to examine the effects (or association) of an intervention on (or exposure with) more than 1 consequence or end point. In this case, a composite end point provides a summary measure for the treatment effect. Composite end points, such as MACE, may also be used when a single outcome of interest (eg, CHD death in a low-risk population) is rare, making it impractical to conduct studies that are adequately powered to demonstrate an effect of an intervention on its occurrence.[2] For rare outcomes, researchers often combine several types of events (CHD death, MI, and stroke) in a single composite end point. Because the frequency of the composite end point is greater than any of its components, this facilitates the design of studies of reasonable size and duration that have sufficient statistical power. If only 1 infrequent outcome were considered, such as CHD death, studies to determine the effect of an intervention on those outcomes could be unreasonably large or take too long to complete.

LIMITATIONS OF COMPOSITE END POINTS

When multiple outcomes are combined into a composite end point, each is given the same importance because the occurrence of any component counts equally within the composite. However, the relative importance of each component to patients, their families, and clinicians may be very different. For example, it is common to count the occurrence of CHD death, nonfatal MI, or stroke equally as a MACE event. If any of these outcomes should occur, the patient is considered to have the outcome event, resulting in each component being weighed equally. However, CHD death is more important to patients than nonfatal MI, especially if the patient recovers from the MI with little or no long-term effects.

If patients perceive the importance of individual component differently (eg, death being a much worse outcome than having an MI), then using a singular composite end point to represent a study result may be misleading. For example, the LIFE trial compared losartan and atenolol for hypertension and showed a statistically significant advantage of losartan for reducing the composite end point of having an ASCVD event (CHD death, MI, or stroke). However, this effect was only observed with stroke (fatal and nonfatal) and not with MI or CHD death.[3] Often, a positive effect on the composite end point is driven by the event with the highest occurrence rate (eg, significant reduction on nonfatal MI). If this component has relatively few consequences for a patient but other outcomes, such as stroke or CHD death, that are more consequential are unaffected or even increased by the intervention, then the apparent benefit of the intervention is misleading. To remedy this limitation, additional analyses, with each component considered individually, are recommended as an adjunct to the analysis of the composite outcome. However, because each individual component is less common than the composite, the power of these analyses is often limited and, further, multiple comparisons increase the risk of a false-positive result.[4]

In addition, if patients can experience the composite outcome more than once, and the number of events is the outcome of interest, then an intervention that increases the incidence of CHD death might incorrectly appear beneficial. This can happen because, when a death occurs, patients are no longer at risk of having a nonfatal MI or stroke. This is known as a competing risk because some of the risks being assessed cannot happen after another, such as death, has occurred. The intervention may not be desirable, even if it shows an overall advantage on the composite of incident ASCVD, because a study participant who would have had 2 mild MIs dies first and has only 1 event that is more serious. Competing risks might therefore result in an underestimate of the occurrence rate of the composite end point that would occur if the mortality rate were not increased by the intervention. The study by Kavousi et al[1] avoided possible bias from competing risks by including only first-incident events in the analysis.

Composite end points can be more useful when a specific weight is assigned to each component that reflects each component's importance or "utility" to patients and clinicians. For example, avoiding CHD death would have a greater utility to patients than avoiding a nonfatal MI. A composite end point with no weights to its components assumes the utilities of all outcomes are equal and, in clinical medicine, this is almost never the case. The relative value of the weights or utilities of each outcome of interest should be scientifically elicited from patients or clinicians. For example, in a study by Ho et al,[5] patient preferences were elicited using a discrete-choice experiment in which 540 obese respondents evaluated the effectiveness, safety, and other attributes of weight-loss devices. The study generated patient utilities for effectiveness, safety, and other device attributes that were subsequently used to inform regulatory decision-making.

Eliciting and assigning utilities can be difficult because individual patients and clinicians are likely to assign different values to each outcome. Equal weighting of each component of a composite outcome avoids this complexity and subjectivity, but the loss of important information can be considerable because this approach ignores the relative importance of markedly different clinical events. Despite the difficulties and subjectivity involved in assigning relative weights or patient utilities, doing so can be advantageous as the weights represent the relative value patients and clinicians place on the individual components of the composite end point.[6]

HOW WERE COMPOSITE END POINTS USED IN THIS STUDY?

Kavousi et al[1] stated that "CAC scanning allows for the detection of subclinical coronary atherosclerosis, and the presence of CAC in asymptomatic individuals is associated with higher risk of coronary heart disease (CHD) and all-cause mortality." They used the composite end point of incident ASCVD (CHD death, nonfatal MI, and stroke) to assess the value of CAC for cardiovascular risk assessment among women with low risk of CVD (<7.5% predicted risk) and concluded that CAC presence was associated with an increased risk of incident ASCVD. The incidence rate difference between CAC presence and CAC absence was 2.92 events (95% CI, 2.02-3.83) per 1000 person-years.

In addition, the composite end point of total CHD (nonfatal MI and CHD death) was examined as a secondary outcome. The incidence rate difference between CAC presence and CAC absence groups was 2.63 events (95% CI, 1.92-3.34) per 1000 person-years.

HOW DOES THE USE OF A COMPOSITE END POINT AFFECT THE INTERPRETATION OF THIS STUDY?

The authors did not separately assess the utility of CAC testing for predicting CHD death, which is the most important component of the ASCVD composite end point to most patients and clinicians. Consequently, the authors' conclusion that "the presence of CAC in asymptomatic individuals is associated with higher risk for coronary heart disease (CHD) and all-cause mortality" could be challenged if the larger incidence of CHD and all-cause mortality in the group in which CAC was present were explained by a higher incidence of nonfatal MI while the group with CAC absence still had a higher incidence of CHD deaths.

Acknowledgment

The following disclosures were reported at the time this original article was first published in *JAMA*.

Conflict of Interest Disclosures: None reported.

Disclaimer: This article reflects the views of the author and should not be construed to represent the Food and Drug Administration's views or policies.

References

1. Kavousi M, Desai CS, Ayers C, et al. Prevalence and prognostic implications of coronary artery calcification in low-risk women: a meta-analysis. *JAMA*. 2016;316(20):2126-2134. Medline:27846641
2. Kleist P. Composite endpoints for clinical trials: current perspectives. *Int J Pharm Med*. 2007;21(3):187-198. doi:10.2165/00124363-200721030-00001
3. Dahlöf B, Devereux RB, Kjeldsen SE, et al. LIFE Study Group. Cardiovascular morbidity and mortality in the Losartan Intervention for Endpoint Reduction in Hypertension Study (LIFE): a randomised trial against atenolol. *Lancet*. 2002;359(9311):995-1003. Medline:11937178
4. Cao J, Zhang S. Multiple comparison procedures. *JAMA*. 2014;312(5):543-544. Medline:25096694
5. Ho MP, Gonzalez JM, Lerner HP, et al. Incorporating patient-preference evidence into regulatory decision making. *Surg Endosc*. 2015;29(10):2984-2993. Medline:25552232
6. Chaisinanunkul N, Adeoye O, Lewis RJ, et al. DAWN Trial and MOST Trial Steering Committees; Additional contributors from DAWN Trial Steering Committee. Adopting a patient-centered approach to primary outcome analysis of acute stroke trials using a utility-weighted Modified Rankin Scale. *Stroke*. 2015;46(8):2238-2243. Medline:26138130

Missing Data: How to Best Account for What Is Not Known

Craig D. Newgard, MD, MPH, and
Roger J. Lewis, MD, PhD

IN THIS CHAPTER

Use of the Method

Why Are These Methods Used?

What Are the Limitations of These Methods?

Why Did the Authors Use This Method in This Particular Study?

How Should This Method's Findings Be Interpreted in This Particular Study?

Caveats to Consider When Looking at the Results in This Study Based on This Method

This JAMA Guide to Statistics and Methods characterizes the strengths and limitations of different approaches for modeling missing data in clinical research using the example of a trial that applied several of these techniques.

Missing data are common in clinical research, particularly for variables requiring complex, time-sensitive, resource-intensive, or longitudinal data collection methods. However, even seemingly readily available information can be missing. There are many reasons for "missingness," including missed study visits, patients lost to follow-up, missing information in source documents, lack of availability (eg, laboratory tests that were not performed), and clinical scenarios preventing collection of certain variables (eg, missing coma scale data in sedated patients). It is particularly challenging to interpret studies when primary outcome data are missing. However, many methods commonly used for handling missing values during data analysis can yield biased results, decrease study power, or lead to underestimates of uncertainty, all reducing the chance of drawing valid conclusions.

For example, Bakris et al[1] evaluated the effect of finerenone on urinary albumin-creatinine ratio (UACR) in patients with diabetic nephropathy in a randomized, phase 2B, dose-finding clinical trial conducted in 148 sites in 23 countries. Because of the logistical complexity of the study, it is not surprising that some of the intended data collection could not be completed, resulting in missing outcome data. Bakris et al used several analysis and imputation techniques (ie, methods for replacing missing data with specific values) to assess the effects of different approaches for handling missing data. These methods included complete case analysis (restricting the analysis to include only patients with observed 90-day UACR values); last observation carried forward (LOCF; typically this involves using the last recorded data point as the final outcome; Bakris et al[1] used the higher of 2 UACR values and, separately, the most recent UACR obtained prior to study discontinuation); baseline observation carried forward (using the baseline UACR value as the outcome UACR value, therefore assuming no treatment effect for that patient); mean value imputation (replacing missing values with the mean of observed UACR values); and random imputation (using randomly selected UACR values to replace missing UACR values).[1] Multiple imputation[2] to handle missing values was also performed. With the exception of multiple imputation, each of the imputation approaches replaces a missing value with a single number (termed "single" or "simple" imputation) and can threaten the validity of study results.[3,4] The authors concluded that finerenone improved the UACR, a result that was consistent regardless of the method for handling missing data.

USE OF THE METHOD

Why Are These Methods Used?

It is rare for a research investigation not to have any missing data. If patients with missing variables are omitted from an analysis, the effective sample size is reduced and the treatment effect estimate may be incorrect.[3] This is known as complete (observed) case analysis and is the default methods used by most statistical software.

Strategies for handling missing values are each based on different assumptions and have different limitations. Key questions to consider when selecting a method for handling missing values include (1) Why are data missing? (2) How do patients with missing and complete data differ? and (3) Do the observed data help predict the missing values? To better understand this last concept, suppose a physician was asked to make a best guess about a characteristic of one of her patients who was missing from their chart; eg, weight, systolic blood pressure, fasting serum cholesterol, or serum creatinine. The chance of guessing a value close to the true value would likely be substantially improved if the physician was given related data about the patient, such as his or her age, comorbidities, and prior laboratory values.

The cause for missing data, called censoring, is "noninformative" when the reason a value could not be measured provides no information for what it should be. Censoring is "informative" when the absence of a value indicates something about what it should be. For example, a patient lost to follow-up may have quit the study because declining health made traveling to follow-up visits more difficult, implying that patients with complete follow-up data may have better health status than those with missing data.

There are 3 ways by which data may be missing.[3,4] The first is that data may be missing completely at random (MCAR), meaning the probability of being missing is completely unrelated to all observed and unobserved patient characteristics. This is the least plausible mechanism but is the only one for which complete case analysis will yield unbiased results.

The next mechanism, missing at random (MAR) or "ignorable," does not assume patients with missing values are similar to those with complete data but instead assumes that observed values can be used to "explain" which values are missing and help predict what the missing values would be.[3] This mechanism of missingness is a more realistic assumption than MCAR, and MAR is assumed by most of the currently used valid techniques for handling missing data. However, most simple imputation methods still yield biased or falsely precise results when MAR is assumed.

Missing not at random (MNAR) is the most problematic censoring mechanism and occurs when missing values are dependent on unobserved or unknown factors. When MNAR is present, statistical adjustment for missing information is virtually impossible.

Because an investigator usually cannot determine the actual mechanism for missingness, statistical analyses usually proceed assuming the data conform to a MAR mechanism.

Collecting information to explain why data are missing (eg, participants' mode of transportation and distance to the clinic) can help predict certain values and make the MAR assumption more plausible.[3,4]

What Are the Limitations of These Methods?

Simple imputation methods (eg, LOCF, complete case analysis, mean value imputation, and random imputation) are considered "naive" because they fail to account for the uncertainty in imputing missing values, do not use information available in observed values, can introduce bias, and artificially increase precision (ie, inappropriately narrow confidence intervals and result in smaller P values).[3,4] Each of these limitations can cause spurious results. Better estimates and measures of uncertainty (eg, confidence intervals) can be obtained by using maximum likelihood–based methods, hot deck imputation, and multiple imputation.[3]

The primary limitation of complete case analysis is bias and reduced sample size, resulting in reduced study power.[4] Unless the data are MCAR (an unlikely event), estimates using observed case analysis will be biased and the direction of the bias unpredictable. Last observation carried forward is a commonly performed simple imputation technique. This strategy requires the tenuous assumption that the final outcome (eg, 90-day UACR) does not change from the last observed value. In mean value imputation, all missing values are replaced with the mean of observed values (eg, 90-day UACR). With an increasing proportion of missing data, mean value imputation results in larger numbers of patients with an identical imputed value, creating smaller measures of variance and greater bias, artificially increasing the apparent precision of inaccurate estimates.[4,5] Random number imputation avoids the repetitive use of the same imputed estimate but fails to use observed values to inform the selected estimate.

Why Did the Authors Use This Method in This Particular Study?

In the study by Bakris et al,[1] the primary outcome had missing values requiring the use of missing data methods. Several imputation methods were used so that results obtained by the various approaches could be compared.

How Should This Method's Findings Be Interpreted in This Particular Study?

Because of the inherent limitations of simple imputation methods, the multiply imputed results provide the most valid results in the study by Bakris et al. Provided the underlying assumptions are met and rigorous imputation methods (eg, multiple imputation) are used, study results can be interpreted as if all values had been observed.

CAVEATS TO CONSIDER WHEN LOOKING AT THE RESULTS IN THIS STUDY BASED ON THIS METHOD

The LOCF method for handling missing values (as used in the primary analysis by Bakris et al[1]) has the same fundamental limitations as other simple imputation methods, generating potentially biased results with inappropriately narrow confidence intervals. Because results from the post hoc multiple imputation analysis were reported to be no different from those of the LOCF analysis,[1] the primary results can be considered valid despite the risks of using simple imputation methods. Nonetheless, results from the multiple imputation analysis are more rigorous (despite the post hoc selection of this strategy) because of the advantages of this method over simple imputation methods.[5] Caution is required when using traditionally defined "conservative" methods for handling missing outcomes (eg, LOCF) over more sophisticated missing data methods. While they may be conservative in assigning the outcome of a participant with missing data, they can lead to both false-positive and false-negative results in measured treatment effects. In general, multiple imputation is the best approach for modeling the effects of missing data in studies.

Acknowledgment

The following disclosures were reported at the time this original article was first published in *JAMA*.

Conflict of Interest Disclosures: None reported.

References

1. Bakris GL, Agarwal R, Chan JCN, et al. Mineralocorticoid Receptor Antagonist Tolerability Study–Diabetic Nephropathy (ARTS-DN) Study Group. Effect of finerenone on albuminuria in patients with diabetic nephropathy: a randomized clinical trial. *JAMA*. 2015;9:884-894. doi:10.1001/jama.2015.10081.
2. Rubin DB. *Multiple Imputation for Nonresponse in Surveys*. New York, NY: Wiley; 1987.
3. Little RJA, Rubin DB. *Statistical Analysis With Missing Data*. 2nd ed. Princeton, NJ: Wiley; 2002.
4. Haukoos JS, Newgard CD. Advanced statistics: missing data in clinical research, I: an introduction and conceptual framework. *Acad Emerg Med*. 2007;14(7):662-668. Medline:17538078
5. Newgard CD, Haukoos JS. Advanced statistics: missing data in clinical research, II: multiple imputation. *Acad Emerg Med*. 2007;14(7):669-678. Medline:17595237

The Intention-to-Treat Principle: How to Assess the True Effect of Choosing a Medical Treatment

Michelle A. Detry, PhD, and
Roger J. Lewis, MD, PhD

IN THIS CHAPTER

Use of the Method

Why Is ITT Analysis Used?

What Are the Limitations of ITT Analysis?

Why Did the Authors Use ITT Analysis in This Particular Study?

Caveats to Consider When Looking at Results Based on ITT Analysis

This JAMA Guide to Statistics and Methods explains the intention-to-treat principle, which defines the study population included in the primary efficacy analysis and how the outcomes are analyzed, including why the intention-to-treat principle is used and its limitations.

The intention-to-treat (ITT) principle is a cornerstone in the interpretation of randomized clinical trials (RCTs) conducted with the goal of influencing the selection of medical therapy for well-defined groups of patients. The ITT principle defines both the study population included in the primary efficacy analysis and how the outcomes are analyzed. Under ITT, study participants are analyzed as members of the treatment group to which they were randomized regardless of their adherence to, or whether they received, the intended treatment.[1-3] For example, in a trial in which patients are randomized to receive either treatment A or treatment B, a patient may be randomized to receive treatment A but erroneously receive treatment B, or never receive any treatment, or not adhere to treatment A. In all of these situations, the patient would be included in group A when comparing treatment outcomes using an ITT analysis. Eliminating study participants who were randomized but not treated or moving participants between treatment groups according to the treatment they received would violate the ITT principle.

Robertson et al conducted an RCT using a factorial design to compare transfusion thresholds of 10 and 7 g/dL and administration of erythropoietin vs placebo in 895 patients with anemia and traumatic brain injury.[4] The primary outcome was the 6-month Glasgow Outcome Scale (GOS), dichotomized so a good or moderate score indicated success. The trial was conducted with high fidelity to the protocol, so only a few patients did not receive the intended treatment strategy. Two patients randomized to the 7-g/dL study group were managed according to the 10-g/dL threshold and an additional 2 patients randomized to the 7-g/dL study group received one transfusion not according to protocol. The authors implemented the ITT principle and the outcomes for these 4 patients were included in the 7-g/dL group.

USE OF THE METHOD

Why Is ITT Analysis Used?

The effectiveness of a therapy is not simply determined by its pure biological effect but is also influenced by the physician's ability to administer, or the patient's ability to adhere to, the intended treatment. The true effect of selecting a treatment is a combination of biological effects, variations in compliance or adherence, and other patient characteristics that influence efficacy. Only by retaining all patients intended to receive a given treatment in their original treatment group can researchers and clinicians obtain an unbiased estimate of the effect of selecting one treatment over another.

Treatment adherence often depends on many patient and clinician factors that may not be anticipated or are impossible to measure and that influence response to treatment. For example, in the study by Robertson et al, some patients randomized to the higher transfusion threshold may not have received the intended therapeutic strategy due to adverse events associated with transfusion, fluid overload, or unwillingness of clinicians to adhere to the strategy for other reasons. These patients are likely to be fundamentally different from those who were actually treated using the 10-g/dL strategy. The characteristics that differ between patients who received the intended therapy and those who did not could easily influence whether a successful GOS score is achieved. If the ITT principle was not followed and patients were removed from their randomized group and either ignored or assigned to the other treatment group, the results of the analysis would be biased and no longer represent the effect of choosing one therapy over the other.

It is common to see alternative analyses proposed, eg, per-protocol or modified intent-to-treat (MITT) analyses.[5] A per-protocol analysis includes only study participants who completed the trial without any major deviations from the study protocol; this usually requires that they successfully receive and complete their assigned treatment(s), complete their study visits, and provide primary outcome data. The requirements to be included in the per-protocol analysis vary from study to study. While the definition of an MITT analysis also varies from study to study, the MITT approach deviates from the ITT approach by eliminating patients or reassigning patients to a study group other than the group to which they were randomized. Neither of these approaches satisfies the ITT principle and may lead to clinically misleading results. It has been observed that studies using MITT analysis are more likely to be positive than those following a strict ITT approach.[5] A comparison of results from ITT and per-protocol or MITT analyses may provide some indication of the potential effect of nonadherence on overall treatment effectiveness.

Noninferiority trials, which are designed to demonstrate that an experimental treatment is no worse than an established one, require special considerations with regard to the ITT principle.[6-8] Consider a noninferiority trial of 2 treatments—treatment A is a biologically ineffective experimental therapy and treatment B is a biologically effective standard therapy—with the goal to demonstrate that treatment A is noninferior to B. Patients may be randomized to receive treatment B, not adhere to the treatment, and fail treatment due to their nonadherence. If this happens frequently, treatment B will appear less efficacious. Thus, the intervention in group A may incorrectly appear noninferior to the intervention in group B, simply as a result of nonadherence rather than because of similar biological efficacy. In this case, the ITT analysis is somewhat misleading because the noninferiority is a result of poor adherence. In a noninferiority trial, both ITT and per-protocol analyses should be conducted and reported. If the per-protocol results are similar to the ITT results, the claim of noninferiority is substantially strengthened.[6-8]

What Are the Limitations of ITT Analysis?

A characteristic of the ITT principle is that poor treatment adherence may result in lower estimates of treatment efficacy and a loss of study power. However, these estimates are clinically relevant because real-world effectiveness is limited by the ability of patients and clinicians to adhere to a treatment.

Because all patients must be analyzed under the ITT principle, it is essential that all patients be followed up and their primary outcomes determined. Patients who discontinue study treatments are often more likely to be lost to follow-up. Following the ITT principle will not eliminate bias associated with missing outcome data; steps must always be taken to keep missing data to a minimum and, when missing data are unavoidable, to use minimally biasing methods for adjusting for missing data (eg, multiple imputation).

Why Did the Authors Use ITT Analysis in This Particular Study?

Robertson et al[4] used an ITT analysis because it allowed the effectiveness of their therapeutic strategies to be evaluated without bias due to differences in adherence. Failure to follow the ITT principle could have led to greater scrutiny of the trial results, especially if adherence to the intended treatments had been poorer.

CAVEATS TO CONSIDER WHEN LOOKING AT RESULTS BASED ON ITT ANALYSIS

Although the ITT principle is important for estimating the efficacy of treatments, it should not be applied in the same way in assessing the safety (eg, medication adverse effects) of interventions. For example, it would not make sense to attribute an apparent adverse effect to an intended treatment when, in fact, the patient was never exposed to the experimental drug. For this reason, safety analyses are generally conducted according to the treatment actually received, even though this may not accurately estimate—and may well overestimate—the burden of adverse effects likely to be seen in clinical practice.

While determining the effect of choosing one treatment over another, or over no treatment at all, is a key goal of trials conducted late in the process of drug and device development, the goals of trials conducted earlier in development are generally focused on narrower questions such as biological efficacy and dose selection. In these cases, MITT and per-protocol analysis strategies have a greater role in guiding the design and conduct of subsequent clinical trials. For example, it would be unfortunate to falsely conclude, based on the ITT analysis of a phase 2 clinical trial, that a novel pharmaceutical agent is not effective when, in fact, the lack of efficacy stems from too high a dose and patients' inability to be adherent because of intolerable adverse effects. In that case, a lower dose may yield clinically important efficacy and a tolerable adverse effect profile. A per-protocol analysis may be helpful in such a case, allowing the detection of the beneficial effect in patients able to tolerate the new therapy.

Acknowledgment

The following disclosures were reported at the time this original article was first published in *JAMA*.

Conflict of Interest Disclosures: None reported.

References

1. Cook T, DeMets DL. *Introduction to Statistical Methods for Clinical Trials*. Boca Raton, FL: Chapman & Hall/CRC; Taylor & Francis Group; 2008:chap 11.

2. Schulz KF, Altman DG, Moher D; CONSORT Group. CONSORT 2010 statement: updated guidelines for reporting parallel group randomized trials. *Ann Intern Med*. 2010;152(11):726-732. Medline:20335313

3. Food and Drug Administration. Guidance for industry e9 statistical principles for clinical trials. http://www.fda.gov/downloads/Drugs/GuidanceCompliance RegulatoryInformation/Guidances/ucm073137.pdf. September 1998. Accessed May 11, 2014.

4. Robertson CS, Hannay HJ, Yamal J-M, et al; and the Epo Severe TBI Trial Investigators. Effect of erythropoietin and transfusion threshold on neurological recovery after traumatic brain injury: a randomized clinical trial. *JAMA*. 2014;312(1):36-47. doi:10.1001/jama.2014.6490.

5. Montedori A, Bonacini MI, Casazza G, et al. Modified versus standard intention-to-treat reporting: are there differences in methodological quality, sponsorship, and findings in randomized trials? a cross-sectional study. *Trials*. 2011;12:58. Medline:21356072

6. Piaggio G, Elbourne DR, Pocock SJ, Evans SJ, Altman DG; CONSORT Group. Reporting of noninferiority and equivalence randomized trials: extension of the CONSORT 2010 statement. *JAMA*. 2012;308(24):2594-2604. Medline:23268518

7. Le Henanff A, Giraudeau B, Baron G, Ravaud P. Quality of reporting of noninferiority and equivalence randomized trials. *JAMA*. 2006;295(10):1147-1151. Medline:16522835

8. Mulla SM, Scott IA, Jackevicius CA, et al. How to use a noninferiority trial: Users' Guides to the Medical Literature. *JAMA*. 2012;308:2605-2611. Medline:23268519

Analyzing Repeated Measurements Using Mixed Models

Michelle A. Detry, PhD, and Yan Ma, PhD

IN THIS CHAPTER

Use of the Method

Why Are Mixed Models Used for Repeated Measures Data?

What Are the Limitations of Mixed Models?

Why Did the Authors Use Mixed Models in This Particular Study?

Caveats to Consider When Looking at Results from Mixed Models

This JAMA Guide to Statistics and Methods discusses analyzing longitudinal studies that use repeated measurements of each participant's status or outcome to assess differences over time using mixed models.

Longitudinal studies often include multiple, repeated measurements of each patient's status or outcome to assess differences in outcomes or in the rate of recovery or decline over time. Repeated measurements from a particular patient are likely to be more similar to each other than measurements from different patients, and this correlation needs to be considered in the analysis of the resulting data. Many common statistical methods, such as linear regression models, should not be used in this situation because those methods assume measurements to be independent of one another.

It is possible to compare outcomes between treatments using only a final measurement to determine whether there was a difference at the end of the study; however, this approach would not include much of the information captured with repeated measurements and there would be no consideration of the pattern of outcomes each patient experienced in reaching his or her final outcome. When outcomes are measured repeatedly over time, a wide variety of clinically important questions may be addressed.

In the EXACT study, Moseley et al[1] examined activity limitations and quality of life (QOL) among patients with ankle fractures to determine if a supervised exercise program with rehabilitation advice was more beneficial than advice alone. Activity limitations and QOL were measured at baseline and at 1, 3, and 6 months of follow-up. The authors used mixed models[2] to compare patient outcomes over time between the 2 intervention groups.

USE OF THE METHOD

Why Are Mixed Models Used for Repeated Measures Data?

Mixed models are ideally suited to settings in which the individual trajectory of a particular outcome for a study participant over time is influenced both by factors that can be assumed to be the same for many patients (eg, the effect of an intervention) and by characteristics that are likely to vary substantially from patient to patient (eg, the severity of the ankle fracture, baseline level of function, and QOL). Mixed models explicitly account for the correlations between repeated measurements within each patient.

The factors assumed to have the same effect across many patients are called fixed effects and the factors likely to vary substantially from patient to patient are called random effects. For example, the effect of a new treatment may be assumed to be the same for all patients and modeled as a fixed effect, whereas patients may have markedly different baseline function or inherent rates of recovery and these may be best modeled as random effects. Mixed models are called "mixed" because they generally contain both fixed and random effects. The ability to consider both fixed and random effects in the model gives flexibility to determine the effects of multiple factors and to address specific questions of clinical importance. In contrast, repeated measures analysis of variance (ANOVA), often used for analyzing longitudinal data, does not have this flexibility and can yield misleading results if its more rigid assumptions (eg, all effects are considered fixed) are not met.

Furthermore, using a mixed model, data from all assessments contribute to the treatment comparisons, resulting in more precise estimates and a more powerful study. A mixed model can also address if outcomes changed over time (eg, the rate of recovery of function or decline) within each treatment group.

Moreover, in addition to population-level comparisons, mixed models can be used to characterize an individual patient's response patterns over time. The specific clinical question motivating the trial determines the structure of the mixed model that is most applicable. For example, if the effect of a treatment on the rate of recovery from a patient-specific baseline is to be determined, then the mixed model is likely to include a random baseline effect and a fixed interaction term between treatment group and time, with the latter term capturing the effect of the treatment on the rate of recovery.

Observations may be correlated with each other in several different ways. These patterns are known as correlation structures and it is important when using mixed models to use the correct structure. For example, if the correlation between each measurement is likely to be the same regardless of the length of time between the measurements, then a "compound symmetry" structure is appropriate. In contrast, if the correlation between measurements decreases as the time between measurements increases, then an "autoregressive" structure should be used. Finally, an "unstructured" correlation can be used if no constraints can be imposed on the correlation pattern, but fitting a model with an unstructured correlation requires a larger data set than the other approaches.

Ideally, the assumed correlation structure should be based on the clinical context in which the repeated measurements were taken. For example, certain longitudinal data (eg, pain scores after joint surgery) at adjacent assessments would tend to be more correlated than those measured farther apart, making an autoregressive structure appropriate. Statistical testing (eg, a likelihood ratio test) may be used when an objective comparison is needed to evaluate competing correlation structures.

Incomplete outcome data, for example, caused by patients missing some visits or dropping out of the study, are common in longitudinal studies.[3] As a result, study participants may have different numbers of available measurements, a situation that cannot be addressed by repeated measures ANOVA.

Mixed models can accommodate unbalanced data patterns and use all available observations and patients in the analysis. Mixed models assume that the missingness is independent of unobserved measurements, but dependent on the observed measurements.[4,5] This assumption is called "missing at random" and is often reasonable.[3,5] Repeated measures ANOVA requires a more unlikely assumption that the missingness is independent of both the observed and unobserved measurements, called "missing completely at random." Using mixed models, reasonably valid estimates of treatment effects can often be obtained even when the missing values are not completely random and additional methods for handling missing data, such as multiple imputation, are generally not required.[3-5]

What Are the Limitations of Mixed Models?

As with any statistical model, a mixed model will have limited validity if its underlying assumptions are not met. For example, if the effect of a treatment varies substantially from patient to patient, for instance, because of genetic differences, then considering the treatment effect as fixed may not be reasonable. Similarly, the assumed correlation structure can adversely impact model results and study conclusions if incorrect. It is important to ensure that the structure of the mixed model matches what is reasonably believed about the clinical setting in which the model is applied.

Because of the larger number of parameters to be estimated from the data, mixed models may be difficult to estimate or "fit" when the available data are limited. This is especially true if an unstructured correlation structure must be used. The precise methods used by different software packages to fit mixed models differ, so the numerical results can vary somewhat based on the statistical software used.

In the presence of missing data, mixed models can provide valid inferences under an assumption that data are missing at random. However, in practice it is often impossible to know that this assumption is met and informative censoring (nonignorable missingness) can never be ruled out. If the investigators suspect deviation from the missing-at-random assumption, sensitivity analyses may be conducted using models appropriate for nonignorable missingness. The models used would depend on the study design, missing data patterns observed, and other study specific considerations.[2]

Why Did the Authors Use Mixed Models in This Particular Study?

The EXACT trial investigators used mixed models in their analyses because they wanted to answer the question of how outcomes changed over time and how they were affected by treatment. The model included fixed effects for treatment group, time of measurement, and baseline score. An interaction term between treatment group and time was also included to determine if the 2 treatment interventions led to different recovery trajectories over time. In addition, the model included a random effect for the baseline value, addressing the variability in the starting point for each patient.

The EXACT trial reported that in each treatment group, 10% to 20% of the patients were lost to follow-up as the study progressed. Thus, it was important for the authors to examine the effects of the missingness. They included a preplanned sensitivity analysis that used multiple imputation[5] to evaluate how sensitive the primary outcome result was to the missing at random data assumption. The results of the main and sensitivity analyses were similar.

CAVEATS TO CONSIDER WHEN LOOKING AT RESULTS FROM MIXED MODELS

As with most statistical models, it is important to consider whether the structure of the data obtained and the clinical setting (eg, repeated measures over time) match the model structure. It is often useful to inspect graphical data summaries (eg, "spaghetti" or "string" plots showing the outcome trajectories of individual study participants over time) to determine whether the observed data patterns appear consistent with model assumptions.

When outcome data are missing, the analyst should consider whether the pattern of missingness is likely to be random, meeting the assumptions inherent in mixed models. The rationale for the chosen correlation structure should be clear and based on study design (eg, the pattern of follow-up visits) rather than based on what allows a model to be fit with the available data.

Acknowledgment

The following disclosures were reported at the time this original article was first published in *JAMA*.

Conflict of Interest Disclosures: Dr Ma receives funding from the Agency for Healthcare Research and Quality. No other disclosures reported.

References

1. Moseley AM, Beckenkamp PR, Haas M, Herbert RD, Lin CW; EXACT Team. Rehabilitation after immobilization for ankle fracture: the EXACT randomized clinical trial. *JAMA*. 2015;314(13):1376-1385. Medline:26441182

2. Fitzmaurice GM, Laird NM, Ware JH. *Applied Longitudinal Analysis*. 2nd ed. Hoboken, NJ: Wiley; 2011.

3. Newgard CD, Lewis RJ. Missing data: how to best account for what is not known. *JAMA*. 2015;314(9):940-941. doi:10.1001/jama.2015.10516. Medline:26325562

4. Ma Y, Mazumdar M, Memtsoudis SG. Beyond repeated-measures analysis of variance: advanced statistical methods for the analysis of longitudinal data in anesthesia research. *Reg Anesth Pain Med*. 2012;37(1):99-105. Medline:22189576

5. Li P, Stuart EA, Allison DB. Multiple imputation: a flexible tool for handling missing data. *JAMA*. 2015;314(18):1966-1967. doi:10.1001/jama.2015.15281. Medline:26547468

JAMAevidence
Using Evidence to Improve Care

Logistic Regression: Relating Patient Characteristics to Outcomes

Juliana Tolles, MD, MHS, and
William J. Meurer, MD, MS

IN THIS CHAPTER

Use of the Method

Why Is Logistic Regression Used?

Description of the Method

What Are the Limitations of Logistic Regression?

Why Did the Authors Use Logistic Regression in This Study?

How Should the Results of Logistic Regression Be Interpreted in This Particular Study?

Caveats to Consider When Assessing the Results of a Logistic Regression Analysis

This JAMA Guide to Statistics and Methods reviews the use of logistic regression methods to quantify associations between patient characteristics and clinical outcomes.

In an article published in *JAMA*, Seymour et al[1] presented a new method for estimating the probability of a patient dying of sepsis using information on the patient's respiratory rate, systolic blood pressure, and altered mentation. The method used these clinical characteristics—called "predictor" or explanatory or independent variables—to estimate the likelihood of a patient having an outcome of interest, called the dependent variable. To determine the best way to use these clinical characteristics, the authors used logistic regression, a common statistical method for quantifying the relationship between patient characteristics and clinical outcomes.[2]

USE OF THE METHOD

Why Is Logistic Regression Used?

One use of logistic regression is to estimate the probability that an event will occur or that a patient will have a particular outcome using information or characteristics that are thought to be related to or influence such events. Logistic regression can show which of the various factors being assessed has the strongest association with an outcome and provides a measure of the magnitude of the potential influence. It also has the ability to "adjust" for confounding factors, ie, factors that are associated with both other predictor variables and the outcome, so the measure of the influence of the predictor of interest is not distorted by the effect of the confounder.

Although logistic regression can be used to evaluate epidemiological associations that do not represent cause and effect, this chapter focuses on the use of logistic regression to create models for predicting patient outcomes. In this context, the term *predictors* is used to refer to the independent factors (variables) for which the influences are being quantified, and the term *outcome* is used for the dependent variable that the logistic regression model is trying to predict.

Description of the Method

Patient outcomes that can only have 2 values (eg, lived vs died) are called binary or dichotomous. The outcomes for groups of patients can be summarized by the fraction of patients experiencing the outcome of interest or, similarly, by the probability that any single patient experiences that outcome. However, to understand the results of a logistic regression model, it is important to understand the difference between probability and odds. The probability that an event will occur divided by the probability that it will not occur is called the odds. For example, if there is a 75% chance of survival and a 25% chance of dying, then the odds of survival is 75%:25%, or 3. Logistic regression quantitatively links one or more predictors thought to influence a particular outcome to the odds of that outcome.[2]

The change in the odds of an outcome—for example, the increase in the odds of mortality associated with tachypnea in a patient with sepsis—is measured as a ratio called the odds ratio (OR). If patients with tachypnea have an odds of mortality of 2.0 and patients without tachypnea have an odds of mortality of 0.5, then the OR associated with tachypnea would be 2.0:0.5, or 4. This is the same as an increase in the probability of mortality from 1/3 to 2/3.

In logistic regression, the weight or coefficient calculated for each predictor determines the OR for the outcome associated with a 1-unit change in that predictor, or associated with a patient state (eg, tachypneic) relative to a reference state (eg, not tachypneic). Through these ORs and their associated 95% confidence intervals, logistic regression provides a measure of the magnitude of the influence of each predictor on the outcome of interest and of the uncertainty in the magnitude of the influence.

Logistic regression also enables "adjustment" for confounding factors—patient characteristics that might also influence the outcome and simultaneously be correlated with 1 or more predictors. To accomplish this, both the confounding factors and the predictors of interest are included in the model. For example, when adjusting for the influence of fever in estimating the influence of tachypnea on mortality, both fever and the presence of tachypnea would be included as predictors in the regression model. The result is that the estimate of the association between tachypnea and mortality would not be confounded by a possible correlation between fever and tachypnea.

What Are the Limitations of Logistic Regression?

First, the validity of a regression model depends on the number and suitability of the measured independent predictor variables. Ideally, all biologically relevant factors should be included. When multiple variables convey closely related information (a situation termed *collinearity*), such as would occur when using both serum lactate and anion gap as predictors in patients with septic shock, this can produce serious errors or great uncertainty in the estimates of the effects of these variables on the outcome of interest. When 2 variables provide overlapping information, minor random variation in the data can greatly and unpredictably influence how much of the association is attributed to one factor vs the other in the model.

A second limitation of logistic regression is that the variables must have a constant magnitude of association across the range of values for that variable. For example, in examining the relationship between age and mortality, if the odds ratio for mortality is 2 for each 10-year increase in age, this association needs to be the same when comparing 30- and 40-year-olds as it is when comparing 70- and 80-year-olds if the model is to be used across this entire age range. If the association is not consistent over the age range, then age may be stratified into ranges (eg, 21-50, 51-65, and ≥66) based on the assumption that within each category, the influence of age will be similar. The age category would then be used as the independent variable, usually with the lowest-risk age group the reference category.

A third limitation is that many logistic regression analyses assume that the effect of one predictor is not influenced by the value of another predictor. When this is not true and the value of one predictor alters the effect of another, there is said to be an "interaction" between the 2 predictors. Such interactions need to be explicitly included in the analysis to ensure the estimated associations are valid.

Why Did the Authors Use Logistic Regression in This Study?

Seymour et al[1] likely selected logistic regression for its familiarity and interpretability. More complex prognostic models may produce algorithms that are difficult to use clinically.

How Should the Results of Logistic Regression Be Interpreted in This Particular Study?

Seymour et al used logistic regression to derive a new clinical tool for assessing the risk of mortality in patients with sepsis, called the quick Sequential [Sepsis-related] Organ Failure Assessment (qSOFA).[1] The qSOFA model is used to estimate the likelihood of in-hospital mortality in patients with suspected infection using respiratory rate, systolic blood pressure, and Glasgow Coma Scale score. Rather than using the precise OR coefficient for each predictor in their final model, the authors simplified the model by assigning the same 1-point value to each predictor. By assigning all coefficients equal value, the authors created a simplified model that could be applied to individual patients by counting the number of positive clinical predictors. The authors then determined how well the qSOFA score estimated mortality relative to other models for estimating mortality in sepsis, demonstrating that a qSOFA score of 2 or more produced a 3- to 14-fold increase in the probability of in-hospital mortality over baseline risk in patients with sepsis. They also found that for patients not in intensive care, the qSOFA predicted mortality in patients with sepsis better than systemic inflammatory response syndrome criteria or the usual Sequential [Sepsis-related] Organ Failure Assessment score.

CAVEATS TO CONSIDER WHEN ASSESSING THE RESULTS OF A LOGISTIC REGRESSION ANALYSIS

The associations found through logistic regression models are intended to provide insights into what might happen in a similar population of future patients. Certain combinations of patient characteristics and factors may have been sparsely represented in the data set (eg, young patients with sepsis and a low Glasgow Coma Scale score but a normal blood pressure and respiratory rate), and the estimates of the model for mortality among such patients should be considered with caution.

Because probabilities are more intuitive than ORs, it is important to avoid confusing them. For example, an increase in probability from 25% to 75% would correspond to a risk ratio (RR) of 3 but an OR of 9. However, when probabilities are very close to zero, the OR and the RR will be nearly equal. Thus, ORs and RRs are practically interchangeable when the outcome of interest is rare. However, when the outcome of interest is a common event (eg, occurring in >20% of patients in any group), it is important to recognize that ORs do not approximate RRs.

Reported ORs for the effects of predictors should be accompanied by 95% confidence intervals; intervals that include an OR of 1 would indicate a non–statistically significant relationship between that predictor and the outcome of interest.

The predictors included in logistic regression models should be selected to avoid redundancy in the information they provide (collinearity). It is also important to consider the possibility that the value of one predictor might alter the effect of another (interactions). Both of these situations can adversely affect the validity of the resulting logistic regression model.

Acknowledgment

The following disclosures were reported at the time this original article was first published in *JAMA*.

Conflict of Interest Disclosures: None reported.

References

1. Seymour CW, Liu VX, Iwashyna TJ, et al. Assessment of Clinical Criteria for Sepsis: For the Third International Consensus Definitions for Sepsis and Septic Shock (Sepsis-3). *JAMA*. 2016;315(8):762-774. Medline:26903335
2. Hosmer DWJr, Lemeshow S, Sturdivant RX. *Applied Logistic Regression*. 3rd ed. Hoboken, NJ: Wiley; 2013.

Logistic Regression Diagnostics: Understanding How Well a Model Predicts Outcomes

William J. Meurer, MD, MS, and
Juliana Tolles, MD, MHS

IN THIS CHAPTER

Use of the Method

Why Are Logistic Regression Model Diagnostics Used?

Description of the Method

What Are the Limitations of Logistic Regression Diagnostics?

Why Did the Authors Use Logistic Regression Diagnostics in This Particular Study?

How Should the Results of Logistic Regression Diagnostics Be Interpreted in This Particular Study?

Caveats to Consider When Assessing the Results of Logistic Regression Diagnostics

This JAMA Guide to Statistics and Methods reviews the use of logistic regression model diagnostics to determine how well a model predicts outcomes.

In 2016, Zemek et al[1] published a study that used logistic regression to develop a clinical risk score for identifying which pediatric patients with concussion will experience prolonged postconcussion symptoms (PPCS). The authors prospectively recorded the initial values of 46 potential predictor variables, or risk factors—selected based on expert opinion and previous research—in a cohort of patients and then followed those patients to determine who developed the primary outcome of PPCS. In the first part of the study, the authors created a logistic regression model to estimate the probability of PPCS using a subset of the variables; in the second part of the study, a separate set of data was used to assess the validity of the model, with the degree of success quantified using regression model diagnostics. The rationale for using logistic regression to develop predictive models was summarized in another JAMA Guide to Statistics and Methods.[2] (See the chapter, Logistic Regression: Relating Patient Characteristics to Outcomes.) In this chapter, we discuss how well a model performs once it is defined.

USE OF THE METHOD

Why Are Logistic Regression Model Diagnostics Used?

Logistic regression models are often created with the goal of predicting the outcomes of future patients based on each patient's predictor variables.[2] Regression model diagnostics measure how well models describe the underlying relationships between predictors and patient outcomes existing within the data, either the data on which the model was built or data from a different population.

The accuracy of a logistic regression model is mainly judged by considering *discrimination* and *calibration*. Discrimination is the ability of the model to correctly assign a higher risk of an outcome to the patients who are truly at higher risk (ie, "ordering them" correctly), whereas calibration is the ability of the model to assign the correct average absolute level of risk (ie, accurately estimate the probability of the outcome for a patient or group of patients). Regression model diagnostics are used to quantify model discrimination and calibration.

Description of the Method

The model developed by Zemek et al discriminates well if it consistently estimates a higher probability of PPCS in patients who develop PPCS vs those who do not; this can be assessed using a receiver operating characteristic (ROC) curve. An ROC curve is a plot of the sensitivity of a model (the vertical axis) vs 1 minus the specificity (the horizontal axis) for all possible cutoffs that might be used to separate patients predicted to have PPCS compared with patients who will not have PPCS (Figure 4).[1] Given any 2 random patients, one with PPCS and one without PPCS, the probability that the model will correctly rank the patient with PPCS as higher risk is equal to the area under the ROC curve (AUROC).[3] This area is also called the *C statistic*, short for "concordance" between model estimates of risk and the observed risk. The C statistic is discussed in detail in another JAMA Guide to Statistics and Methods chapter.[4] (See the chapter, Evaluating Discrimination of Risk Prediction Models: The C Statistic.) A model with perfect sensitivity and specificity would have an AUROC of 1. A model that predicts who has PPCS no better than chance would have an AUROC of 0.5. While dependent on context, C statistic values higher than 0.7 are generally considered fair and values higher than 0.9 excellent; those less than 0.7 generally are not clinically useful.[5]

A particular model might discriminate well, correctly identifying patients who are at higher risk than others, but fail to accurately estimate the absolute probability of an outcome. For example, the model might estimate that patients with a high

FIGURE 4

Receiver Operating Characteristic Curves

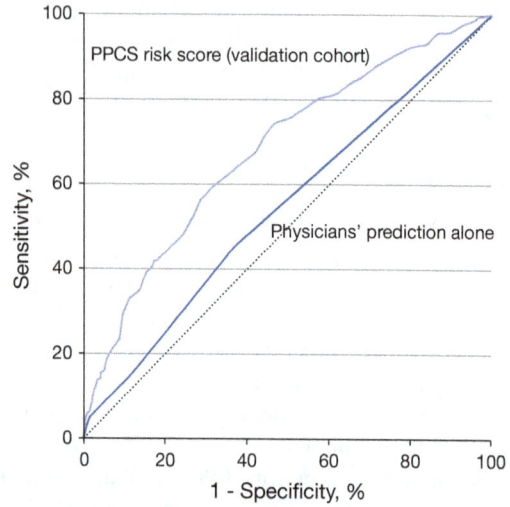

PPCS indicates persistent postconcussion symptoms. The area under the curve was 0.71 (95% CI, 0.69-0.74) for the derivation cohort and 0.68 (95% CI, 0.65-0.72) for the validation cohort. Based on Figure 2 from Zemek et al.[1]

risk of PPCS have a 99% chance of developing the condition, whereas their actual risk is only 80%. Although this hypothetical model would correctly discriminate, it would be poorly calibrated. One method to assess calibration is to compare the average predicted and average observed probabilities of an outcome both for the population as a whole and at each level of risk across a population. The patients are commonly divided into 10 groups based on their predicted risk, so-called deciles of risk. In a well-calibrated model, the observed and predicted proportions of patients with the outcome of interest will be the same within each risk category, at least within the expected random variability (see Table 6 in the article by Zemek et al[1]).

The Hosmer-Lemeshow test measures the statistical significance of any differences between the observed and predicted outcomes over the risk groups; when there is good agreement, the Hosmer-Lemeshow statistic will not show a statistically significant difference, suggesting that the model is well calibrated.[6] Another way to assess calibration is through a calibration plot (eFigure 3 in the article by Zemek et al[1]) in which the observed proportion of the outcome of interest is plotted against the predicted probability.

Some statistical programs also report a *pseudo-R^2* regression diagnostic for logistic regression models. The pseudo-R^2 is meant to mimic the R^2 calculated for linear regression models, a measure of the fraction of the variability in the outcome that is explained by the model. However, because there is no direct equivalent to R^2 in logistic regression, many variations of pseudo-R^2 have been developed by different statisticians, each with a slightly different interpretation.[7]

What Are the Limitations of Logistic Regression Diagnostics?

It is easy to interpret extreme values of the AUROC statistic—those close to 1 or 0.5—but it is a matter of judgment to decide whether a value of 0.75, for example, represents acceptable discrimination. The AUROC is therefore subject to interpretation and comparison with the AUROC values of competing diagnostic tests. Additionally, using the AUROC alone as a metric assumes that a false-positive result is just as bad as a false-negative result. This assumption is often not appropriate in clinical scenarios, and more sophisticated metrics such as a *decision curve analysis* may be needed to appropriately account for the different costs of different types of misclassification.[8]

With large sample sizes the Hosmer-Lemeshow statistic can yield false-positive results and thus falsely suggest that a model is poorly calibrated. In addition, the Hosmer-Lemeshow statistic depends on the number of risk groups into which the study population is divided. There is no theoretical basis for the "correct" number of risk groups into which a population should be divided. Also, with sample sizes smaller than 500, the test has low power and can fail to identify poorly calibrated models.[9]

Why Did the Authors Use Logistic Regression Diagnostics in This Particular Study?

Logistic regression model diagnostics, and model diagnostics generally, are essential for judging the usefulness of any new prediction instrument. A model is unlikely to improve practice if it performs no better than chance or currently available tests. However, in particular clinical applications, physicians may be interested in using models that perform well on only one of these metrics or perform well only at a particular cut point. For example, consider a clinical screening test for which the intended use is to discriminate between patients with very low risk of a particular outcome and all others. Such a model might discriminate well at a particular screening cut point but have poor calibration, or it may have inaccurate estimation of risk for patients who are not classified as very low risk but still be completely appropriate for its intended use.

How Should the Results of Logistic Regression Diagnostics Be Interpreted in This Particular Study?

The ROC curve plotted by Zemek et al (Figure 4) demonstrates modest discrimination; in the initial derivation cohort, the AUROC was 0.71. In the validation cohort, the combination of physician judgment with the final prediction model produced an AUROC of 0.68. While this AUROC value might seem low, it was substantially better than physician estimation alone for predicting PPCS (AUROC of 0.55). As the authors pointed out, this difference indicated that the model generally outperformed clinical judgment alone, although it provided only fair discrimination at best.

The model used by Zemek et al appears well calibrated. The Hosmer-Lemeshow statistic associated with the comparison between predicted and observed rates of PPCS (Table 6 in the article by Zemek et al[1]) across all deciles of risk was not significant. Furthermore, the sample size in this study is large enough that the Hosmer-Lemeshow statistic should have reasonable power to detect poor calibration. The intercept and slope of the calibration plot on the validation cohort were 0.07 and 0.90, respectively, closely approaching their respective ideals of 0 and 1.

CAVEATS TO CONSIDER WHEN ASSESSING THE RESULTS OF LOGISTIC REGRESSION DIAGNOSTICS

Whenever possible, all metrics of model quality should be measured on a data set separate from the data set used to build the model. Independence of test data is crucial because reusing the data on which a model was built (the "training data") to measure accuracy will overestimate the accuracy of the model in future clinical applications. Zemek et al used an independent validation cohort, recruited from the same centers as the training cohort. Therefore, although the model was tested against data other than from which it was derived, it still may lack external validity in patient populations seen in other settings.[10]

Acknowledgment

The following disclosures were reported at the time this original article was first published in *JAMA*.

Conflict of Interest Disclosures: None reported.

References

1. Zemek R, Barrowman N, Freedman SB, et al; Pediatric Emergency Research Canada (PERC) Concussion Team. Clinical risk score for persistent postconcussion symptoms among children with acute concussion in the ED. *JAMA*. 2016;315(10):1014-1025. Medline:26954410

2. Tolles J, Meurer WJ. Logistic regression: relating patient characteristics to outcomes. *JAMA*. 2016;316(5):533-534. Medline:27483067

3. Hanley JA, McNeil BJ. The meaning and use of the area under a receiver operating characteristic (ROC) curve. *Radiology*. 1982;143(1):29-36. Medline:7063747

4. Pencina MJ, D'Agostino RB Sr. Evaluating discrimination of risk prediction models: the C statistic. *JAMA*. 2015;314(10):1063-1064. Medline:26348755

5. Swets JA. Measuring the accuracy of diagnostic systems. *Science*. 1988;240(4857):1285-1293. Medline:3287615

6. Hosmer DW Jr, Lemeshow S, Sturdivant RX. *Applied Logistic Regression*. 3rd ed. New York, NY: Wiley; 2013.

7. Cameron AC, Windmeijer FAG. An R-squared measure of goodness of fit for some common nonlinear regression models. *J Econom*. 1997;77(2):329-342. doi:10.1016/S0304-4076(96)01818-0

8. Fitzgerald M, Saville BR, Lewis RJ. Decision curve analysis. *JAMA*. 2015;313(4):409-410. Medline:25626037

9. Hosmer DW, Hosmer T, Le Cessie S, Lemeshow S. A comparison of goodness-of-fit tests for the logistic regression model. *Stat Med*. 1997;16(9):965-980. Medline:9160492

10. Efron B. How biased is the apparent error rate of a prediction rule? *J Am Stat Assoc*. 1986;81(394):461-470. doi:10.2307/2289236

… evidence

Number Needed to Treat: Conveying the Likelihood of a Therapeutic Effect

Jeffrey L. Saver, MD, and
Roger J. Lewis, MD, PhD

IN THIS CHAPTER

Explanation of the Concept

What Is the NNT?

Why Is the NNT Important?

Limitations and Alternatives to the NNT

How Was the Concept of NNT Applied in This Particular Study?

How Should the NNT Be Interpreted in the Study by Zhao et al?

This JAMA Guide to Statistics and Methods explains the calculations and concepts underlying the number needed to treat (NNT) as a summary statistic of effect, and the assumptions underlying the measure that affect its interpretation.

Effectively communicating clinical trial results to patients and clinicians is a requirement for appropriate application in clinical practice. In a recent issue of *JAMA*, Zhao et al[1] reported the results from a randomized clinical trial comparing dual antiplatelet therapy with aspirin monotherapy for preserving saphenous vein graft patency in 500 patients undergoing coronary artery bypass grafting. Dual antiplatelet therapy was found to be superior to aspirin monotherapy. The authors[1] used the number needed to treat (NNT) to communicate effect size, reporting that for every 8 patients treated with dual agents rather than aspirin alone, 1 additional patient would achieve saphenous graft patency at 1 year. The NNT may be defined as the number of patients who need to be treated with one therapy vs another for 1 additional patient to have the desired outcome. Since its first description 30 years ago,[2] the NNT has become an important means to express the magnitude of benefit conferred by a therapy.[3]

EXPLANATION OF THE CONCEPT

What Is the NNT?

When a clinical trial is completed, the fraction or proportion of patients experiencing the desired outcome is reported for the active and control groups. The NNT is derived from these values and indicates the magnitude of the therapy's treatment effect on the disease observed in the clinical trial. The NNT is computed by dividing 100 by the difference between the percentage response of the treatment group from that of the control group.

Alternatively, the NNT is calculated by taking the reciprocal of the absolute risk reduction between the groups. The NNT indicates how many patients must be managed on average with active rather than control therapy to achieve 1 additional good outcome.

The number needed concept may be applied to many types of outcomes from both therapeutic and diagnostic studies. When a therapy increases desirable outcomes, the resulting value is the number needed to benefit (more often denoted as just NNT). When a therapy increases adverse events, the resulting value is the number needed to harm. When applied to diagnostic strategies, the resulting values are the number needed to screen for tests in asymptomatic individuals, and the number needed to diagnose for tests in symptomatic individuals.

Why Is the NNT Important?

The NNT is intuitively understandable by patients and clinicians. It is also quantitative, facilitating decision making when selecting among available therapeutic strategies. By including a 95% confidence interval (CI) around the observed NNT, the uncertainty in the benefit also can be communicated effectively.

Other well-established indices of treatment effect are not well suited for this purpose. For example, a statistically significant P value conveys statistical rather than clinical significance. The P value suggests there will be a difference in outcomes associated with choice of therapy, but not how large that difference will be.

Risk ratios and odds ratios convey the relative rather than the absolute differences in outcomes with different treatments.[4] They are interpretable only if the event rate in the control comparator group is also stated, and then require mental calculation not readily performable by many decision makers. For example, a treatment that increases by 1.5-fold the frequency of a desirable outcome (risk ratio = 1.5) will help only 1 of every 100 patients if the base rate of the desirable outcome in the control group is 2% (increased in the active group to 3%), but will help 20 of every 100 patients if the base rate of the desirable outcome in the control group is 40% (increased in the active group to 60%). In contrast, the NNT conveys the absolute size of differences in outcome proportions with different treatments in a readily interpretable manner.

LIMITATIONS AND ALTERNATIVES TO THE NNT

Despite its several advantages, the NNT metric does have important limitations, and alternative indices of treatment effect magnitude are available that provide helpful complementary information. First, the NNT combines 2 proportions (the fraction of treatment success in each treatment group) into a single number, which sacrifices information. For example, the same NNT may represent increases in treatment success (eg, from 5% to 15% or from 85% to 95%) that may be viewed differently by patients and clinicians.

A second limitation is that it can be challenging to compare and integrate different NNTs because their values are expressed as fractions with different denominators. In contrast, the natural frequency metric (most often stated as benefit per hundred and harm per hundred) more readily facilitates comparisons because it expresses the treatment effect magnitude using a uniform (100) and familiar (from percentages) denominator.[5,6]

For example, consider the following statements describing the same treatment effect. The NNT to prevent 1 myocardial infarction is 25 patients, to prevent 1 ischemic stroke is 50, and to cause 1 major bleeding event is 33. For every 100 patients treated, 4 fewer will have a myocardial infarction, 2 fewer an ischemic stroke, and 3 more a major bleeding event. The different framing of the clinical trial result provided by the NNT and benefit per hundred can influence decision making despite the fact that they are numerically equivalent.

The NNT aligns more closely with the patient perspective because the patient will often be making a particular treatment decision only once ("my chance of benefit is 1 in X"). The benefit per hundred aligns more closely with the perspective of the clinician, who will often be making the same treatment decision tens of times during a career ("out of 100 patients I treat, I will help X").[7]

A limitation of the NNT shared by the natural frequency is that randomized clinical trial results fully specify NNT values only for binary outcomes (such as the occurrence of an infection, a rash, or death), but not for ordinal or continuous outcomes (such as reduced pain or degree of disability). This drawback has been partially mitigated by the development of methods that provide estimated NNT values for ordinal or continuous outcomes using automated or content expert–informed derivation techniques.[8] However, these methods require additional, often untestable, assumptions to estimate the distribution of an observed treatment group benefit among individual patients because the same clinical trial result can arise when many patients experience a small individual benefit or when fewer patients experience a large individual benefit.

Another limitation is that the NNT reflects the number not the importance of events. Different types of events are each given their own separate NNT values and the resulting quantitative statements may encourage overweighting of less important outcomes. For example, a therapy is clearly of substantial net benefit even if it has a nominally lower NNT to harm of 3 for a minor adverse effect (such as transient mild headache) accompanying a nominally higher NNT to benefit of 5 for a major beneficial effect (such as fatal cardiac failure). An alternative approach is to integrate multiple outcomes into a single measure of treatment effect using health-related utility values for each of the outcomes.[9,10] Once event values are converted to this single consistent measure, an NNT to achieve any given magnitude of benefit on the utility scale can be derived.[6]

For example, the "number needed to save one life" was recently used to express the number of patients with acute ischemic stroke treated with thrombectomy required to achieve the same total benefit as saving the life of 1 patient who would have died and achieving a normal neurological outcome.[6]

Further limitations include that the NNT does not convey the financial costs and benefits of treatments and only expresses the magnitude of effect expected for a prototypical patient, reflecting the aggregate characteristics of the population enrolled in a particular clinical trial. In contrast, each individual patient has distinctive features modifying the baseline risk and treatment response. In addition, when patient outcomes vary over time, the reported NNT reflects the benefit at a particular time point and several different NNT values might be needed to capture varying benefits (eg, at early, middle, or late stages of the treatment course).

How Was the Concept of NNT Applied in This Particular Study?

In the Results section of the study by Zhao et al,[1] the primary efficacy end point findings were reported including each group's individual outcome proportions and 95% CIs, the relative treatment effect magnitude (relative risk, 0.48 [95% CI, 0.31-0.74]), the absolute treatment effect magnitude (risk difference, 12.2% [95% CI, 5.2%-19.2%]), and the statistical significance ($P < .001$). The authors restated this result as an NNT of 8 (the approximate reciprocal of 12.2%). Reporting the findings this way conveyed the probability of benefit in a clinically useful manner. The authors did not provide the 95% CI around the NNT value. The absence of a 95% CI around the NNT improves readability, but somewhat obscures the degree of uncertainty around the estimated value. An NNT to harm value was not provided for the increase in minor bleeding events that also was observed with double antiplatelet therapy. However, it is prudent in primary trial reports to state NNT values only for the lead efficacy and safety end points that were the prespecified focus of hypothesis testing.

How Should the NNT Be Interpreted in the Study by Zhao et al?

The absolute risk difference of 12.2% with the 95% CI of 5.2% to 19.2% reported by Zhao et al[1] indicates that approximately 8 patients (given by the reciprocal of 0.122) need to be treated with dual antiplatelet therapy as opposed to aspirin monotherapy to avoid 1 case of saphenous vein graft occlusion. However, the data are also consistent with this number being as low as 5 or as high as 19 (given by the reciprocals of 0.192 and 0.052, respectively). These values capture both the probability of benefit for the individual patient (approximately 1 in 8) and the uncertainty in that probability.

Acknowledgment

The following disclosures were reported at the time this original article was first published in *JAMA*.

Conflict of Interest Disclosures: None reported.

References

1. Zhao Q, Zhu Y, Xu Z, et al. Effect of ticagrelor plus aspirin, ticagrelor alone, or aspirin alone on saphenous vein graft patency 1 year after coronary artery bypass grafting: a randomized clinical trial. *JAMA*. 2018;319(16):1677-1686. Medline:29710164
2. Laupacis A, Sackett DL, Roberts RS. An assessment of clinically useful measures of the consequences of treatment. *N Engl J Med*. 1988;318(26):1728-1733. Medline:3374545
3. Mendes D, Alves C, Batel-Marques F. Number needed to treat (NNT) in clinical literature. *BMC Med*. 2017;15(1):112. Medline:28571585
4. Norton EC, Dowd BE, Maciejewski ML. Odds ratios—current best practice and use. *JAMA*. 2018;320(1):84-85. Medline:29971384
5. Hoffrage U, Lindsey S, Hertwig R, Gigerenzer G. Medicine: communicating statistical information. *Science*. 2000;290(5500):2261-2262. Medline: 11188724

6. Nogueira RG, Jadhav AP, Haussen DC, et al. Thrombectomy 6 to 24 hours after stroke with a mismatch between deficit and infarct. *N Engl J Med*. 2018; 378(1):11-21. Medline:29129157

7. Peng J, He F, Zhang Y, et al. Differences in simulated doctor and patient medical decision making. *PLoS One*. 2013;8(11):e79181. Medline:24244445

8. Saver JL. Optimal end points for acute stroke therapy trials. *Stroke*. 2011; 42(8):2356-2362. Medline:21719772

9. Irony TZ. The "utility" in composite outcome measures. *JAMA*. 2017;318(18): 1820-1821. Medline:29136430

10 Hong KS, Ali LK, Selco SL, et al. Weighting components of composite end points in clinical trials. *Stroke*. 2011;42(6):1722-1729. Medline:21527766

Multiple Comparison Procedures

Jing Cao, PhD, and Song Zhang, PhD

IN THIS CHAPTER

Use of Method

Why Are Multiple Comparison Procedures Used?

What Are the Limitations of Multiple Comparison Procedures?

Why Did the Authors Use Multiple Comparison Procedures in This Particular Study?

How Should This Method's Findings Be Interpreted in This Particular Study?

Caveats to Consider When Looking at Multiple Comparison Procedures

To Adjust or Not

Confirmatory vs Exploratory

FWER vs FDR

Definition of Family

This JAMA Guide to Statistics and Methods explains when adjustment for multiple comparisons is appropriate and outlines the limitations, interpretations, and cautions to be aware of when using these adjustments.

Problems can arise when researchers try to assess the statistical significance of more than 1 test in a study. In a single test, statistical significance is often determined based on an observed effect or finding that is unlikely (<5%) to occur due to chance alone. When more than 1 comparison are made, the chance of falsely detecting a nonexistent effect increases. This is known as the problem of multiple comparisons (MCs), and adjustments can be made in statistical testing to account for this.[1]

Saitz et al[2] reported results of a randomized trial evaluating the efficacy of 2 brief counseling interventions (ie, a brief negotiated interview and an adaptation of a motivational interview, referred to as MOTIV) in reducing drug use in primary care patients when compared with not having an intervention. Because MCs were made, the authors adjusted how they determined statistical significance. In this chapter, we explain why adjustment for MCs is appropriate in this study and point out the limitations, interpretations, and cautions when using these adjustments.

USE OF METHOD

Why Are Multiple Comparison Procedures Used?

When a single statistical test is performed at the 5% significance level, there is a 5% chance of falsely concluding that a supposed effect exists when in fact there is none. This is known as making a false discovery or having a false-positive inference. The significance level represents the risk of making a false discovery in an individual test, denoted as the individual error rate (IER).

If 20 such tests are conducted, there is a 5% chance of making a false-positive inference with each test so that, on average, there will be 1 false discovery in the 20 tests.

Another way to view this is in terms of probabilities. If the probability of making a false conclusion (ie, false discovery) is 5% for a single test in which the effect does not exist, then 95% of the time, the test will arrive at the correct conclusion (ie, insignificant effect). With 2 such tests, the probability of finding an insignificant effect with the first test is 95%, as it is for the second. However, the probability of finding insignificant effects in the first and the second test is 0.95×0.95, or 90%. With 20 such tests, the probability that all of the 20 tests correctly show insignificance is $(0.95)^{20}$ or 36%. So there is a 100% − 36%, or 64%, chance of at least 1 false-positive test occurring among the 20 tests. Because this probability quantifies the risk of making any false-positive inference by a group, or family, of tests, it is referred to as the family-wise error rate (FWER). The FWER generally increases as the number of tests performed increases. For example, assuming IER = 5% and denoting the number of multiple tests performed as K, then for $K = 2$ independent tests, FWER $= 1 - (0.95)^2 = 10\%$; for $K = 3$, FWER $= 1 - (0.95)^3 = 14\%$; and for $K = 20$, FWER $= 1 - (0.95)^{20} = 64\%$. This shows that the risk of making at least 1 false discovery in MCs can be greatly inflated even if the error rate is well controlled in each individual test.

When MCs are made, to control FWER at a certain level, the threshold for determining statistical significance in individual tests must be adjusted.[1] The simplest approach is known as the Bonferroni correction. It adjusts the statistical significance threshold by the number of tests. For example, for an FWER fixed at 5%, the IER in a group of 20 tests is set at $0.05/20 = 0.0025$; ie, an individual test would have to have a P value less than .0025 to be considered statistically significant. The Bonferroni correction is easy to implement, but it sets the significance threshold too rigidly, reducing the statistical procedure's power to detect true effects.

The Hochberg sequential procedure, which was used in the study by Saitz et al,[2] takes a different approach.[3] All of the tests (the multiple comparisons) are performed and the resultant P values are ordered from largest to smallest on a list. If the FWER is fixed at 5% and the largest observed P value is less than .05, then all the tests are considered significant. Otherwise, if the next largest P value is less than 0.05/2 (.025), then all the tests except the one with the largest P value are considered significant. If not, and the third P value in the list is less than 0.05/3 (.017), then all the tests except those with the largest 2 P values are considered significant. This is continued until all the comparisons are made. This approach uses progressively more stringent statistical thresholds with the most stringent one being the Bonferroni threshold, and thus the approach can achieve a greater power to detect true effect than the Bonferroni procedure under appropriate conditions. An example in Table 1 consists of 6 tests in MCs; given an FWER of 5%, none of the tests are significant with the Bonferroni procedure. By comparison, 3 tests are significant with the Hochberg sequential procedure.

What Are the Limitations of Multiple Comparison Procedures?

Statistical procedures to control FWER in MCs were developed to reduce the risk of making any false-positive discovery. This is offset by having a lower test power to detect true effects. For example, when $K = 10$, the Bonferroni-corrected IER is $0.05/10 = 0.005$ to control FWER at 0.05. Under the conventional 2-sided t test, for a single test in the group to be considered significant, the observed effect needs to be 43% larger than that with an IER $= 0.05$. When $K = 20$, the Bonferroni-corrected IER is $0.05/20 = 0.0025$, and the observed effect needs to be 54% larger than that with an IER $= 0.05$. This limitation of reduced test power by controlling FWER becomes more apparent as the number of tests in MCs increases.

TABLE 1

An Example to Compare the Bonferroni Procedure and the Hochberg Sequential Procedure

Test	P Value	Bonferroni		Hochberg	
		Threshold	Result	Threshold	Result
1	.40	0.05/6 = 0.008	Not significant	0.05	Not significant
2	.027	0.05/6 = 0.008	Not significant	0.05/2 = 0.025	Not significant
3	.020	0.05/6 = 0.008	Not significant	0.05/3 = 0.017	Not significant
4	.012	0.05/6 = 0.008	Not significant	0.05/4 = 0.0125	Significant
5	.011	0.05/6 = 0.008	Not significant	NA	Significant
6	.010	0.05/6 = 0.008	Not significant	NA	Significant

Abbreviation: NA, not applicable.

Why Did the Authors Use Multiple Comparison Procedures in This Particular Study?

In the study by Saitz et al, 2 tests were performed (brief negotiated interview vs no brief interview and MOTIV vs no brief interview) to determine if interventions with brief counseling were more effective in reducing drug use than interventions without counseling. With 2 tests and the IER set at 5%, the risk of falsely concluding at least 1 treatment is effective because of chance alone is 10%. To avoid the inflated FWER, the authors used the Hochberg sequential procedure.[3]

How Should This Method's Findings Be Interpreted in This Particular Study?

Saitz et al[2] found that the adjusted P value[4] based on the Hochberg procedure was .81 for both the brief negotiated interview and MOTIV vs no brief interview. The study did not provide sufficient evidence to claim that interventions with brief counseling were more effective than the one without brief counseling in reducing drug use among primary care patients. However, the absence of evidence does not mean there is an absence of an effect. The interventions may be effective, but this study did not have the statistical power to detect the effect.

CAVEATS TO CONSIDER WHEN LOOKING AT MULTIPLE COMPARISON PROCEDURES

To Adjust or Not

If researchers conduct multiple tests, each addressing an unrelated research question, then adjusting for MCs is unnecessary. Suppose in a different study, brief negotiated interview was intended to treat alcohol use and MOTIV was intended to treat drug use. Then there is no need to adjust for MCs. This is in contrast to performing a family of tests from which the results as a whole address a single research question; then adjusting for MCs is necessary. As in the report by Saitz et al,[2] both the brief negotiated interview and MOTIV were compared with the control to draw a single conclusion about the efficacy of brief counseling interventions for drug use.

Confirmatory vs Exploratory

Bender and Lange[5] suggested that MC procedures are only required for confirmatory studies for which the goal is the definitive proof of a predefined hypothesis to support final decision making. For exploratory studies seeking to generate hypotheses that will be tested in future confirmatory studies, the number of tests is usually large and the choice of hypotheses is likely data dependent (ie, selecting hypotheses after reviewing data), making MC adjustments unnecessary or even impossible at this stage of research. "Significant" results based on exploratory studies, however, should be clearly labeled so readers can correctly assess their scientific strength.

FWER vs FDR

The main approaches to MC adjustment include controlling FWER, which is the probability of making at least 1 false discovery in MCs, or controlling the false discovery rate (FDR), which is the expected proportion of false positives among all discoveries. When using the FDR approaches, a small proportion of false positives are tolerated to improve the chance of detecting true effects.[6] In contrast, the FWER approaches avoid any false positives even at the cost of increased false negatives. The FDR and FWER represent 2 extremes of the relative importance of controlling for false positive or false negatives. The decision whether to control FWER or FDR should be made by carefully weighing the relative benefits between false-positive and false-negative discoveries in a specific study.

Definition of Family

Both FWER and FDR are defined for a particular family of tests. This "family" should be prespecified at the design stage of a study. Test bias can occur in MCs when selecting hypothesis to be tested after reviewing the data.

Acknowledgment

The following disclosures were reported at the time this original article was first published in *JAMA*.

Conflict of Interest Disclosures: None reported.

References

1. Hsu JC. *Multiple Comparisons: Theory and Methods*. London, UK: Chapman & Hall; 1996.
2. Saitz R, Palfai TPA, Cheng DM, et al. Screening and brief intervention for drug use in primary care: the ASPIRE randomized clinical trial. *JAMA*. 2014;312(5): 502-513. doi:10.1001/jama.2014.7862.
3. Hochberg Y. A sharper Bonferroni procedure for multiple tests of significance. *Biometrika*. 1988;75(4):800-802.
4. Wright SP. Adjusted P value for simultaneous inference. Biometrics. 1992;48(4): 1005-1013.
5. Bender R, Lange S. Adjusting for multiple testing: when and how? *J Clin Epidemiol*. 2001;54(4):343-349. Medline:11297884
6. Benjamini Y, Hochberg Y. Controlling the false discovery rate: a practical and powerful approach to multiple testing. *J R Stat Soc B*. 1995;57(1):289-300.

Gatekeeping Strategies for Avoiding False-Positive Results in Clinical Trials With Many Comparisons

Kabir Yadav, MDCM, MS, MSHS, and
Roger J. Lewis, MD, PhD

IN THIS CHAPTER

Use of the Method
   Why Is Serial Gatekeeping Used?
   Description of the Method
What Are the Limitations of Gatekeeping Strategies?
How Was Gatekeeping Used in This Case?
How Should the Results Be Interpreted?

This JAMA Guide to Statistics and Methods explains the gatekeeping approach to evaluating the statistical significance of secondary outcomes by not pursuing analysis once a primary finding or a higher order secondary outcome is rendered nonsignificant.

Clinical trials characterizing the effects of an experimental therapy rarely have only a single outcome of interest. For example, the CLEAN-TAVI investigators evaluated the benefits of a cerebral embolic protection device for stroke prevention during transcatheter aortic valve implantation.[1] The primary end point was the reduction in the number of ischemic lesions observed 2 days after the procedure. The investigators were also interested in 16 secondary end points involving measurement of the number, volume, and timing of cerebral lesions in various brain regions. Statistically comparing a large number of outcomes using the usual significance threshold of .05 is likely to be misleading because there is a high risk of falsely concluding that a significant effect is present when none exists.[2] If 17 comparisons are made when there is no true treatment effect, each comparison has a 5% chance of falsely concluding that an observed difference exists, leading to a 58% chance of falsely concluding at least 1 difference exists. The formula $1 - [1 - \alpha]^N$ can be used to calculate the chance of obtaining at least 1 falsely significant result, when there is no true underlying difference between the groups (in this case α is .05 and N is 17 for the number of tests).

To avoid a false-positive result, while still comparing the multiple clinically relevant end points used in the CLEAN-TAVI study, the investigators used a serial gatekeeping approach for statistical testing. This method tests an outcome, and if that outcome is statistically significant, then the next outcome is tested. This minimizes the chance of falsely concluding a difference exists when it does not.

USE OF THE METHOD

Why Is Serial Gatekeeping Used?

Many methods exist for conducting multiple comparisons while keeping the overall trial-level risk of a false-positive error at an acceptable level. The Bonferroni approach[3] requires a more stringent criterion for statistical significance (a smaller P value) for each statistical test, but each is interpreted independently of the other comparisons. This approach is often considered to be too conservative, reducing the ability of the trial to detect true benefits when they exist.[4] Other methods leverage additional knowledge about the trial design to allow only the comparisons of interest. In the Dunnett method for comparing multiple experimental drug doses against a single control, the number of comparisons is reduced by never comparing experimental drug doses against each other.[5] Multiple comparison procedures, including the Hochberg procedure, have been discussed in a prior JAMA Guide to Statistics and Methods.[2]

Description of the Method

A serial gatekeeping procedure controls the false-positive risk by requiring the multiple end points to be compared in a predefined sequence and stopping all further testing once a nonsignificant result is obtained. A given comparison might be considered positive if it were placed early in the sequence, but the same analysis would be considered negative if it were positioned in the sequence after a negative result. By restricting the pathways for obtaining a positive result, gatekeeping controls the risk of false-positive results but preserves greater power for the earlier, higher-priority end points. This approach works well to test a sequence of secondary end points as in the CLEAN-TAVI study or to test a series of branching secondary end points (Figure 5).

FIGURE 5

Criteria for Statistical Significance That Would Be Used in a Hypothetical Gatekeeping Strategy

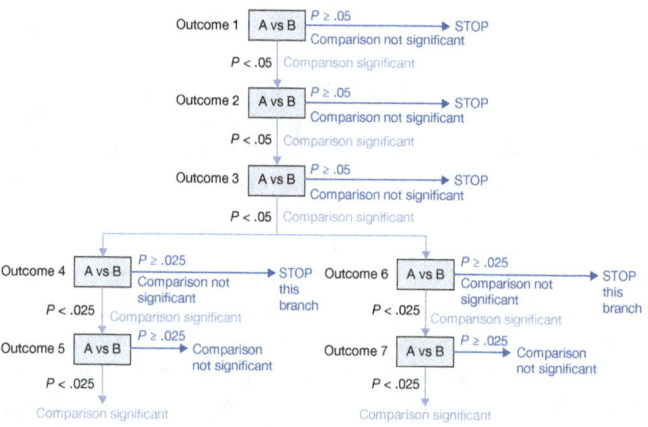

This Figure shows the criteria for statistical significance that would be used in a hypothetical gatekeeping strategy in which there are 3 levels each with a single end point, followed by 2 levels with 2 end points each. The 3 end points are each tested in order against a criterion of .05. All testing stops as soon as 1 result is nonsignificant. If all are significant then a pair of fourth-level end points is tested, and to preserve the required significance of .05 at that level across 2 end points, the criterion for statistical significance is adjusted with a Bonferroni correction value of .025 for each. If 1 or both of these end points is significant at .025, then the next end point in the branch is tested, against a criterion of .025. If 1 or both are nonsignificant, no further testing occurs. If any outcome tested along a given pathway is not statistically significant, no further outcomes along that branch are tested because they are assumed to be nonsignificant.

Steps in serial gatekeeping are as follows: (1) determine the order for testing multiple end points, considering their relative importance and the likelihood that there is a difference in each; (2) test the first end point against the desired global false-positive rate (ie, .05) and, if the finding does not reach statistical significance, then stop all further testing and declare this and all downstream end points nonsignificant. If testing the first end point is significant, then declare this difference significant and proceed with the testing of the next end point; (3) test the next end point using a significance threshold of .05; if not significant, stop all further testing and declare this and all downstream end points nonsignificant. If significant, then declare this difference significant and proceed with the testing of the next end point; and (4) repeat the prior step until obtaining a first nonsignificant result, or until all end points have been tested.

As shown in Figure 5, this approach can be extended to test 2 or more end points at the same step by using a Bonferroni adjustment to evenly split the false-positive error rate within the step. In that case, testing is continued until either all branches have obtained a first nonsignificant result or all end points have been tested. For example, a neuroimaging end point could be used as a single end point for the first level, reflecting the assumption that if an improvement in an imaging outcome is not achieved then an improvement in a patient-centered functional outcome is highly unlikely, followed by a split to allow the testing of motor functions on one branch and verbal functions on the other. This avoids the need to prioritize either motor or verbal function over the other and may increase the ability to demonstrate an improvement in either domain.

Serial gatekeeping provides strict control of the false-positive error rate because it restricts multiple comparisons by sequentially testing hypotheses until the first nonsignificant test is found, and, no matter how significant later end points appear to be, they are never tested. The advantage is increased power for detecting effects on the end points that appear early in the sequence because they are tested against .05 rather than, eg, .05 divided by the total number of outcomes tested using a traditional Bonferroni adjustment. By accounting for the importance of certain hypotheses over others and by grouping hypotheses into primary and secondary groups, gatekeeping allocates the trial's power to be consistent with the investigators' priorities.[6]

WHAT ARE THE LIMITATIONS OF GATEKEEPING STRATEGIES?

Gatekeeping strategies are a powerful way to incorporate trial-specific clinical information to create prespecified ordering of hypotheses and mitigate the need to adjust for multiple comparisons at each stage of testing. The primary challenge in using gatekeeping is the need to prespecify and truly commit to the order of testing. The resulting limitation is that if, in retrospect, the order of outcome testing appears ill chosen (eg, if an early end point is negative and important end points later in the sequence appear to suggest large treatment effects), then there is no rigorous, post hoc method for statistically evaluating the later end points. This highlights the importance of having a clear data analysis strategy determined before the trial is started, and maintaining transparency (eg, publishing the study design and analysis plan on public websites or in journals).

HOW WAS GATEKEEPING USED IN THIS CASE?

The CLEAN-TAVI investigators used a gatekeeping strategy to compare several magnetic resonance imaging end points along with neurological and neurocognitive performance.[1] The first was the primary study end point, the number of brain lesions 2 days after TAVI. Secondary end points were only tested if the primary one was positive. Then, up to 16 secondary end points were tested in a defined sequence. The study was markedly positive, with the primary and many secondary end points demonstrating benefit. The first 8 comparisons were reported in detail in the publication—in their prespecified order—retaining the structure of the gatekeeping strategy.[1]

HOW SHOULD THE RESULTS BE INTERPRETED?

The CLEAN-TAVI clinical trial demonstrated the efficacy of a cerebral protection strategy with respect to multiple imaging measures of ischemic damage. The use of the prespecified gatekeeping strategy should provide assurance that the large number of imaging end points that were compared was unlikely to have led to false-positive results.

Acknowledgment

The following disclosures were reported at the time this original article was first published in *JAMA*.
    Conflict of Interest Disclosures: None reported.

References

1. Haussig S, Mangner N, Dwyer MG, et al. Effect of a cerebral protection device on brain lesions following transcatheter aortic valve implantation in patients with severe aortic stenosis. *JAMA*. 2016;316(6):592-601. Medline:27532914
2. Cao J, Zhang S. Multiple comparison procedures. *JAMA*. 2014;312(5):543-544. Medline:25096694
3. Bland JM, Altman DG. Multiple significance tests: the Bonferroni method. *BMJ*. 1995;310(6973):170-170. Medline:7833759
4. Hommel G, Bretz F, Maurer W. Powerful short-cuts for multiple testing procedures with special reference to gatekeeping strategies. *Stat Med*. 2007;26(22):4063-4073. Medline:17348083
5. Holm S. A simple sequentially rejective multiple test procedure. *Scand J Stat*. 1979;6(2):65-70.
6. Dmitrienko A, Millen BA, Brechenmacher T, Paux G. Development of gatekeeping strategies in confirmatory clinical trials. *Biom J*. 2011;53(6):875-893. Medline:22069199

# Multiple Imputation: A Flexible Tool for Handling Missing Data

Peng Li, PhD, Elizabeth A. Stuart, PhD, and David B. Allison, PhD

IN THIS CHAPTER

Use of the Method

Why Is Multiple Imputation Used?

What Are the Limitations of Multiple Imputation?

Why Did the Authors Use Multiple Imputation in This Particular Study?

How Should Multiple Imputation Findings Be Interpreted in This Particular Study?

Caveats to Consider When Looking at Results Based on Multiple Imputation

This JAMA Guide to Statistics and Methods discusses the use of multiple imputation in statistical analyses when data are missing for some participants in a clinical trial.

In a study published in *JAMA*, Asch et al[1] reported results of a cluster randomized clinical trial designed to evaluate the effects of physician financial incentives, patient incentives, or shared physician and patient incentives on low-density lipoprotein cholesterol (LDL-C) levels among patients with high cardiovascular risk. Because 1 or more follow-up LDL-C measurements were missing for approximately 7% of participants, Asch et al used multiple imputation (MI) to analyze their data and concluded that shared financial incentives for physicians and patients, but not incentives to physicians or patients alone, resulted in the patients having lower LDL-C levels. Imputation is the process of replacing missing data with 1 or more specific values, to allow statistical analysis that includes all participants and not just those who do not have any missing data.

Missing data are common in research. In another JAMA Guide to Statistics and Methods, Newgard and Lewis[2] reviewed the causes of missing data. (See the chapter Missing Data: How to Best Account for What Is Not Known.) These are divided into 3 classes: (1) missing completely at random, the most restrictive assumption, indicating that whether a data point is missing is completely unrelated to observed and unobserved data; (2) missing at random, a more realistic assumption than missing completely at random, indicating whether a missing data point can be explained by the observed data; or (3) missing not at random, meaning that the missingness is dependent on the unobserved values. Common statistical methods used for handling missing values were reviewed.[2] When missing data occur, it is important to not exclude cases with missing information (analyses after such exclusion are known as complete case analyses). Single-value imputation methods are those that estimate what each missing value might have been and replace it with a single value in the data set. Single-value imputation methods include mean imputation, last observation carried forward, and random imputation. These approaches can yield biased results and are suboptimal. Multiple imputation better handles missing data by estimating and replacing missing values many times.

USE OF THE METHOD

Why Is Multiple Imputation Used?

Multiple imputation fills in missing values by generating plausible numbers derived from distributions of and relationships among observed variables in the data set.[3] Multiple imputation differs from single imputation methods because missing data are filled in many times, with many different plausible values estimated for each missing value. Using multiple plausible values provides a quantification of the uncertainty in estimating what the missing values might be, avoiding creating false precision (as can happen with single imputation). Multiple imputation provides accurate estimates of quantities or associations of interest, such as treatment effects in randomized trials, sample means of specific variables, correlations between 2 variables, as well as the related variances. In doing so, it reduces the chance of false-positive or false-negative conclusions.

Multiple imputation entails 2 stages: (1) generating replacement values ("imputations") for missing data and repeating this procedure many times, resulting in many data sets with replaced missing information, and (2) analyzing the many imputed data sets and combining the results. In stage 1, MI imputes the missing entries based on statistical characteristics of the data, for example, the associations among and distributions of variables in the data set. After the imputed data sets are obtained, in stage 2, any analysis can be conducted within each of the imputed data sets as if there were no missing data. That is, each of the "filled-in" complete data sets is simply analyzed with any method that would be valid and appropriate for addressing a scientific question in a data set that had no missing data.

After the intended statistical analysis (regression, *t* test, etc) is run separately on each imputed data set (stage 2), the estimates of interest (eg, the mean difference in outcome between a treatment and a control group) from all the imputed data sets are combined into a single estimate using standard combining rules.[3] For example, in the study by Asch et al,[1] the reported treatment effect is the average of the treatment effects estimated from each of the imputed data sets. The total variance or uncertainty of the treatment effect is obtained, in part, by seeing how much the estimate varies from one imputed data set to the next, with greater variability across the imputed data sets indicating greater uncertainty due to missing data. This imputed-data-set-to-imputed-data-set variability is built into a formula that provides accurate standard errors and, thereby, confidence intervals and significance tests for the quantities of interest, while allowing for the uncertainty due to the missing data. This distinguishes MI from single imputation.

Combining most parameter estimates, such as regression coefficients, is straightforward,[4] and modern software (including R, SAS, Stata, and others) can do the combining automatically. There are some caveats as to which variables must be included in the statistical model in the imputation stage, which are discussed extensively elsewhere.[5]

Another advantage of adding MI to the statistical toolbox is that it can handle interesting problems not conventionally thought of as missing data problems. Multiple imputation can correct for measurement error by treating the unobserved true scores (eg, someone's exact degree of ancestry from a particular population when there are only imperfect estimates for each person) as missing,[6] generate data appropriate for public release while ensuring confidentiality,[7] or make large-scale sampling more efficient through planned missing data (ie, by intentionally measuring some variables on only a subset of participants in a study to save money).[8]

What Are the Limitations of Multiple Imputation?

As with any statistical technique, the validity of MI depends on the validity of its assumptions. But when those assumptions are met, MI rests on well-established theory.[3,5] Moreover, substantial empirical support exists for the validity of MI in simulations, including those based on real data patterns.[9] In principle, computational speed can be a problem because each analysis must be run multiple times, but in practice, this is rarely an issue with modern computers.

Many nonstatisticians chafe at "making up data" as is done in MI and note that the validity of MI depends on an assumption about which factors relate to the probability that a data point is missing. Because of concern this assumption may be violated, it is tempting to retreat to the safe haven of complete case analysis, ie, only analyze the participants without missing values. This safe haven is, however, illusory. Although rarely made explicit by users, complete case analysis requires a far more restrictive assumption: that any data point missing is missing completely at random. Other common strategies—mean imputation, last observation carried forward, and other single imputation approaches—underestimate standard errors by ignoring or underestimating the inherent uncertainty created by missing data, a problem MI helps overcome.

Why Did the Authors Use Multiple Imputation in This Particular Study?

In the study by Asch et al,[1] the primary outcome, LDL-C levels, had missing values. Thus, a method to handle missingness was needed to maintain the validity of the statistical inferences. Complete case analysis would have inappropriately not included 7% of their sample, leading to less study power, results restricted to those individuals without missing values, violation of the intent-to-treat principle, possible nonrandom loss and therefore a loss of the ability to rely on the fact of randomization to justify causal inferences, and ultimately to results that may not apply to the original full sample.

How Should Multiple Imputation Findings Be Interpreted in This Particular Study?

Provided that the underlying assumptions of MI are met, the results from this study can be interpreted as if all the participants had no missing entries. That is, both the estimates of quantities like means and measures of association and the estimates of their uncertainty (standard errors) on which formal statistical testing is based will not be biased by the fact that some data were missing. There would have been greater precision of the estimates and study power had there been no missing data. But imputation at least appropriately reflects the amount of information there actually is in the data available.

CAVEATS TO CONSIDER WHEN LOOKING AT RESULTS BASED ON MULTIPLE IMPUTATION

When the missing data are not missing at random, results from MI may not be reliable. Generally, reasons for missingness cannot be fully identified. In practice, collecting more information about study participants may help identify why data are missing. These "auxiliary variables" can then be used in the imputation process and improve MI's performance. All other things being equal, imputation models with more variables included and a large number of imputations improve MI's performance. Multiple imputation is arguably the most flexible valid missing data approach among those that are commonly used.

Acknowledgment

The following disclosures were reported at the time this original article was first published in *JAMA*.

Conflict of Interest Disclosures: None reported.

Funding/Support: This work was supported in part by grants from the National Institutes of Health (NIH) (R25HL124208, R25DK099080, R01MH099010, and P30DK056336).

Role of the Funder/Sponsor: The funding sources had no role in the preparation, review, or approval of the manuscript.

Disclaimer: The opinions expressed are those of the authors and do not necessarily represent those of the NIH or any other organization.

References

1. Asch DA, Troxel AB, Stewart WF, et al. Effect of financial incentives to physicians, patients, or both on lipid levels: a randomized clinical trial. *JAMA*. 2015;314(18):926-1935. doi:10.1001/jama.2015.14850.

2. Newgard CD, Lewis RJ. Missing data: how to best account for what is not known. *JAMA*. 2015;314(9):940-941. Medline:26325562

3. Rubin DB. *Multiple Imputation for Nonresponse in Surveys*. New York, NY: Wiley; 1987.

4. White IR, Royston P, Wood AM. Multiple imputation using chained equations: issues and guidance for practice. *Stat Med*. 2011;30(4):377-399. Medline:21225900

5. Schafer JL. *Analysis of Incomplete Multivariate Data*. New York, NY: Chapman & Hall; 1997.

6. Padilla MA, Divers J, Vaughan LK, Allison DB, Tiwari HK. Multiple imputation to correct for measurement error in admixture estimates in genetic structured association testing. *Hum Hered*. 2009;68(1):65-72. Medline:19339787

7. Wang H, Reiter JP. Multiple imputation for sharing precise geographies in public use data. *Ann Appl Stat*. 2012;6(1):229-252. Medline:23990852

8. Capers PL, Brown AW, Dawson JA, Allison DB. Double sampling with multiple imputation to answer large sample meta-research questions: introduction and illustration by evaluating adherence to two simple CONSORT guidelines. *Front Nutr*. 2015;2:6. Medline:25988135

9. Elobeid MA, Padilla MA, McVie T, et al. Missing data in randomized clinical trials for weight loss: scope of the problem, state of the field, and performance of statistical methods. *PLoS One*. 2009;4(8):e6624. Medline:19675667

Interpretation of Clinical Trials That Stopped Early

Kert Viele, PhD, Anna McGlothlin, PhD, and Kristine Broglio, MS

IN THIS CHAPTER

Use of the Method

Why Is Early Stopping Used?

What Are the Limitations of Early Stopping?

Why Did the Authors Use Early Stopping in This Study?

How Should Early Stopping Be Interpreted in This Particular Study?

Caveats to Consider When Looking at a Trial That Stopped Early

This JAMA Guide to Statistics and Methods discusses how to interpret the results of clinical trials that are stopped early based on formal, prespecified stopping rules.

Clinical trials require significant resources to complete in terms of patients, investigators, and time and should be carefully designed and conducted so that they use the minimum amount of resources necessary to answer the motivating clinical question. The size of a clinical trial is typically based on the minimum number of patients required to have high probability of detecting the anticipated treatment effect. However, it is possible that strong evidence could emerge earlier in the trial either in favor of or against the benefit of the novel treatment. If early trial results are compelling, stopping the trial before the maximum planned sample size is reached presents ethical advantages for patients inside and outside the trial and can save resources that can be redirected to other clinical questions. This advantage must be balanced against the potential for overestimation of the treatment effect and other limitations of smaller trials (eg, limited safety data, less information about treatment effects in subgroups).

Many methods have been proposed to allow formal incorporation of early stopping into a clinical trial.[1,2] All of these methods allow a trial to stop at a prespecified interim analysis while maintaining good statistical properties. Data monitoring committees or other similar governing bodies may also monitor the progress of a trial and recommend stopping the trial early in the absence of a prespecified formal rule. An overwhelmingly positive treatment effect might lead to a recommendation for unplanned early stopping but, more commonly, unplanned early stopping results from concerns for participant safety, lack of observed benefit, or concerns about the feasibility of continuing the trial due to slow patient accrual or new external information. Trials stopped for success in an ad hoc manner are challenging to interpret rigorously. In this chapter, we focus on early stopping for success or futility based on formal, prespecified stopping rules.

In 2015, Stupp et al[3] reported the results of a trial assessing electric tumor-treating fields plus temozolomide vs temozolomide alone in patients with glioblastoma. The trial design included a preplanned interim analysis defined according to an early stopping procedure. The trial was stopped for success at the interim analysis, reporting a hazard ratio of 0.62 for the primary end point of progression-free survival.

USE OF THE METHOD

Why Is Early Stopping Used?

When 2 treatments are compared in a randomized clinical trial, the treatment effects observed both during the trial and when the trial ends are subject to random highs and lows that depart from the true treatment effect. Sample sizes for trials are selected to reliably detect an anticipated treatment effect even if a modest, random low observed treatment effect occurs at the final analysis. If such a random low value does not occur or the true treatment effect is larger than anticipated, the extra study participants required to provide this protection against a false-negative result may not be necessary. During the course of a trial, strong evidence may accumulate that the experimental treatment offers a benefit. This may be from a large observed treatment effect emerging early in a trial or from the anticipated treatment effect being observed as early as two-thirds of the way through a trial.

Conversely, evidence could accumulate early in a trial that the experimental treatment performs no better than the control. In a trial with no provision for early stopping, patients would continue to be exposed to the potential harms of the experimental therapy with no hope of benefit. Interim analyses to stop trials early for futility may avoid this risk. Trials may also stop early for futility if there is a limited likelihood of eventual success.[4]

What Are the Limitations of Early Stopping?

One key statistical issue with early stopping, particularly early stopping for success, is accounting for multiple "looks" at the data. Accumulating data, particularly early in the trial with a smaller number of observations, is likely to exhibit larger random highs and lows of values for the treatment effects. The more frequently the data are analyzed as they accumulate, the greater the chance of observing one of these fluctuations. Rules allowing early stopping therefore require a higher level of evidence, such as a lower P value, at each interim analysis than would be required at the end of a trial with no potential for early stopping. Taken together, the multiple looks at the data, each requiring a higher bar for success, lead to the same overall chance of falsely declaring success (type I error) as a trial with the usual criterion for success (eg, a $P < .05$) and no potential for early stopping.

Early stopping for futility requires no such adjustment. There are no added opportunities to declare a success; thus, no statistical adjustment to the success threshold is required. However, futility stopping may reduce the power of the trial by stopping trials based on a random low value for the treatment effect that could have gone on to be successful. This reduction in power is usually quite small.

Success thresholds are typically chosen to be more conservative for interim analyses than for the final analysis should the trial continue to completion. The O'Brien-Fleming method, for example, requires very small P values to declare success early in the trial and then maintains a final P value very close to the traditional .05 level at the final analysis.[1] Using this method, very few trials could be successful at the interim analyses that would not have been successful at the final analysis. Thus, there is a minimal "penalty" for the interim analyses. The more conservative the early stopping criteria, the more assurance there is that an early stop for success is not a false-positive result.

While methods such as O'Brien-Fleming protect against falsely declaring an ineffective drug successful, the accuracy of estimates of the treatment effect in trials that have stopped early for success remains a concern.[5] When considering the true effect of a treatment, bias is introduced when considering only trials that have observed a large enough treatment effect to meet the critical value for success. By definition, successful trials have larger treatment effects than unsuccessful trials; thus, successful trials include more random highs than random lows. As such, small trials that end in success, either at the end or early, are prone to overestimating the treatment effect. The larger the observed treatment effect, the more likely it is an extreme random high, and the greater the chance for overestimation. If the trial were continued, with the enrollment of additional patients, it is likely that there would be a reduction of the observed treatment effect. In other words, trials with very impressive early results are likely to become less impressive after observing more data, and this should be taken into account when monitoring and interpreting such trials. Extreme attenuation, such as a complete disappearance of the observed treatment benefit, however, is less likely.

Why Did the Authors Use Early Stopping in This Study?

Glioblastoma is an aggressive cancer with few treatment options. In the report by Stupp et al,[3] enrollment was largely complete at the time of the interim analysis. However, the interim analysis allowed the possibility that a beneficial result could be disseminated many months (potentially years) earlier in advance of the fully mature data.

How Should Early Stopping Be Interpreted in This Particular Study?

The primary analysis in this study found a hazard ratio of 0.62 ($P = .001$) based on 18 months of follow-up from the first 315 patients enrolled. This is strong evidence of a treatment benefit for tumor-treating fields plus temozolomide in this population.

However, care should be taken when interpreting the estimated benefit corresponding to a hazard ratio of 0.62. Given the potential for an overestimated treatment effect, combined with the general intractability of treating glioblastoma, there is good reason to suspect that the actual benefit of tumor-treating fields, while present, might be smaller than that observed in the study. A robustness analysis (ie, a supplementary or supporting analysis conducted to see how consistent the results are if different approaches were taken in conducting the analysis), based on the then-available data from all participants, illustrates this pattern. That analysis resulted in a hazard ratio of 0.69 (95% CI, 0.55−0.86), also with a $P < .001$. The result remained statistically significant, but the magnitude of the treatment effect was smaller.

CAVEATS TO CONSIDER WHEN LOOKING AT A TRIAL THAT STOPPED EARLY

It is important to consider trial design, quality of trial conduct, safety and secondary end points, and other supplementary data when interpreting the results of any clinical trial. For trials that stop early for success, the statistical superiority of an experimental treatment is straightforward when the early stopping was preplanned and it is reasonable to preserve patient resources and time once the primary objective of a trial has been addressed. Early stopping procedures protect against a false conclusion of superiority. However, if the result seems implausibly good, there is a high likelihood that the true effect is smaller than the observed effect. In that light, the benefits of early stopping, to patients both in and out of the trial, must be weighed against how much potential additional knowledge would be gained if the trial were continued.

Acknowledgment

The following disclosures were reported at the time this original article was first published in JAMA.
Conflict of Interest Disclosures: None reported.

References

1. Jennison C, Turnbull BW. *Group Sequential Methods With Applications to Clinical Trials*. Boca Raton, FL: Chapman & Hall; 2000.
2. Broglio KR, Connor JT, Berry SM. Not too big, not too small: a Goldilocks approach to sample size selection. *J Biopharm Stat*. 2014;24(3):685-705. Medline:24697532
3. Stupp R, Taillibert S, Kanner AA, et al. Maintenance therapy with tumor-treating fields plus temozolomide vs temozolomide alone for glioblastoma: a randomized clinical trial. *JAMA*. 2015;314(23):2535-2543. Medline:26670971
4. Saville BR, Connor JT, Ayers GD, Alvarez J. The utility of Bayesian predictive probabilities for interim monitoring of clinical trials. *Clin Trials*. 2014;11(4):485-493. Medline:24872363
5. Zhang JJ, Blumenthal GM, He K, Tang S, Cortazar P, Sridhara R. Overestimation of the effect size in group sequential trials. *Clin Cancer Res*. 2012;18(18):4872-4876. Medline:22753584

Bayesian Analysis: Using Prior Information to Interpret the Results of Clinical Trials

Melanie Quintana, PhD, Kert Viele, PhD, and Roger J. Lewis, MD, PhD

IN THIS CHAPTER

Prior Information

What Is Prior Information?

Why Is Prior Information Important?

Limitations of Prior Information

How Was Prior Information Used?

How Should the Trial Results Be Interpreted in Light of the Prior Information?

This JAMA Guide to Statistics and Methods discusses the Bayesian approach to integrating or updating information from previous studies with newly obtained data to yield a final quantitative summary of the information.

In a study published in *JAMA*, Laptook et al[1] reported the results of a clinical trial investigating the effect of hypothermia administered between 6 and 24 hours after birth on death and disability from hypoxic-ischemic encephalopathy (HIE). Hypothermia is beneficial for HIE when initiated within 6 hours of birth but administering hypothermia that soon after birth is impractical.[2] The study by Laptook et al[1] addressed the utility of inducing hypothermia 6 or more hours after birth because this is a more realistic time window given the logistics of providing this therapy. Performing this study was difficult because of the limited number of infants expected to be enrolled. To overcome this limitation, the investigators used a Bayesian analysis of the treatment effect to ensure that a clinically useful result would be obtained even if traditional approaches for defining statistical significance were impractical. The Bayesian approach allows for the integration or updating of prior information with newly obtained data to yield a final quantitative summary of the information. Laptook et al[1] considered several options for the representation of prior information—termed neutral, skeptical, and optimistic priors—generating different final summaries of the evidence.

PRIOR INFORMATION

What Is Prior Information?

Prior information is the evidence or beliefs about something that exist prior to or independently of the data to be analyzed. The mathematical representation of prior information (eg, of beliefs regarding the likely efficacy of hypothermia for HIE 6-24 hours after birth) must summarize both the known information and the remaining uncertainty. Some prior information is quite strong, such as data from many similar patients, and might have little remaining uncertainty or it can be weak or uninformative with substantial uncertainty.

Clinicians routinely interpret the results of a new study in the context of prior work. Are the new results consistent? How can new information be synthesized with the old? Often this synthesis is done by clinicians when they consider the totality of evidence used to treat patients or interpret research studies.

Prior information may be formally incorporated in trial analysis using Bayes theorem, which provides a mechanism for synthesizing information from multiple sources.[3,4] Clear specification of the prior information used and assumptions made need to be reported in the article or appendix to allow transparency in the analysis and reporting of outcomes.

Why Is Prior Information Important?

When large quantities of patient outcome data are available, traditional non-Bayesian (frequentist) and Bayesian approaches for quantifying observed treatment effects will yield similar results because the contribution of the observed data will outweigh that of the prior information. This is not the case for evaluating HIE treatments because very few neonates are affected. Despite a large research network, Laptook et al[1] were only able to enroll 168 eligible newborns in 8 years.

Prior information facilitates more efficient study design, allowing stronger, more definitive conclusions without requiring additional patients to be included in the study or analysis. As such, the use of prior information is particularly relevant and important for the study of rare diseases where patient resources are limited.

Prior information can take a number of forms. For example, for binary outcomes, the knowledge that an adverse outcome occurs in 15% to 40% of cases is worth the equivalent of having to enroll 30 or more patients into the trial (depending on the certainty attached to this knowledge). Another form of prior information could be beliefs held regarding the effect of a delay beyond 6 hours in instituting therapeutic hypothermia, ie, that the treatment effect at 7 hours is similar to that at 6 hours and the longer it takes to begin treatment, the less effective the treatment is likely to be.

LIMITATIONS OF PRIOR INFORMATION

Prior information is a form of assumption. As with any assumption, incorrect prior information can result in invalid or misleading conclusions. For instance, if prior information used the assumption that hypothermia becomes less effective with increasing postnatal age and, in fact, waiting until 12 to 24 hours was associated with the greatest benefit, the resulting inferences would likely be incompatible with the data, less accurate, or biased. If the statistical model uses prior information derived from neonates 0 to 6 hours old in evaluating the treatment effect in neonates 6 to 24 hours of age, and is based on the assumption that the patients respond similarly, the results may be biased or less accurate if the 2 age groups actually respond differently to treatment.

These assumptions can be assessed. Just as the modeling assumptions made in logistic regression can be checked through goodness-of-fit tests,[5] there are tests that can be used to verify agreement between prior and current data. More importantly, some methods for incorporating prior information can explicitly adjust to conflict between the prior and the data, decreasing the reliance on prior information when the new data appear to be inconsistent with the proposed prior information.[6]

HOW WAS PRIOR INFORMATION USED?

Laptook et al[1] incorporated prior information by allowing for the outcome to vary across time windows of 6 to 12 hours and

12 to 24 hours and prespecifying 3 separate prior distributions on the overall treatment effect (see Description of Bayesian Analyses and Implementation Details section of the eAppendix in Supplement 2 in the Laptook et al article). The neutral prior assumes that the treatment effect diminishes completely after 6 hours, the enthusiastic prior assumes that effect does not diminish at all after 6 hours, and the skeptical prior assumes that the treatment is detrimental after 6 hours. Primary results are presented based on the neutral prior and, as such, the authors' approach is transparent and easily interpretable. The authors found a 76% probability of benefit with the neutral prior, a 90% probability of benefit with the enthusiastic prior, and a 73% probability of benefit with the skeptical prior.[1]

An alternative to this approach might include specifying a model that relates postnatal age at the start of therapeutic hypothermia to the magnitude of the treatment effect, assuming that the effect does not increase over time. This model would explicitly account for a possible decrease in treatment benefit with increasing age at initiation, while still allowing the effect at each age to inform the effects at other ages. Additionally, this model could be heavily informed or anchored in the 0 to 6–hour range using data from previous studies.[2] With this anchor, inferences would be improved across the range of 6 to 24 hours, with a particular increase in precision for the time intervals closer to 6 hours. This may have allowed more definitive conclusions to be drawn from the same set of data.

HOW SHOULD THE TRIAL RESULTS BE INTERPRETED IN LIGHT OF THE PRIOR INFORMATION?

Laptook et al[1] used a prespecified Bayesian analysis, using prior information, to allow quantitatively rigorous conclusions to be drawn regarding the probability that therapeutic hypothermia is effective 6 to 24 hours after birth in neonates with HIE. Conclusions of the analysis were given as probabilities that benefit exists. For example, the statement that there is "a 76% probability of any reduction in death or disability, and a 64% probability of at least 2% less death or disability" is easily understood by clinicians and can be used to inform clinical care. The use of several options for prior information allows clinicians with different perspectives to have the data interpreted over a range of prior beliefs.

Acknowledgment

The following disclosures were reported at the time this original article was first published in JAMA.

Conflict of Interest Disclosures: None reported.

References

1. Laptook AR, Shankaran S, Tyson JE, et al; Eunice Kennedy Shriver National Institute of Child Health and Human Development Neonatal Research Network. Effect of therapeutic hypothermia initiated after 6 hours of age on death or disability among newborns with hypoxic-ischemic encephalopathy: a randomized clinical trial. *JAMA*. 2017;318(16):1550-1560. doi:10.1001/jama.2017.14972

2. Jacobs SE, Morley CJ, Inder TE, et al; Infant Cooling Evaluation Collaboration. Whole-body hypothermia for term and near-term newborns with hypoxic-ischemic encephalopathy: a randomized controlled trial. *Arch Pediatr Adolesc Med*. 2011;165(8):692-700. Medline:21464374

3. Food and Drug Administration. Guidance for the use of Bayesian statistics in medical device clinical trials. https://www.fda.gov/MedicalDevices/ucm071072.htm. Published February 5, 2010. Accessed September 20, 2017.

4. Spiegelhalter DJ, Abrams KR, Myles JP. *Bayesian Approaches to Clinical Trials and Health-Care Evaluation*. Chichester, England: Wiley; 2004.

5. Meurer WJ, Tolles J. Logistic regression diagnostics: understanding how well a model predicts outcomes. *JAMA*. 2017;317(10):1068-1069. Medline:28291878

6. Viele K, Berry S, Neuenschwander B, et al. Use of historical control data for assessing treatment effects in clinical trials. *Pharm Stat*. 2014;13(1):41-54. Medline:23913901

Decision Curve Analysis

Mark Fitzgerald, PhD, Benjamin R. Saville, PhD, and Roger J. Lewis, MD, PhD

IN THIS CHAPTER

Use of the Method

Why Is DCA Used?

What Are the Limitations of the DCA Method?

Why Did the Authors Use DCA in This Particular Study?

How Should DCA Findings Be Interpreted in This Particular Study?

Caveats to Consider When Looking at Results Based on DCA

This JAMA Guide to Statistics and Methods describes how a decision curve analysis can be used to evaluate the benefits of a diagnostic test, such as 3 prostate biopsy strategies.

Decision curve analysis (DCA) is a method for evaluating the benefits of a diagnostic test across a range of patient preferences for accepting risk of undertreatment and overtreatment to facilitate decisions about test selection and use.[1] For example, Siddiqui and colleagues[2] used DCA to evaluate 3 prostate biopsy strategies: targeted magnetic resonance/ultrasound fusion biopsy, standard extended-sextant biopsy, or a combination, for establishing the diagnosis of intermediate- to high-risk prostate cancer. Their goal was to identify the best biopsy strategy to ensure prostatectomy is offered to patients with intermediate- and high-risk tumors and avoided for patients with low-risk tumors.

USE OF THE METHOD

Why Is DCA Used?

When patients have signs or symptoms suggestive of but not diagnostic of a disease, they and their physician must decide whether to (1) treat empirically, (2) not treat, or (3) perform further diagnostic testing before deciding between options 1 and 2. The decision to treat depends on how confident the clinician is that the disease is present, the effectiveness and complications of treatment if the disease is present, and the patient's willingness to accept the risks and burden of a treatment that might not be necessary. A diagnostic test may provide additional information on whether the disease is present.[3] Decision curve analysis is a method to assess the value of information provided by a diagnostic test by considering the likely range of a patient's risk and benefit preferences, without the need for actually measuring these preferences for a particular patient.[1]

A key concept in DCA is that of a *probability threshold*, namely, a level of diagnostic certainty above which the patient would choose to be treated. The probability threshold used in DCA captures the relative value the patient places on receiving treatment for the disease, if present, to the value of avoiding treatment if the disease is not present. If the treatment has high efficacy and minimal cost, inconvenience, and adverse effects (eg, oral antibiotics for community-acquired pneumonia), then the probability threshold will be low; conversely, if the treatment is minimally effective or associated with substantial morbidity (eg, radiation for a malignant brain tumor), then the probability threshold will be high.

The net benefit, or "benefit score," is determined by calculating the difference between the expected benefit and the expected harm associated with each proposed testing and treatment strategy. The expected benefit is represented by the number of patients who have the disease and who will receive treatment (true positives) using the proposed strategy.

The expected harm is represented by number of patients without the disease who would be treated in error (false positives) multiplied by a weighting factor based on the patient's threshold probability. The weighting factor captures the patient's values regarding the risks of undertreatment and overtreatment. Specifically, the false-positive rate is multiplied by the ratio of the threshold probability divided by 1 − the threshold probability. For example, if the treatment threshold is 10% (0.1) for a patient with possible pneumonia, then the weighting factor applied to the number of patients without pneumonia treated in error would be 0.1/0.9, or one-ninth, minimizing the effect of false-positive results because the burden of unnecessary treatment is low. Conversely, for a patient with a brain mass that is possibly malignant, the probability threshold might be 90% (0.9), leading to a weighting factor of 0.9/0.1, or 9, and greatly increasing the effect of the risk of false-positive results with any proposed testing and treatment strategy.

Graphically, the DCA is expressed as a curve, with benefit score on the vertical axis and probability thresholds on the horizontal axis. A curve is drawn for each approach that might be taken to establish a diagnosis. Another line is drawn to show what happens when no treatment is ever given (ie, no net benefit), and another curve is drawn as if all patients receive treatment irrespective of test results. For any given patient's probability threshold, the curve with the highest benefit score at that threshold is the best choice.[1]

If one curve is highest over the full range of probability thresholds, then the associated diagnostic approach would be the best decision for all patients, regardless of individual values, and a clinician can use this approach uniformly. If the curves cross, then the optimal approach will depend on the patient's risk tolerance, expressed through their probability threshold.

What Are the Limitations of the DCA Method?

For diseases that are not well studied, there may be insufficient knowledge regarding patient preferences to determine the relevant range of threshold probabilities. Even when the likely range of probability thresholds is known, if the decision curves cross within that range, then the clinician must delve deeper into individual patient preferences to choose a testing and treatment strategy.[3]

Caution should be used in interpreting DCAs based on published ranges of threshold probabilities, particularly when there are many treatment options available to a patient. A patient is likely to have a different threshold probability if treatment is, for example, radiation rather than prostatectomy. The threshold probability needs to apply to a well-defined path of treatment.

Decision curve analysis does not explicitly account for the costs (monetary costs, time lost, physical or psychological discomfort, etc) associated with the diagnostic test. Further, if the diagnostic test provides information about how to treat as well as whether to treat (eg, a biopsy that yields both a cancer diagnosis and tumor type, allowing the selection of a specific therapy), the decision curve does not incorporate the value of this additional information.

Another challenge in correct implementation of DCA is that the data required for establishing the curve are often difficult to obtain. There must be sufficient study data for the population of interest to whom the diagnostic test has been applied and the true state of the disease known for each patient at the time of the test. A fairly large patient study may be needed to establish estimates of traditional measures of accuracy (sensitivity, specificity).

Why Did the Authors Use DCA in This Particular Study?

There is controversy surrounding the benefits of screening and intervention relative to the costs of unnecessarily treating low-risk prostate cancers.[4,5] Justification for use of MR/ultrasound fusion–guided biopsy with ultrasound-guided biopsy to diagnose prostate cancer must be shown to benefit a broad range of patients.

How Should DCA Findings Be Interpreted in This Particular Study?

The DCA reported by Siddiqui et al[2] showed that for patients with threshold probabilities of 0% to 30%, representing a relative preference for empirical treatment, the net benefit is greatest if all patients are treated and that the diagnostic tests do not add sufficient information to improve care (Figure 6). In this range of threshold probabilities, patients appear to be more concerned about missing a diagnosis of cancer than about receiving unnecessary treatment. For midrange threshold probabilities of 30% to 75%, the targeted biopsy approach is superior to other strategies, including the 2 other diagnostic approaches evaluated. For higher thresholds (>75%) at which patients may be more concerned about unnecessary treatment than missed cancer, the option to not treat is preferred and neither diagnostic test has value.

FIGURE 6

Net Benefit as a Function of a Threshold Probability of Intermediate- to High-Risk Prostate Cancer

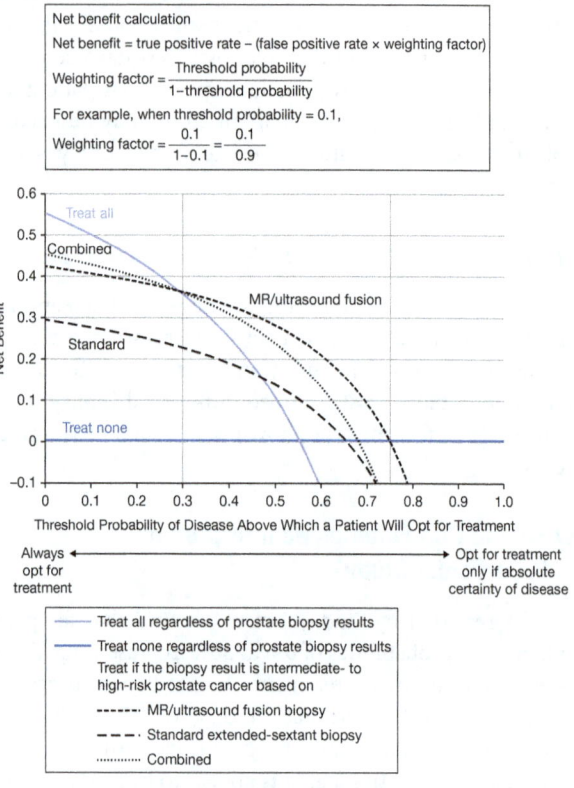

Threshold probability refers to the point at which a patient considers the benefit of treatment for intermediate- to high-risk prostate cancer equivalent to the harm of overtreatment for low-risk disease and thus reflects how the patient weights the benefits and harms associated with this decision. The highest curve at any given threshold probability is the optimal decision-making strategy to maximize net benefit. Net benefit was maximized with threshold probabilities of 0%-30% by the "treat all" approach; with threshold probabilities of 30%-75%, net benefit was maximized by the targeted magnetic resonance (MR)/ultrasound fusion approach; and with 75%-100%, net benefit was maximized by the "treat none" approach. (Adapted from Supplement, Siddiqui et al.[2])

CAVEATS TO CONSIDER WHEN LOOKING AT RESULTS BASED ON DCA

One shortcoming of this study was the use of a subset of 170 patients who underwent prostatectomy in constructing the DCA. These patients self-selected for prostatectomy after learning the results of their targeted and standard biopsies. This group primarily comprised men who had higher cancer risk, resulting in potential bias when estimating false positives, false negatives, and other diagnostic measures. The patients classified as low risk who still opted for prostatectomy are patients with low probability thresholds, who might also be different from the broader population of men with symptoms or findings suggesting prostate cancer.

Acknowledgment

The following disclosures were reported at the time this original article was first published in JAMA.
Conflict of Interest Disclosures: None reported.

References

1. Vickers AJ, Elkin EB. Decision curve analysis. *Med Decis Making*. 2006;26(6):565-574. Medline:17099194
2. Siddiqui MM, Rais-Bahrami S, Turkbey B, et al. Comparison of MR/ultrasound fusion–guided biopsy with ultrasound-guided biopsy for the diagnosis of prostate cancer. *JAMA*. 2015;313(4):390-397. doi:10.1001/jama.2014.17942.
3. Sox HC, Higgins MC, Owens DK. *Medical Decision Making*. 2nd ed. West Sussex, UK: John Wiley & Sons; 2013.
4. Froberg DG, Kane RL. Methodology for measuring health-state preferences. *J Clin Epidemiol*. 1989;42(4-7):345-354. Medline:2723695
5. Hoffman RM. Clinical practice: screening for prostate cancer. *N Engl J Med*. 2011;365(21):2013-2019. Medline:22029754

Methods for Evaluating Changes in Health Care Policy— The Difference-in-Differences Approach

Justin B. Dimick, MD, MPH, and
Andrew M. Ryan, PhD

IN THIS CHAPTER

Use of the Method

Why Was the Difference-in-Differences Method Used?

What Are the Limitations of the Difference-in-Differences Method?

Why Did the Authors Use the Difference-in-Differences Method?

How Should the Findings Be Interpreted?

Caveats to Consider When Assessing the Results of a Difference-in-Differences Analysis

This JAMA Guide to Statistics and Methods describes when to use a difference-in-differences analysis to evaluate changes in health care before and after changes in health care policy.

Observational studies are commonly used to evaluate the changes in outcomes associated with health care policy implementation. An important limitation in using observational studies in this context is the need to control for background changes in outcomes that occur with time (eg, secular trends affecting outcomes). The difference-in-differences approach is increasingly applied to address this problem.[1]

Two studies by Rajaram and colleagues[2] and Patel and colleagues[3] used the difference-in-differences approach to evaluate the changes that occurred following the 2011 Accreditation Council for Graduate Medical Education (ACGME) duty hour reforms. These 2 studies were conducted with different data sources and study populations but used similar methods.

USE OF THE METHOD

Why Was the Difference-in-Differences Method Used?

The association between policy changes and subsequent outcomes is often evaluated by pre-post assessments. Outcomes after implementation are compared with those before. This design is valid only if there are no underlying time-dependent trends in outcomes unrelated to the policy change. If clinical outcomes were already improving before the policy, then using a pre-post study would lead to the erroneous conclusion that the policy was associated with better outcomes.

The difference-in-differences study design addresses this problem by using a comparison group that is experiencing the same trends but is not exposed to the policy change.[4] Outcomes after and before the policy are compared between the study group and the comparison group without the exposure (group A) and the study group with the exposure (group B), which allows the investigator to subtract out the background changes in outcomes. Two differences in outcomes are important: the difference after vs before the policy change in the group exposed to the policy (B2−B1, Figure 7) and the difference after vs before the date of the policy change in the unexposed group (A2−A1). The change in outcomes that are related to implementation of the policy beyond background trends can then be estimated from the difference-in-differences analysis as follows: (B2−B1) − (A2−A1). If there is no relationship between policy implementation and subsequent outcomes, then the difference-in-differences estimate is equal to 0 (Figure 7, A). In contrast, if the policy is associated with beneficial changes, then the outcomes following implementation will improve to a greater extent in the exposed group. This will be shown by the difference-in-differences estimate (Figure 7, B).

These estimates are derived from regression models rather than simple subtraction. Using regression modeling allows the estimates to be adjusted for other factors (eg, patient or hospital characteristics) that may differ between the groups.[4] Regression models also offer a way to estimate the statistical significance of the association between policy change and outcomes, by including a variable that indicates if the observation is in the pre or post period and another variable that divides the groups into those exposed and unexposed to the policy.

Statistically, the association between policy implementation and outcomes is estimated by examining the interaction between the pre-post and exposed-unexposed variables. If the association exists, this interaction term will be significantly different from zero. Other design and statistical issues should be considered when performing difference-in-differences analysis and are considered in detail elsewhere.[1,5]

FIGURE 7

Conceptual Illustration of a Difference-in-Differences Analysis for 2 Scenarios

A No association between exposure and measured outcome

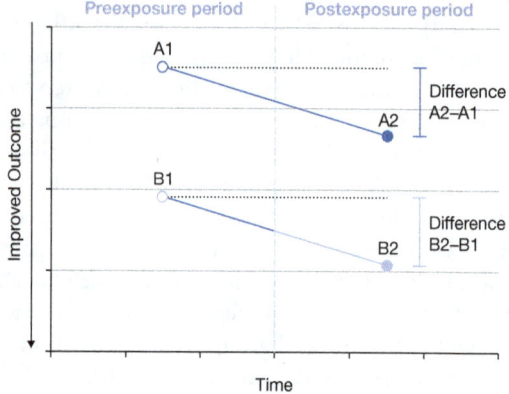

B Association of exposure and measured outcome

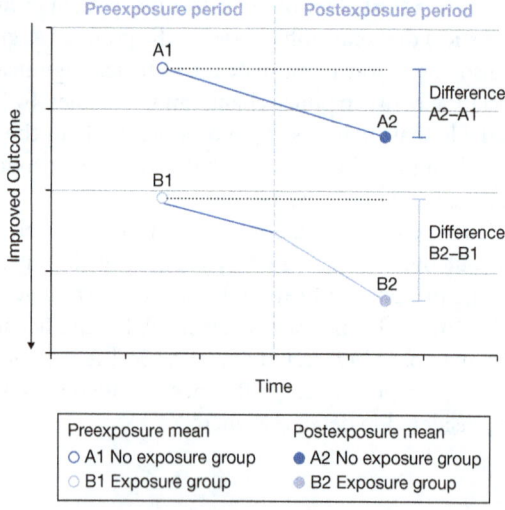

Preexposure mean	Postexposure mean
○ A1 No exposure group	● A2 No exposure group
○ B1 Exposure group	● B2 Exposure group

What Are the Limitations of the Difference-in-Differences Method?

The 2 main assumptions of difference-in-differences analysis are parallel trends and common shocks.[4] The *parallel trends assumption* states that the trends in outcomes between the treated and comparison groups are the same prior to the intervention (Figure 7). If true, it is reasonable to assume that these parallel trends would continue for both groups even if the program was not implemented. This is tested empirically by examining the trends in both groups before the policy was implemented. In a regression model, this is evaluated by assessing the significance of the interaction term between time and policy exposure in the preintervention period. If the trends are significantly different prior to the intervention, a difference-in-differences analysis would be biased and a different comparison group should be sought.

In economics, a *shock* is an unexpected or unpredictable event (unrelated to the policy) that affects a system. The *common shocks assumptions* state that any events occurring during or after the time the policy changed will equally affect the treatment and comparison groups. A key limitation to implementing difference-in-differences design is finding a control group for which these assumptions are met. Ideally, the only difference between the comparison group and the study group would be exposure to the policy. In practice, such a group may be difficult to find.

Why Did the Authors Use the Difference-in-Differences Method?

The studies by Rajaram et al[2] and Patel et al[3] both used the difference-in-differences method to control for background trends in patient outcomes. The study by Rajaram et al, conducted using a large clinical registry for surgical patients (American College of Surgeons National Surgical Quality Improvement Program), evaluated several clinical outcomes (mortality, serious morbidity, readmission, failure to rescue) and American Board of Surgery pass rates after vs before the 2011 ACGME duty hour reforms.[2] The authors chose to use nonteaching hospitals as a control group, which makes the assumption that teaching and nonteaching hospitals have similar trends for improved outcomes prior to the ACGME policy changes. Similarly, the study by Patel et al, conducted using Medicare claims data, evaluated mortality and readmissions after vs before the ACGME duty hour reforms, also using a comparison group of nonteaching hospitals.[3]

How Should the Findings Be Interpreted?

Both studies found no association of the 2011 ACGME duty hour reform with clinical outcomes. After accounting for the slight background trend for improved outcomes among these populations using the difference-in-differences method, there was no additional improvement (or worsening) in outcomes associated with the ACGME policy. Both studies had strong comparison groups and neither appeared to violate the key assumptions of this approach. The rigorous approach and the consistency of the finding across outcomes make a compelling case that there was no association between implementation of the policy and the measured outcomes.

CAVEATS TO CONSIDER WHEN ASSESSING THE RESULTS OF A DIFFERENCE-IN-DIFFERENCES ANALYSIS

Difference-in-differences analyses must also account for spillover effects. Spillovers occur when some aspect of the policy spills over and influences clinical care in the hospitals unexposed to the policy (eg, nonteaching hospitals improved quality in some way in reaction to the ACGME duty hour reforms).

Spillover can be evaluated by examining whether there is a measurable change in outcomes in the comparison group of hospitals at the time of the policy implementation. In the studies[2,3], the lack of a change in outcomes among nonteaching hospitals at the time of the duty hour reforms suggests there were no associated spillover effects.

Acknowledgment

The following disclosures were reported at the time this original article was first published in JAMA.

Conflict of Interest Disclosures: Dr Dimick reported that he receives grant funding from the National Institutes of Health, the Agency for Healthcare Research and Quality, and BlueCross BlueShield of Michigan Foundation; and is a cofounder of ArborMetrix Inc, a company that makes software for profiling hospital quality and efficiency. Dr Ryan reported that he receives grant funding from Agency for Healthcare Research and Quality.

References

1. Ryan AM, Burgess J, Dimick JB. Why we shouldn't be indifferent to specification in difference in-differences analysis [published online December 9, 2014]. *Health Serv Res*. doi:10.1111/1475-6773.12270.
2. Rajaram R, Chung JW, Jones AT, et al. Association of the 2011 ACGME resident duty hour reform with general surgery patient outcomes and with resident examination performance. *JAMA*. 2014;312:2374-2384. doi:10.1001/jama.2014.15277.
3. Patel MS, Volpp KG, Small DS, et al. Association of the 2011 ACGME resident duty hour reforms with mortality and readmissions among hospitalized Medicare patients. *JAMA*. 2014;312:2364-2373. doi:10.1001/jama.2014.15273.
4. Angrist JD, Pischke JS. *Mostly Harmless Econometrics: An Empiricist's Companion*. Princeton, NJ: Princeton University Press; 2008.
5. Bertrand M, Duflo E, Mullainathan S. How much should we trust differences-in-differences estimates? *Q J Econ*. 2004;119:249-275.

/ # Case-Control Studies: Using "Real-world" Evidence to Assess Association

Telba Z. Irony, PhD

IN THIS CHAPTER

Explanation of the Method

What Are Case-Control and Nested Case-Control Studies?

Why Are Case-Control Studies Used?

Limitations of Case-Control Studies

How Was the Method Applied in This Case?

How Does the Case-Control Design Affect the Interpretation of the Study?

This JAMA Guide to Statistics and Methods explains the construction and utility of case-control studies to find associations between risk factors, including treatments, and patient outcomes.

Associations between patient characteristics or treatments received and clinical outcomes are often first described using observational data, such as data arising through usual clinical care without the experimental assignment of treatments that occurs in a randomized clinical trial (RCT). These data based on usual clinical care are referred to by some as "real-world" data. A key strategy for efficiently finding such associations is to use a case-control study.[1] In a recent issue of *JAMA Internal Medicine*, Wang et al[2] assessed the association between cardiovascular disease (CVD) and use of inhaled long-acting β_2-agonists (LABAs) or long-acting antimuscarinic antagonists (LAMAs) in chronic obstructive pulmonary disease (COPD), utilizing a nested case-control study.

EXPLANATION OF THE METHOD

What Are Case-Control and Nested Case-Control Studies?

A case-control study compares individuals who had the outcome of interest (cases) vs individuals who did not have that outcome (controls) with respect to exposure to a potential risk factor. The goal is to determine if there is an association between the risk factor and the outcome. The risk factor may be a behavior such as tobacco use, a patient characteristic, or a treatment. The idea is to define a population or cohort, identify the cases and controls in the population, and retrospectively determine which patients in each group were exposed to the risk factor; the case-control study works backward from outcome to exposure (Figure 8). A higher proportion of individuals with exposure to the risk factor among cases than among controls suggests that

FIGURE 8

Hypothetical Example of a Case-Control Study

Example of Case-Control Study Analysis

1. **Study population** selected for patients with chronic obstructive pulmonary disease (COPD) Patients with COPD

2. **Cases** selected for disease outcome of interest (recent cardiac event) Recent cardiac event

3. **Controls** selected for similar distribution of hypertension and/or diabetes as the cases H Hypertension / D Diabetes

4. **Exposure** to risk factor of treatment compared between cases and controls New use of COPD inhaler

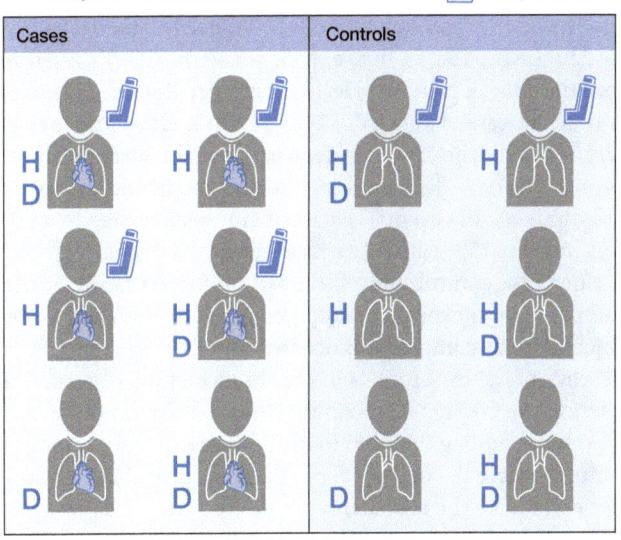

Exposure to a risk factor (in this case, new COPD inhaler use) changes the chance of subsequently developing the outcome of interest. However, in conducting a case-control study, the outcome (in this case, a cardiovascular event) is used initially to define cases and controls, and then the distribution of the exposure is assessed.

the risk factor is associated with the outcome. The term *control* refers to an individual who did not have the outcome; in contrast, the same term in a clinical trial refers to a study participant who receives the standard (or placebo) treatment.

In a nested case-control study, the cases are identified in a large cohort and, for each case, a specified number of controls matching the case are selected from the cohort. The selected controls should match the cases with respect to characteristics, other than the risk factor, that are likely related to the outcome of interest. Because it is easier to find controls than cases when the outcome is rare, increasing the number of controls beyond the number of cases (eg, 2:1 or 3:1 matching) may be used to improve study precision.

The nested case-control study by Wang et al[2] used data from 284 220 LABA-LAMA–naive patients with COPD retrieved from the Taiwan National Health Insurance Research Database with health care claims from 2007 to 2011. Cases (n = 37 719) were patients who had inpatient or emergency care visits for coronary artery disease, heart failure, ischemic stroke, or arrhythmia (CVD events). Each patient was matched to 4 controls (n = 146 139) without visits for these disorders.

In a case-control study, the most common measure of association between exposure and outcome is the odds ratio (OR), which aims to compare the occurrence of the outcome in the presence of the exposure vs in the absence of the exposure.[3] In practice, the OR in a case-control study is the ratio of the odds of exposure among the cases to the odds of exposure among the controls, where the odds of exposure is the probability of exposure divided by the probability of no exposure. The prevalence of the exposure is compared between cases and controls and not the other way around. However, because the OR treats outcome and exposure symmetrically, it provides the desired measure of association. If the OR is greater than 1, the exposure is associated with the outcome, ie, having the exposure increases the odds of having an outcome (and vice versa). The OR is a measure of effect size; the larger the OR, the stronger the association.

In the study by Wang et al,[2] new use of LABA occurred in 520 cases (1.4%) and 1186 controls (0.8%), resulting in an adjusted odds ratio of 1.50 (95% CI, 1.35-1.67). New use of LAMA occurred in 190 cases (0.5%) and 463 controls (0.3%), resulting in an adjusted odds ratio of 1.52 (95% CI, 1.28-1.80). An OR of 1.5 represents a modest association[4] between outcome (CVD) and exposure (LABA and LAMA). Thus, the authors found that new use of LABAs or LAMAs was associated with a modest increase in cardiovascular risk in patients with COPD, within 30 days of therapy initiation.

Why Are Case-Control Studies Used?

Case-control studies are time-efficient and less costly than RCTs, particularly when the outcome of interest is rare or takes a long time to occur, because the cases are identified at study onset and the outcomes have already occurred with no need for a long-term follow-up. The case-control design is useful in exploratory studies to assess a possible association between an exposure and an outcome. Nested case-control studies are less expensive than full cohort studies because the exposure is only assessed for the cases and for the selected controls, not for the full cohort.

LIMITATIONS OF CASE-CONTROL STUDIES

Case-control studies are retrospective and data quality must be carefully evaluated to avoid bias. For instance, because individuals included in the study and evaluators need to consider exposures and outcomes that happened in the past, these studies may be subject to recall bias and observer bias. Because the controls are selected retrospectively, such studies are also subject to selection bias, which may make the case and control groups not comparable. For a valid comparison, appropriate controls must be used, ie, selected controls must be representative of the population that produced the cases. The ideal control group would be generated by a random sample from the general population that generated the cases. If controls are not representative of the population, selection bias may occur.

Case-control studies provide less compelling evidence than RCTs. Due to randomization, treatment and control groups in RCTs tend to be similar with respect to baseline variables, including unmeasured ones.[5] Because the only difference between treatment and control groups is the treatment, RCTs can demonstrate causation between treatment and outcome. In case-control studies, case and control groups are similar with respect to the matching variables, but are not necessarily similar with respect to unmeasured variables. Such studies are susceptible to confounding, which occurs when the exposure and the outcome are both associated with a third unmeasured variable.[6] Unlike RCTs, case-control studies demonstrate association between exposure and outcome but do not demonstrate causation.

The objective of case-control studies is to compare the occurrence of an outcome with and without an exposure. The relative risk (RR), which is the ratio between the probability of the outcome when exposed and the probability of the outcome when not exposed, provides a straightforward comparison measure but, because the case-control study design does not allow for the estimation of the occurrence of the outcome in the population (ie, incidence or prevalence), the RR cannot be determined from a case-control study. A case-control study can only estimate the OR, which is the ratio of odds and not the ratio of probabilities. The OR approximates the RR for rare outcomes, but differs substantially when the outcome of interest is common. In addition, case-control studies are limited to the examination of one outcome, and it is difficult to examine the temporal sequence between exposure and outcome.

Despite these limitations, case-control studies and other "real-world" evidence can provide valuable empirical evidence to complement RCTs. Additionally, case-control studies may be able to address questions for which an RCT is either not feasible or not ethical.[7]

HOW WAS THE METHOD APPLIED IN THIS CASE?

In the case-control study by Wang et al,[2] the exposure to LABA and LAMA use for both cases and controls in the year preceding the occurrence of the CVD event was measured and stratified by duration since initiation of LABA or LAMA into 4 groups: current (≤30 days), recent (31-90 days), past (91-180 days), and remote (>180 days). Additional stratification on concomitant COPD medications and other factors was also conducted. The data source used in the study (Taiwan National Health Insurance Research Database) mitigates data quality concerns because it is national, universal, compulsory, and subject to periodic audits. Overall, the authors found that new use of LABAs or LAMAs was associated with a modest increase in cardiovascular risk in patients with COPD, within 30 days of therapy initiation, and this finding was strengthened by the steps taken to ensure data quality and comparability of cases and controls.

HOW DOES THE CASE-CONTROL DESIGN AFFECT THE INTERPRETATION OF THE STUDY?

Causality cannot be established in a case-control study because there is no way to control for unmeasured confounders. In the study by Wang et al,[2] the use of the disease risk score for predicting CVD events was helpful to control for measured confounders but could not adjust for unmeasured confounders. The authors mitigated further possible confounding effects by conducting extensive sensitivity analyses.

Acknowledgment

The following disclosures were reported at the time this original article was first published in *JAMA*.

Conflict of Interest Disclosures: None reported.

Disclaimer: This article reflects the views of the author and should not be construed to represent FDA's views or policies.

References

1. Breslow NE. Statistics in epidemiology: the case-control study. *J Am Stat Assoc*. 1996;91(433):14-28. Medline:12155399 doi:10.1080/01621459.1996.10476660
2. Wang MT, Liou JT, Lin CW, et al. Association of cardiovascular risk with inhaled long-acting bronchodilators in patients with chronic obstructive pulmonary disease: a nested case-control study. *JAMA Intern Med*. 2018;178(2):229-238. Medline:29297057 doi:10.1001/jamainternmed.2017.7720
3. Norton EC, Dowd BE, Maciejewski ML. Odds ratios: current best practice and use. *JAMA*. 2018;320(1):84-85. Medline:29971384 doi:10.1001/jama.2018.6971
4. Chen H, Cohen P, Chen S. How big is a big odds ratio? interpreting the magnitudes of odds ratios in epidemiological studies. *Commun Stat Simul Comput*. 2010;39(4):860-864.
5. Broglio K. Randomization in clinical trials: permuted blocks and stratification. *JAMA*. 2018;319(21):2223-2224. Medline:29872845 doi:10.1001/jama.2018.6360
6. Kyriacou DN, Lewis RJ. Confounding by indication in clinical research. *JAMA*. 2016;316(17):1818-1819. Medline:27802529 doi:10.1001/jama.2016.16435
7. Corrigan-Curay J, Sacks L, Woodcock J. Real-world evidence and real-world data for evaluating drug safety and effectiveness [published online August 13, 2018]. *JAMA*. 2018. Medline:30105359 doi:10.1001/jama.2018.10136

Meta-analyses Can Be Credible and Useful: A New Standard

John P. A. Ioannidis, MD, DSc

IN THIS CHAPTER

Overview

The Existing Evidence

Improvements

Conclusions

This JAMA Guide to Statistics and Methods contends that meta-analyses can become the new prototype for original research.

OVERVIEW

Carefully done meta-analyses constitute a major advance compared with expert opinion and nonsystematic attempts at summarizing, synthesizing, and integrating information. Meta-analyses serve many fields in summarizing an increasing stream of data and, for clinical purposes, streamlining information for decision making. However, there are flaws and caveats that threaten the validity and utility of meta-analyses.[1]

Most of these efforts are retrospective exercises that try to piece together fragments of information from multiple completed studies. They depend on information that is already published (or at least retrievable) with all the accompanying errors and biases and rarely correct these problems. For example, 8 meta-analyses of imaging in unipolar depression have reached inconsistent conclusions because they have used different studies with diverse protocols and methods that are difficult to standardize post hoc and different errors that other meta-analyses may or may not correct for. A meta-analysis should systematically probe, detect, dissect, and highlight major errors and biases (instead of sanctifying flawed studies by their inclusion). Careful bias scrutiny alone can be a major service to a field. However, it is always tempting to take a shortcut to talk about summary effects and forget about the deficiencies of the evidence.

THE EXISTING EVIDENCE

Bias is inflated when meta-analyses are done by authors and/or sponsors with financial or other conflicts of interest. Authorship by company employees and/or sponsorship by companies was the strongest risk factor for reporting no caveats for antidepressants among a body of 185 meta-analyses on antidepressants for depression published between 2007 and 2014.[2] Allegiance bias may be an equivalent problem for evidence on psychotherapies.[3] Conflicted meta-analyses compound the distortion that exists in the publication process of primary studies, including a publication bias against negative results, the selective reporting of negative trials as positive,[4] and other spins (eg, changing the analysis plan or the focus of interpretation) that lead to more favorable results and interpretations.

Of approximately 20 000 meta-analyses performed annually,[1] well over 1000 have relevance for mental health. In an empirical survey using stringent criteria for labeling meta-analyses,[5] 7% pertained to mental and behavior disorders. Most of these meta-analyses look only at published data and circumscribed, small fractions of the evidence that might be relevant for the question of interest. For example, in therapeutics research, of 822 network meta-analyses of clinical trials published until May 2015, only 39 pertained to mental health. Moreover, to my knowledge, there are few meta-analyses in mental health that have been able to use individual-level data. In a database of 829 meta-analyses with individual-level data published until 2012,[6] only 52 (6.3%) pertained to mental and behavioral disorders. Most of them either pertained to nontherapeutic questions (eg, prognostic, biomarker, imaging, and association studies) that mostly had no clinical relevance or lacked systematic searches. I found only 7 meta-analyses that addressed therapeutic questions and had performed a systematic search to retrieve trials, and 4 of these dealt with only a single drug. What is more common is pooling projects done by the industry in which a few trials on a specific sponsored drug have their individual-level data combined. Typically, these pooling exercises work as marketing efforts reassuring, by default, that the drug is effective and safe. Typically, they do not perform a systematic review for the assessed drug, nor do they consider drugs from other competitors. While meta-analyses with individual-level data have become more common in other popular applications of the method beyond therapeutics—in particular for imaging studies—most imaging meta-analyses still depend on published group-level data and examine narrow questions.

Therefore, almost all meta-analyses with systematic searches depend on published group-level data and/or examine small fragments of the evidence space. However, when there are dozens of therapeutic options, as is the case with antidepressants or antipsychotics, a meta-analysis focusing on 1 agent has limited use because it says nothing about the relative benefits and harms of this agent compared with other competitors. Similarly, when data are combined from only a few imaging studies, the emerging picture will be uncertain and possibly misleading depending on what factors have shaped data availability.

The few network meta-analyses published to date in the field offer a wider view of the evidence by considering multiple treatments and understanding better their relative benefits and harms. However, those efforts are still in an exploratory phase and may disagree on the final conclusions. For example, network meta-analyses on antidepressants for depression have yielded radically different conclusions on the relative ranking of various antidepressants. Differences may be caused by variability in the eligibility criteria, efforts (or lack of efforts) to overcome publication and other selective reporting bias, the choice of outcomes, and analytical methods, among other factors.

IMPROVEMENTS

Improvements in meta-analyses may stem from improvements in the primary studies that they synthesize and improvement in the design, conduct, and reporting of meta-analyses themselves.

First, there is encouraging news that after many years of inertia, protocols and individual-level data from randomized clinical trials may start becoming more routinely available for use in reanalyses, meta-analyses, or other purposes.

Similarly, several efforts try to promote the availability of raw data from other studies, such as brain imaging (eg, NeuroVault [neurovault.org] and OpenfMRI [openfmri.org]). The use of individual-level data may become more convenient, and thus meta-analyses of individual-level data may offer advantages and bypass the shortcomings of partial, biased coverage of the evidence by the available raw data.[7]

Second, there are ongoing efforts to increase the proportion of registered clinical trials and the completeness of information provided on registration.

Third, constructive criticism on the poor standards of many mental health trials—eg, the use of short follow-up, nonrelevant, extremely diverse, and nonstandardized outcomes, and use of inappropriate statistical methods such as the last observation carried forward—may start improving the primary material that meta-analyses assess and combine. This also applies to improved methods and standardized protocols for other types of studies, such as imaging.

Fourth, the wider adoption of reporting standards for meta-analyses, including the Preferred Reporting Items for Systematic Reviews and Meta-analyses (PRISMA) and its extensions for harms and networks, may couple with the adoption of standards for meta-analysis protocols, such as the Preferred Reporting Items for Systematic Reviews and Meta-analyses Protocols (PRISMA-P).

Fifth, the preregistration of systematic reviews and meta-analyses in registries such as PROSPERO may also enhance transparency. It should also become easier to update meta-analyses with new data and to consider systematic reviews as "living documents"[8] able to incorporate new evidence in real time. Otherwise, numerous meta-analyses on the same question are an avoidable redundancy.

Sixth, network meta-analyses should also become more inclusive and should be considered routinely, whenever appropriate, in therapeutic topics in which multiple intervention choices are available. Finally, systematic reviews and meta-analyses also need to strengthen their editorial independence and protection from conflicts of interest.

CONCLUSIONS

Primary studies and meta-analyses should eventually become more confluent and, whenever possible, they should coincide. For many topics of prognostic, biomarker, and association research, the consortia of multiple teams can work with pre-agreed protocols and statistical, clinical, and laboratory methods to generate data prospectively and integrate them in a single meta-analysis. To my knowledge, the consortium paradigm has always been very successful in omics fields and is immediately relevant to imaging and biomarker studies. For therapeutics research, meta-analyses may also be designed upfront with the intention to summarize a research agenda of multiple primary trials. The research agenda is constructed with the anticipation that all of the studies will provide full detailed data to an ongoing updated meta-analysis.[9] The meta-analysis update can also inform the need for future studies, as well as the sample size and comparisons that they should address.[10] Sufficient safeguards should be in place to guarantee the independence of these large living individual-level network data syntheses from conflicts of interest. Meta-analysis can become the new prototype of robust, primary, original research.

Acknowledgment

The following disclosures were reported at the time this original article was first published.
    Conflict of Interest Disclosures: None reported.

References

1. Ioannidis JPA. The mass production of redundant, misleading, and conflicted systematic reviews and meta-analyses. *Milbank Q.* 2016;94(3):485-514. Medline:27620683

2. Ebrahim S, Bance S, Athale A, Malachowski C, Ioannidis JP. Meta-analyses with industry involvement are massively published and report no caveats for antidepressants. *J Clin Epidemiol*. 2016;70:155-163. Medline:26399904

3. Cuijpers P, Cristea IA. How to prove that your therapy is effective, even when it is not: a guideline. *Epidemiol Psychiatr Sci*. 2016;25(5):428-435. Medline:26411384

4. Turner EH, Matthews AM, Linardatos E, Tell RA, Rosenthal R. Selective publication of antidepressant trials and its influence on apparent efficacy. *N Engl J Med*. 2008;358(3):252-260. Medline:18199864

5. Page MJ, Shamseer L, Altman DG, et al. Epidemiology and reporting characteristics of systematic reviews of biomedical research: a cross-sectional study. *PLoS Med*. 2016;13(5):e1002028. Medline:27218655

6. Huang Y, Mao C, Yuan J, et al. Distribution and epidemiological characteristics of published individual patient data meta-analyses. *PLoS One*. 2014;9(6):e100151. Medline:24945406

7. Ahmed I, Sutton AJ, Riley RD. Assessment of publication bias, selection bias, and unavailable data in meta-analyses using individual participant data: a database survey. *BMJ*. 2012;344:d7762. Medline:22214758

8. Page MJ, Moher D. Mass production of systematic reviews and meta-analyses: an exercise in mega-silliness? *Milbank Q*. 2016;94(3):515-519. Medline:27620684

9. Ioannidis JPA, Karassa FB. The need to consider the wider agenda in systematic reviews and meta-analyses: breadth, timing, and depth of the evidence. *BMJ*. 2010;341:c4875. Medline:20837576

10. Nikolakopoulou A, Mavridis D, Salanti G. Planning future studies based on the precision of network meta-analysis results. *Stat Med*. 2016;35(7):978-1000. Medline:26250759

Mendelian Randomization

Connor A. Emdin, DPhil, Amit V. Khera, MD, and Sekar Kathiresan, MD

IN THIS CHAPTER

Use of the Method
Why Is Mendelian Randomization Used?
What Are the Limitations of Mendelian Randomization?
How Did the Authors Use Mendelian Randomization?

Caveats to Consider When Evaluating Mendelian Randomization Studies

This JAMA Guide to Statistics and Methods reviews the concepts underlying mendelian randomization and provides examples of its application to clinical trial design.

Mendelian randomization uses genetic variants to determine whether an observational association between a risk factor and an outcome is consistent with a causal effect.[1] Mendelian randomization relies on the natural, random assortment of genetic variants during meiosis yielding a random distribution of genetic variants in a population.[1] Individuals are naturally assigned at birth to inherit a genetic variant that affects a risk factor (eg, a gene variant that raises low-density lipoprotein [LDL] cholesterol levels) or not inherit such a variant. Individuals who carry the variant and those who do not are then followed up for the development of an outcome of interest. Because these genetic variants are typically unassociated with confounders, differences in the outcome between those who carry the variant and those who do not can be attributed to the difference in the risk factor. For example, a genetic variant associated with higher LDL cholesterol levels that also is associated with a higher risk of coronary heart disease would provide supportive evidence for a causal effect of LDL cholesterol on coronary heart disease.

One way to explain the principles of mendelian randomization is through an example: the study of the relationship of high-density lipoprotein (HDL) cholesterol and triglycerides with coronary heart disease. Increased HDL cholesterol levels are associated with a lower risk of coronary heart disease, an association that remains significant even after multivariable adjustment.[2] By contrast, an association between increased triglyceride levels and coronary risk is no longer significant following multivariable analyses. These observations have been interpreted as HDL cholesterol being a causal driver of coronary heart disease, whereas triglyceride level is a correlated bystander.[2] To better understand these relationships, researchers have used mendelian randomization to test whether the observational associations between HDL cholesterol or triglyceride levels and coronary heart disease risk are consistent with causal relationships.[3-5]

USE OF THE METHOD

Why Is Mendelian Randomization Used?

Basic principles of mendelian randomization can be understood through comparison with a randomized clinical trial. To answer the question of whether raising HDL cholesterol levels with a treatment will reduce the risk of coronary heart disease, individuals might be randomized to receive a treatment that raises HDL cholesterol levels and a placebo that does not have this effect. If there is a causal effect of HDL cholesterol on coronary heart disease, a drug that raises HDL cholesterol levels should eventually reduce the risk of coronary heart disease. However, randomized trials are costly, take a great deal of time, and may be impractical to carry out, or there may not be an intervention to test a certain hypothesis, limiting the number of clinical questions that can be answered by randomized trials.

What Are the Limitations of Mendelian Randomization?

Mendelian randomization rests on 3 assumptions: (1) the genetic variant is associated with the risk factor; (2) the genetic variant is not associated with confounders; and (3) the genetic variant influences the outcome only through the risk factor. The second and third assumptions are collectively known as independence from pleiotropy. *Pleiotropy* refers to a genetic variant influencing the outcome through pathways independent of the risk factor. The first assumption can be evaluated directly by examining the strength of association of the genetic variant with the risk factor. The second and third assumptions, however, cannot be empirically proven and require both judgment by the investigators and the performance of various sensitivity analyses.

If genetic variants are pleiotropic, mendelian randomization studies may be biased. For example, if genetic variants that increase HDL cholesterol levels also affect the risk of coronary heart disease through an independent pathway (eg, by decreasing inflammation), a causal effect of HDL cholesterol on coronary heart disease may be claimed when the true causal effect is due to the alternate pathway.

Another limitation is statistical power. Determinants of statistical power in a mendelian randomization study include the frequency of the genetic variant(s) used, the effect size of the variant on the risk factor, and study sample size. Because any given genetic variant typically explains only a small proportion of the variance in the risk factor, multiple variants are often combined into a polygenic risk score to increase statistical power.

How Did the Authors Use Mendelian Randomization?

In a study reported in *JAMA*, Frikke-Schmidt et al[4] applied mendelian randomization to HDL cholesterol and coronary heart disease using gene variants in the *ABCA1* gene. When compared with noncarriers, carriers of loss-of-function variants in the *ABCA1* gene displayed a 17-mg/dL lower HDL cholesterol level but did not have an increased risk of coronary heart disease (odds ratio, 0.93; 95% CI, 0.53-1.62). The observed 17-mg/dL decrease in HDL cholesterol level is expected to increase coronary heart disease by 70% and this study had more than 80% power to detect such a difference; thus, the lack of a genetic association of *ABCA1* gene variants and coronary heart disease was unlikely to be due to low statistical power. These data were among the first to cast doubt on the potential causal role of HDL cholesterol for coronary heart disease. In other mendelian randomization studies, genetic variants that raised HDL cholesterol levels were not associated with reduced risk of coronary heart disease, a result consistent with HDL cholesterol as a noncausal factor.[5]

Low HDL cholesterol levels track with high plasma triglyceride levels, and triglyceride levels reflect the concentration of triglyceride-rich lipoproteins in blood. Using multivariable mendelian randomization, Do et al[3] examined the relationship among correlated risk factors such as HDL cholesterol and triglyceride levels. In an analysis of 185 polymorphisms that altered plasma lipids, a 1-SD increase in HDL cholesterol level (approximately 14 mg/dL) due to genetic variants was not associated with risk of coronary heart disease (odds ratio, 0.96; 95% CI, 0.89-1.03; Figure 9). In contrast, a 1-SD increase in triglyceride level (approximately 89 mg/dL) was associated

FIGURE 9

Comparison of Observational Estimates and Mendelian Randomization Estimates of the Association of Low-Density Lipoprotein (LDL) Cholesterol, High-Density Lipoprotein (HDL) Cholesterol, and Triglycerides With Coronary Heart Disease

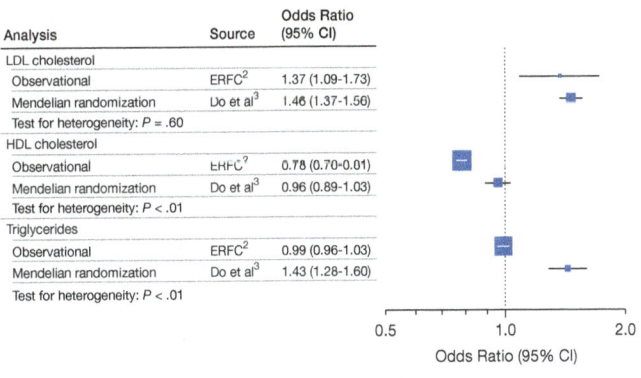

Analysis	Source	Odds Ratio (95% CI)
LDL cholesterol		
Observational	ERFC[2]	1.37 (1.09-1.73)
Mendelian randomization	Do et al[3]	1.46 (1.37-1.56)
Test for heterogeneity: $P = .60$		
HDL cholesterol		
Observational	ERFC[2]	0.78 (0.70-0.81)
Mendelian randomization	Do et al[3]	0.96 (0.89-1.03)
Test for heterogeneity: $P < .01$		
Triglycerides		
Observational	ERFC[2]	0.99 (0.96-1.03)
Mendelian randomization	Do et al[3]	1.43 (1.28-1.60)
Test for heterogeneity: $P < .01$		

Observational estimates are derived from the Emerging Risk Factors Collaboration (ERFC).[2] Mendelian randomization estimates are derived from Do et al[3] based on an analysis of 185 genetic variants that alter plasma lipids and mutually adjusted for other lipid fractions (eg HDL cholesterol and triglycerides for LDL cholesterol). A formal test of heterogeneity (Cochran Q test) shows that the observational and mendelian randomization estimates are consistent for LDL cholesterol but not so for HDL cholesterol or triglycerides.

with an elevated risk of coronary heart disease (odds ratio, 1.43; 95% CI, 1.28-1.60). LDL cholesterol and triglyceride-rich lipoprotein levels, but not HDL cholesterol level, may be the causal drivers of coronary heart disease risk as demonstrated by these mendelian randomization studies.

CAVEATS TO CONSIDER WHEN EVALUATING MENDELIAN RANDOMIZATION STUDIES

The primary concern when evaluating mendelian randomization studies is whether genetic variants used in the study are likely to be pleiotropic. Variants in a single gene that affects an individual risk factor are most likely to affect the outcome only through the risk factor and do not have pleiotropic effects. For example, variants in *CRP*, the gene encoding C-reactive protein, have been used in a mendelian randomization study to exclude a direct causal effect of C-reactive protein on coronary heart disease.[6] However, variants in single genes that encode a risk factor of interest are often not available. In these cases, pleiotropy can be examined by testing whether the gene variants used are associated with known confounders such as diet, smoking, and lifestyle factors.[7] More advanced statistical techniques, including median regression[8] and use of population-specific instruments,[7] have recently been proposed to protect against pleiotropic variants biasing results.

A second concern relates to whether the mendelian randomization study has adequate statistical power to detect an association. Consequently, an estimate from a mendelian randomization study that is nonsignificant should be accompanied by a power analysis based on the strength of the genetic instrument and the size of the study. Furthermore, mendelian randomization estimates should be compared with results from traditional observational analyses using a formal test for heterogeneity.

Acknowledgment

The following disclosures were reported at the time this original article was first published in *JAMA*.
Conflict of Interest Disclosures: None reported.

References

1. Smith GD, Ebrahim S. 'Mendelian randomization': can genetic epidemiology contribute to understanding environmental determinants of disease? *Int J Epidemiol*. 2003;32(1):1-22. Medline:12689998
2. Di Angelantonio E, Sarwar N, Perry P, et al. Emerging Risk Factors Collaboration. Major lipids, apolipoproteins, and risk of vascular disease. *JAMA*. 2009;302(18):1993-2000. Medline:19903920
3. Do R, Willer CJ, Schmidt EM, et al. Common variants associated with plasma triglycerides and risk for coronary artery disease. *Nat Genet*. 2013;45(11):1345-1352. Medline:24097064
4. Frikke-Schmidt R, Nordestgaard BG, Stene MCA, et al. Association of loss-of-function mutations in the ABCA1 gene with high-density lipoprotein cholesterol levels and risk of ischemic heart disease. *JAMA*. 2008;299(21):2524-2532. Medline:18523221
5. Voight BF, Peloso GM, Orho-Melander M, et al. Plasma HDL cholesterol and risk of myocardial infarction: a mendelian randomisation study. *Lancet*. 2012;380(9841):572-580. Medline:22607825
6. Zacho J, Tybjaerg-Hansen A, Jensen JS, Grande P, Sillesen H, Nordestgaard BG. Genetically elevated C-reactive protein and ischemic vascular disease. *N Engl J Med*. 2008;359(18):1897-1908. Medline:18971492
7. Emdin CA, Khera AV, Natarajan P, et al. Genetic association of waist-to-hip ratio with cardiometabolic traits, type 2 diabetes, and coronary heart disease. *JAMA*. 2017;317(6):626-634. Medline:28196256
8. Bowden J, Davey Smith G, Haycock PC, Burgess S. Consistent estimation in mendelian randomization with some invalid instruments using a weighted median estimator. *Genet Epidemiol*. 2016;40(4):304-314. Medline:27061298

JAMAevidence
Using Evidence to Improve Care

Using the E-Value to Assess the Potential Effect of Unmeasured Confounding in Observational Studies

Sebastien Haneuse, PhD,
Tyler J. VanderWeele, PhD, and
David Arterburn, MD

IN THIS CHAPTER

Why Is the E-Value Used?

What Are the Limitations of the E-Value?

Why Did the Authors Use the E-Value in This Particular Study?

How Should the E-Value Findings Be Interpreted in This Particular Study?

Caveats to Consider When Looking at Results Based on the E-Value

This JAMA Guide to Statistics and Methods discusses E-value analysis, an alternative approach to sensitivity analyses for unmeasured confounding in observational studies that specifies the degree of unmeasured confounding that would need to be operative to negate observed results in a study.

Randomized trials serve as the standard for comparative studies of treatment effects. In many settings, it may not be feasible or ethical to conduct a randomized study,[1] and researchers may pursue observational studies to better understand clinical outcomes. A central limitation of observational studies is the potential for confounding bias that arises because treatment assignment is not random. Thus, the observed associations may be attributable to differences other than the treatment being investigated and causality cannot be assumed.

In the October 16, 2018, issue of *JAMA*, results from a large, multisite observational study of the association between bariatric surgery and long-term macrovascular disease outcomes among patients with severe obesity and type 2 diabetes were reported by Fisher et al.[2] Using data from 5301 patients aged 19 to 79 years who underwent bariatric surgery at 1 of 4 integrated health systems in the United States between 2005 and 2011 and 14 934 matched nonsurgical patients, they found that bariatric surgery was associated with a 40% lower incidence of macrovascular disease at 5 years (2.1% in the surgical group and 4.3% in the nonsurgical group; hazard ratio [HR], 0.60 [95% CI, 0.42-0.86]).

Two strategies were used to mitigate confounding bias. In the first, a matched cohort design was used where nonsurgical patients were matched to surgical patients on the basis of a priori–identified potential confounders (study site, age, sex, body mass index, hemoglobin A_{1c} level, insulin use, observed diabetes duration, and prior health care use). In the second strategy used to adjust for confounding bias, the primary results were based on the fit of a multivariable Cox model that adjusted for all of the factors used in the matching as well as a broader range of potential confounders (Table 1 in the article[2]). Thus, any imbalances in the observed potential confounders that remained after the matching process were controlled for by the statistical analysis. Despite these efforts, however, given the observational design, the potential for unmeasured confounding remained.

WHY IS THE E-VALUE USED?

While matching and regression-based analysis provide some control of confounding, it can only be with respect to factors that are measured. The potential for confounding from factors that were not measured in the study still exists. To assess how much of a problem unmeasured confounding factors may pose, researchers may conduct a sensitivity or bias analysis.[3] Common to most of these sensitivity analysis methods is the use of a formula for which 2 inputs are required: (1) the strength and direction of the association between the unmeasured confounder and treatment choice and (2) the strength and direction of association between the unmeasured confounder and outcome.[4]

Furthermore, additional inputs or information may be needed, such as the prevalence of the unmeasured confounder and how it is associated with measured confounders. When it is known what the unmeasured confounder is, these could potentially be obtained from published studies and/or through other data sources. For example, smoking is a known risk factor for developing cardiovascular disease but the smoking status for an individual patient may not be included in a database. In this case, an assumption about the prevalence of smoking could be made based on prior research where smoking status was considered in similar clinical conditions. However, the prevalence cannot be estimated for a true unknown confounder. Additionally, many approaches require making simplifying assumptions such as that the unmeasured confounder is binary. Thus, sensitivity analyses of this type can only proceed once additional information, typically in the form of a series of inputs for some formulas, has been specified by investigators. Because decisions about each of the assumptions can affect the analysis results, the most rigorous approach to these types of sensitivity analyses would involve investigators considering a broad range of values for each input and then examining how the results are influenced.

While achievable in principle, this approach has limitations. First, the approach has been criticized as being susceptible to misuse, in the sense that an investigator could choose to focus on assumptions that make the original result seem robust. Second, if many scenarios are considered, there is potential for conflicting results within the sensitivity analysis, which may make it difficult to draw firm conclusions.

The E-value is an alternative approach to sensitivity analyses for unmeasured confounding in observational studies that avoids making assumptions that, in turn, require subjective assignment of inputs for some formulas.[4] Specifically, an E-value analysis asks the question: how strong would the unmeasured confounding have to be to negate the observed results?[5] The E-value itself answers this question by quantifying the minimum strength of association on the risk ratio scale that an unmeasured confounder must have with both the treatment and outcome, while simultaneously considering the measured covariates, to negate the observed treatment–outcome association. If the strength of unmeasured confounding is weaker than indicated by the E-value, then the main study result could not be overturned to one of "no association" (ie, moving the estimated risk ratio to 1.0) by the unmeasured confounder. E-values can therefore help assess the robustness of the main study result by considering whether unmeasured confounding of this magnitude is plausible. The E-value provides a measure related to the *evidence* for potential causality, hence the name "E-value."

The E-value has many appealing features. First, in contrast to standard methods for sensitivity, it requires no assumptions from investigators. Second, it is intuitive because the lowest possible number is 1. The higher the E-value is, the stronger the unmeasured confounding must be to explain the observed association. Third, the calculation is also readily applied to the bounds of a 95% CI. Thus, investigators can assess the extent of unmeasured confounding that would be required to shift the confidence interval so that it includes a risk ratio of 1.0 (ie, no association). Fourth, the E-value is simple to calculate for a range of effect measures, including relative risks, HRs, and risk differences, and study designs. The formulas for the E-value for different effect measures, including continuous outcomes, are available[4] and the E-value has been implemented in freely available software and an online calculator (https://evalue.hmdc.harvard.edu/app/).[6]

WHAT ARE THE LIMITATIONS OF THE E-VALUE?

The E-value is a general tool for sensitivity analyses that does not require assumptions about the nature of the unmeasured confounder. In some settings, investigators may be amenable to making assumptions (eg, about the prevalence of an unmeasured confounder) so that their sensitivity analyses can be tailored to their specific study design and/or statistical analyses. Such analyses, however, should always be considered in the context of the plausibility of the assumptions made.

WHY DID THE AUTHORS USE THE E-VALUE IN THIS PARTICULAR STUDY?

The data used by Fisher and colleagues[2] were abstracted retrospectively from the medical record databases of 4 integrated health care systems and, as such, are representative of clinical decisions and care at these institutions. Because the investigative team did not have control over whether patients underwent bariatric surgery (ie, treatment was not randomly assigned), the potential for unmeasured confounding bias needed to be acknowledged and thoroughly investigated.

HOW SHOULD THE E-VALUE FINDINGS BE INTERPRETED IN THIS PARTICULAR STUDY?

Fisher and colleagues[2] found that bariatric surgery was associated with a lower composite incidence of macrovascular events at 5 years (2.1% in the surgical group vs 4.3% in the nonsurgical group) that had an HR of 0.60 (95% CI, 0.42-0.86). The E-value for this was 2.72, meaning that residual confounding could explain the observed association if there exists an unmeasured covariate having a relative risk association at least as large as 2.72 with both macrovascular events and bariatric surgery. The E-value for the upper limit of the confidence interval was 1.60. In the Fisher et al[2] study, the HRs for some of the known, powerful macrovascular disease risk factors were 1.09 (95% CI, 0.85-1.41) for hypertension, 1.88 (95% CI, 1.34-2.63) for dyslipidemia, and 1.48 (95% CI, 1.17-1.87) for being a current smoker. It is not likely that an unmeasured or unknown confounder would have a substantially greater effect on macrovascular disease development than these known risk factors by having a relative risk exceeding 2.72.

CAVEATS TO CONSIDER WHEN LOOKING AT RESULTS BASED ON THE E-VALUE

E-values must be interpreted, and indeed only have meaning, within the context of the study at hand. In particular, its magnitude may be large or small depending on the magnitude of the associations of other risk factors. For example, if most other risk factors have an HR of 1.1, then an E-value of 1.3 will be relatively large because unmeasured confounding would have to have much larger effects than most risk factors to explain away the reported association. In contrast, if many risk factors have an HR of 2.0, then an E-value of 1.3 will be relatively modest. The adjustments that have been performed (ie, for the observed confounders) should also be considered.

Acknowledgment

The following disclosures were reported at the time this original article was first published in *JAMA*.

Conflict of Interest Disclosures: Drs Haneuse and VanderWeele reported receiving grants from the National Institutes of Health. Dr Arterburn reported receiving grants from the National Institutes of Health and Patient-Centered Outcomes Research Institute. No other disclosures were reported.

References

1. Courcoulas AP, Yanovski SZ, Bonds D, et al. Long-term outcomes of bariatric surgery: a National Institutes of Health symposium. *JAMA Surg*. 2014;149(12):1323-1329. Medline:25271405 doi:10.1001/jamasurg.2014.2440
2. Fisher DP, Johnson E, Haneuse S, et al. Association between bariatric surgery and macrovascular disease outcomes in patients with type 2 diabetes and severe obesity. *JAMA*. 2018;320(15):1570-1582. Medline:30326126 doi:10.1001/jama.2018.14619
3. Lash TL, Fox MP, Fink AK. *Applying Quantitative Bias Analysis to Epidemiologic Data*. Berlin, Germany: Springer Science & Business Media; 2011.
4. Ding P, VanderWeele TJ. Sensitivity analysis without assumptions. *Epidemiology*. 2016;27(3):368-377. Medline:26841057 doi:10.1097/EDE.0000000000000457
5. VanderWeele TJ, Ding P. Sensitivity analysis in observational research: introducing the E-value. *Ann Intern Med*. 2017;167(4):268-274. Medline:28693043 doi:10.7326/M16-2607
6. Mathur MB, Ding P, Riddell CA, VanderWeele TJ. Web site and R Package for computing E-values. *Epidemiology*. 2018;29(5):e45-e47. Medline:29912013 doi:10.1097/EDE.0000000000000864

Confounding by Indication in Clinical Research

Demetrios N. Kyriacou, MD, PhD, and
Roger J. Lewis, MD, PhD

IN THIS CHAPTER

Addressing Confounding in Clinical Research

Use of Methods to Control Confounding

What Are the Limitations of Methods to Control for Confounding?

How Should the Results Be Interpreted?

Caveats to Consider When Interpreting an Analysis Intended to Adjust for Confounding by Indication

This JAMA Guide to Statistics and Methods reviews the use of methods to control for confounding by indication in clinical studies that assess the potential effect of a treatment of risk factor on a patient outcome.

In the assessment of the effect of a treatment or potential risk factor—termed an exposure—on a patient outcome, the possibility of confounding by other factors must be considered.[1] For example, if researchers studied the effect of coffee drinking on the development of lung cancer, they might observe an apparent association between these 2 variables. However, because drinking coffee is also related to smoking, the observed association between coffee drinking and lung cancer does not represent a true causal relationship but is rather the result of the association of coffee drinking with smoking—the confounder—which is the true cause of lung cancer.

This illustration is a simple example of the very complicated and multifaceted phenomenon of confounding. Distortion from a confounder can appear to strengthen, weaken, or completely reverse the true effect of an exposure. In addition, multiple factors can interact to cause confounding in both epidemiologic and clinical research. Notwithstanding these complexities, a confounding variable can be readily identified if it meets 3 important criteria.[1] First, a confounder must be an independent risk factor for the outcome, either a causal factor or a surrogate for a casual factor (eg, smoking for lung cancer). Second, a confounder must be associated with the exposure (eg, smoking and coffee drinking). Third, a confounder cannot be an intermediate variable between the exposure and the outcome (eg, smoking is not caused by drinking coffee).

A particularly important type of confounding in clinical research is "confounding by indication," which occurs when the clinical indication for selecting a particular treatment (eg, severity of the illness) also affects the outcome. For example, patients with more severe illness are likely to receive more intensive treatments and, when comparing the interventions, the more intensive intervention will appear to result in poorer outcomes. This is called "confounding by severity" to emphasize that the degree of illness is the confounder. Because the degree of severity affects both treatment selection and patient outcome and is not an intermediate between the treatment and outcome, it fulfills the criteria for confounding.

As an example, the nonrandomized assessment of tracheal intubation vs bag-valve-mask ventilation for pediatric cardiopulmonary arrest reported by Andersen et al[2] is likely to be complicated by confounding by indication. Clinical conditions (eg, asthma, cystic fibrosis, and upper airway obstruction) existing before and during a patient's cardiopulmonary resuscitation will both affect the patient's outcome and influence the type of airway management.[2] In other words, it is likely that children with more severe disease and worse overall prognosis for survival had a greater probability to be intubated.[2] This possibility is especially great because severity of illness is both a strong predictor of mortality and a strong predictor of the clinical decision to intubate.

Not all confounding by indication is related to severity of illness. Other factors that affect both the type of intervention and the outcome can result in this form of confounding. For example, patients with health insurance may receive different interventions for their illness compared with patients without insurance. Furthermore, patients with insurance also tend to be healthier and have access to better overall medical care, thus improving their overall measured outcomes. In this case, having health insurance may act as a confounder when estimating the effect of the treatment on the outcome.

ADDRESSING CONFOUNDING IN CLINICAL RESEARCH

The primary goal of clinical research, whether observational or interventional, is to obtain valid measures of the effects of treatments or potential risk factors on patient outcomes. Because confounding distorts the true relationship between the exposure of interest and the outcome, investigators attempt to control confounding to provide valid measures of the observed associations or treatment effects.[3] In particular, randomized clinical trials (RCTs) use randomized treatment assignment to balance potential confounding factors—whether measured, unmeasured, or unknown—that might affect the outcome to ensure that those factors are unrelated to the assigned intervention. Thus, RCTs do not typically require use of statistical methods to adjust for confounding, as the randomization process is meant to limit all forms of confounding.

In some settings, RCTs may be inappropriate, impossible, or not feasible.[4] In these situations, observational studies are often used to investigate causal relationships in which the treatment assignment for each patient is not randomized but instead is determined by clinical indications. These types of observational studies are generally more difficult to interpret than RCTs. Without an opportunity to randomize the exposure, potential confounding frequently exists. Failing to adjust for confounding during the statistical analysis could result in inaccurate estimates of the relationship between the exposure and the outcome.

USE OF METHODS TO CONTROL CONFOUNDING

To control confounding, clinical researchers implement study design procedures to prevent confounding (eg, randomization, restriction, and matching) and conduct statistical procedures in the analysis to remove confounding (eg, stratified analyses, regression modeling, and propensity scoring) for both clinical trials and observational studies. Other JAMA Guide to Statistics and Methods chapters have summarized the use of logistic regression models and propensity score methods.[5,6] (See the chapter, Logistic Regression: Relating Patient Characteristics to Outcomes, and the chapter, The Propensity Score.)

Andersen et al used propensity score matching to statistically adjust for confounding.[6] The propensity score is the probability that a patient receives a specific treatment based on his or her characteristics and the clinical indications determined by the treating physician. This probability is used to match patients receiving the treatment of interest with those receiving the comparison treatment to control confounding by balancing potential confounding factors between these groups.

What Are the Limitations of Methods to Control for Confounding?

Incompletely controlled "residual" confounding may persist in clinical investigations despite study design and statistical procedures aimed at eliminating this form of bias.[1,7,8] This can occur in RCTs when the randomization process fails (typically in smaller trials) to completely balance confounders between the treatment groups. More likely, residual confounding occurs in observational studies of interventions when statistical analyses do not adequately adjust for confounding. Reasons for failure of statistical adjustments include the following: (1) failure to measure the confounding variable so that it cannot be included in the statistical analysis (ie, "unmeasured confounding"); (2) use of a measure for the confounding variable that does not accurately reflect or capture the characteristic it is supposed to represent (eg, the variable used to describe the confounder is an imperfect or misclassified measure of the characteristic); and (3) use of overly broad categories for the confounder (ie, even for patients with the same value for the confounding variable there is important variability in the likelihood of receiving each treatment and in experiencing the outcome).

How Should the Results Be Interpreted?

In the study by Andersen et al,[2] some degree of confounding by indication exists in the comparison between tracheal intubation and bag-valve-mask ventilation. Confounding by indication is evident because inclusion in the propensity score–matched statistical analysis of certain clinical conditions that might influence a clinician's decision to intubate a patient (eg, illness category, preexisting conditions, whether the arrest was witnessed; see Supplement in Andersen et al[2]) reduced the strength of the estimated deleterious effect of tracheal intubation. For example, in the unadjusted statistical analysis, tracheal intubation during pediatric cardiopulmonary resuscitation was associated with decreased survival to hospital discharge, with a risk ratio of 0.64 (95% CI, 0.59-0.69; $P < .001$). However, in the propensity score–matched adjusted statistical analysis, the risk ratio effect estimate was only 0.89 (95% CI, 0.81-0.99; $P = .03$). This change in estimate with statistical adjustment is evidence of confounding by 1 or more clinical conditions that were included in the multivariable analyses.[9] Furthermore, if all of the important confounding variables were not included in the adjusted analyses, then residual confounding could still persist. Although Andersen et al implemented sophisticated statistical methods to specifically limit confounding by indication, their observational cohort study may not have included measures of all potential confounding, such as factors concerned with the resuscitation phase that influenced the decision to intubate the patients.

CAVEATS TO CONSIDER WHEN INTERPRETING AN ANALYSIS INTENDED TO ADJUST FOR CONFOUNDING BY INDICATION

When assessing an observational study of treatment effects for confounding by indication, the reader should consider why clinicians select specific interventions and how those decisions might be influenced by factors that also directly affect outcomes. Conversely, investigators must know and understand the causal and noncausal relationships among the intervention, potential confounders, and the outcome to ensure potential confounding is controlled. Underlying pathophysiologic processes must also be considered when determining what variables should be measured and included in any statistical analysis. Any assessment of a clinical intervention should include an evaluation of confounding by indication that is best accomplished by the following: (1) understanding the underlying pathophysiologic mechanisms leading to specific outcomes; (2) understanding the criteria for confounding and describing the relationships between potential confounders and both intervention and outcome variables; and (3) understanding effective study designs and statistical methods that reduce or eliminate confounding by indication.

Acknowledgment

The following disclosures were reported at the time this original article was first published in *JAMA*.
Conflict of Interest Disclosures: None reported.

References

1. Rothman KJ, Greenland S, Lash T, eds. *Modern Epidemiology.* 3rd ed. Philadelphia, PA: Lippincott Williams & Wilkins; 2008.
2. Andersen LW, Raymond TT, Berg RA, et al. The association between tracheal intubation during pediatric in-hospital cardiac arrest and survival. *JAMA*. 2016;316(17):1786-1797. doi:10.1001/jama.2016.14486
3. Greenland S, Morgenstern H. Confounding in health research. *Annu Rev Public Health*. 2001;22:189-212. Medline:11274518
4. Black N. Why we need observational studies to evaluate the effectiveness of health care. *BMJ*. 1996;312(7040):1215-1218. Medline:8634569
5. Tolles J, Meurer WJ. Logistic regression: relating patient characteristics to outcomes. *JAMA*. 2016;316(5):533-534. Medline:27483067
6. Haukoos JS, Lewis RJ. The propensity score. *JAMA*. 2015;314(15):1637-1638. Medline:26501539
7. Szklo M, Nieto FJ, eds. *Epidemiology: Beyond the Basics*. 3rd ed. Burlington, MA: Jones & Bartlett; 2014.
8. Fewell Z, Davey Smith G, Sterne JA. The impact of residual and unmeasured confounding in epidemiologic studies: a simulation study. *Am J Epidemiol*. 2007;166(6):646-655. Medline:17615092
9. McNamee R. Confounding and confounders. *Occup Environ Med*. 2003;60(3):227-234. Medline:12598677

Mediation Analysis

Hopin Lee, PhD, Robert D. Herbert, PhD, and James H. McAuley, PhD

IN THIS CHAPTER

Use of the Method

Why Is Mediation Analysis Used?

Description of Mediation Analysis

What Are the Limitations of Mediation Analysis?

Why Did the Authors Use Mediation Analysis?

Caveats to Consider When Assessing the Results of Mediation Analysis

This JAMA Guide to Statistics and Methods reviews the use of mediation analysis to evaluate possible mechanisms that the effects of interventions are presumed to work through.

In a study published in *JAMA Network Open*, Silverstein et al[1] used mediation analysis to investigate how a problem-solving educational program prevented depressive symptoms in low-income mothers. Using data from a randomized trial, the authors tested 8 plausible mechanisms by which the intervention could have its effects. They concluded that problem-solving education reduced the risk of depressive symptoms in low-income mothers primarily by reducing maternal stress.

USE OF THE METHOD

Why Is Mediation Analysis Used?

The effects of health and medical interventions are often presumed to work through specific biological or psychosocial mechanisms. Possible mechanisms can be evaluated using mediation analysis.

Description of Mediation Analysis

In mediation analysis, the effect of an intervention on an outcome is partitioned into indirect and direct effects. Indirect effects work through mediators of interest, whereas direct effects work through other mechanisms. These effects are often shown in a diagram (Figure 10). Mediation analysis can estimate indirect and direct effects and the proportion mediated, a statistical measure estimating how much of the total intervention effect works through a particular mediator.

Two broad analytical approaches are used to conduct a mediation analysis: statistical and causal. Statistical mediation analysis uses regression models to estimate the strength of

Mediation Analysis Applied to a Study of Problem-Solving Education (PSE) to Prevent Maternal Depression

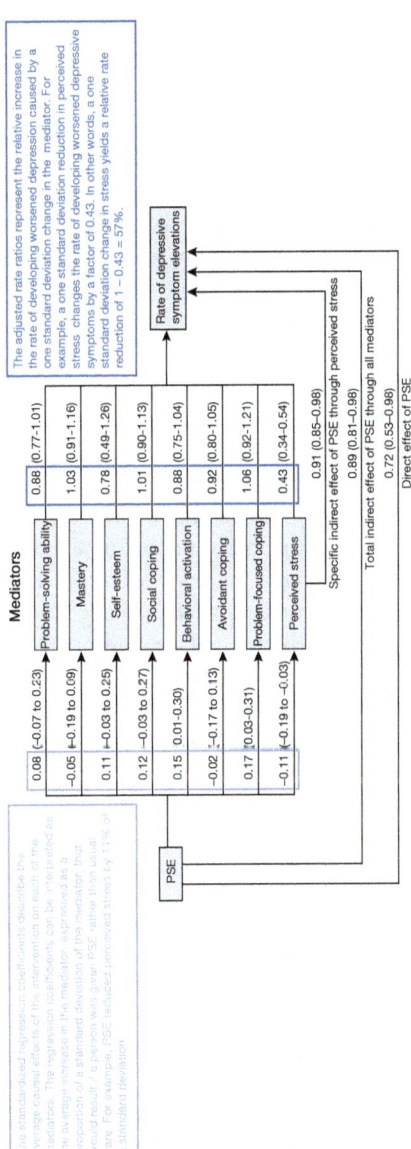

Mediation analysis exploring how PSE reduced depressive symptoms in low-income mothers. The numbers on the arrows connecting PSE to each of the mediators are standardized regression coefficients (with 95% CIs). The numbers on the arrows linking mediators to the rate of worsened depression are adjusted rate ratios. The indirect and direct effects derived from the mediation analysis are reported in the lower right corner. The rate ratio of the specific indirect effect of PSE through perceived stress is 0.91, indicating that on average, PSE reduced the rate of worsened depression by 1 − 0.91 = 9% through its effect on perceived stress. PSE also reduced the rate of worsened depression through other mechanisms in the model, including stress (rate ratio for the total indirect effect of PSE through all mediators = 0.89). The direct effect rate ratio of 0.72 indicates that a substantial effect of PSE on the rate of worsened depression worked through unmeasured mechanisms. Adapted from Silverstein et al.[1]

intervention-mediator and mediator-outcome effects. These regression coefficients can then be multiplied to estimate the indirect effect.[2] Statistical mediation analysis is limited by its inability to accurately model situations in which there are nonlinear relationships between the intervention, mediator, and outcome or when there is an interaction between the intervention and the mediator.[2] Causal mediation analysis is more general and rigorous. It is more general because it allows for nonlinear relationships and interactions,[3] and more rigorous because it explicitly outlines the assumptions that are necessary for making causal claims and includes sensitivity analyses to assess these assumptions.[2,3] Causal mediation analysis uses linear or nonlinear regression techniques to model the intervention-mediator and mediator-outcome effects. The regression models are used to simulate potential values of the mediator and outcome for each study participant under hypothetical and observed scenarios of receiving and not receiving the intervention. These estimates are then used to calculate the average indirect and direct effects.[3]

Statistical and causal mediation analyses produce similar estimates when linear models are used for continuous variables and there are no interactions between the intervention and the mediator. When mediators or outcomes are binary variables or when nonlinear models are used or interactions are present, statistical mediation can produce biased estimates and the causal mediation approach is preferred.[2]

What Are the Limitations of Mediation Analysis?

The explicit objective of all mediation analyses is to demonstrate causal relationships. This objective requires that specific assumptions are met. In a mediation analysis, the intervention-outcome, intervention-mediator, and mediator-outcome effects must be unconfounded to permit valid causal inferences. This requirement is often called the no confounding, or ignorability, assumption.[2] In a randomized trial, participants are randomly assigned to intervention groups, so the intervention-outcome and intervention-mediator effects can be assumed to be unconfounded. However, trial participants are not usually randomly assigned to receive or not receive the mediator, so the mediator-outcome effect may be confounded, even in randomized trials. To overcome this potential source of bias, investigators can control for known confounders of the mediator-outcome effect by using techniques such as regression adjustment. However, as highlighted in another JAMA Guide to Statistics and Methods chapter,[4] unmeasured confounding may still introduce bias even if known confounders have been adjusted for. (See the chapter, The Propensity Score.) Sensitivity analyses can and should be used to assess the potential bias caused by unmeasured confounding in mediation analyses.[3]

The risk of confounding in mediation analyses is greater in observational studies than in randomized trials[3] because participants in observational studies are not randomly allocated to receive the exposure. In observational studies, unlike randomized trials, it cannot be assumed that either the exposure-mediator or exposure-outcome effects are unconfounded. Therefore, estimates of all effects in the mediation model of an observational study could be biased, and control of confounding may be required for all effects. An example is provided by an observational study in which Cheng et al[5] used mediation analysis to test whether functional brain connectivity mediated the effect of depression on sleep quality. Because participants were not randomly allocated to levels of depression (the exposure) or functional brain connectivity (the mediator), the investigators adjusted for known confounders of all effects in the mediation models. Despite these efforts, it is possible that in this study, as in all observational studies, unmeasured confounding could have biased the estimates of indirect and direct effects.

Why Did the Authors Use Mediation Analysis?

Although the effectiveness of problem-solving education on depression is well established, the psychological mechanisms mediating this effect are not known. Silverstein et al[1] conducted a planned mediation analysis of their randomized trial to understand the mechanisms by which problem-solving education reduced depressive symptoms (Figure 10). Knowledge of the mediating mechanisms may be useful in creating more efficient or effective problem-solving educational interventions.

CAVEATS TO CONSIDER WHEN ASSESSING THE RESULTS OF MEDIATION ANALYSIS

If a mediation analysis has not adjusted for confounding or explored the effects of unmeasured confounding using sensitivity analysis techniques, the findings should be interpreted with caution. Mediation analyses of randomized or nonrandomized studies can only demonstrate causal effects if confounding can be confidently ruled out. If there are multiple mediators of the intervention that affect one another, mediators may act as postrandomization confounders of the effects of other mediators.[6] In these cases, caution is necessary when interpreting estimates of indirect and direct effects derived from mediation analyses of single mediators. The timing of measurements of the mediator and outcome are also important. If the mediator is measured at the same time as the outcome, there could be reverse causation. That is, the outcome could cause the mediator rather than the mediator causing the outcome.

Acknowledgment

The following disclosures were reported at the time this original article was first published in *JAMA*.

Conflict of Interest Disclosures: None reported.

References

1. Silverstein M, Cabral H, Hegel M, et al. Problem-solving education to prevent depression among low-income mothers. *JAMA Netw Open*. 2018;1(2):e180334. doi:10.1001/jamanetworkopen.2018.0334

2. VanderWeele TJ. *Explanation in Causal Inference: Methods for Mediation and Interaction*. New York, NY: Oxford University Press; 2015.
3. Imai K, Keele L, Yamamoto T. Identification, inference and sensitivity analysis for causal mediation effects. *Stat Sci*. 2010;25(1):51-71.
4. Haukoos JS, Lewis RJ. The propensity score. *JAMA*. 2015;314(15): 1637-1638. Medline:26501539 doi:10.1001/jama.2015.13480
5. Cheng W, Rolls ET, Ruan H, Feng J. Functional connectivities in the brain that mediate the association between depressive problems and sleep quality. *JAMA Psychiatry*. 2018;75(10):1052-1061. Medline:PMC6233808 doi:10.1001/jamapsychiatry.2018.1941
6. VanderWeele TJ, Vansteelandt S. Mediation analysis with multiple mediators. *Epidemiol Methods*. 2014;2(1):95-115. Medline:25580377

Odds Ratios—Current Best Practice and Use

Edward C. Norton, PhD, Bryan E. Dowd, PhD, and Matthew L. Maciejewski, PhD

IN THIS CHAPTER

Why Report Odds Ratios From Logistic Regression?

What Are the Limitations of Odds Ratios?

How Did the Authors Use Odds Ratios?

How Should the Findings Be Interpreted?

What Caveats Should the Reader Consider?

This JAMA Guide to Statistics and Methods explains the correct usage of odds ratios in the clinical literature to report the strength of the association between binary outcomes.

Odds ratios frequently are used to present strength of association between risk factors and outcomes in the clinical literature. Odds and odds ratios are related to the probability of a binary outcome (an outcome that is either present or absent, such as mortality). The *odds* are the ratio of the probability that an outcome occurs to the probability that the outcome does not occur. For example, suppose that the probability of mortality is 0.3 in a group of patients. This can be expressed as the odds of dying: $0.3/(1 - 0.3) = 0.43$. When the probability is small, odds are virtually identical to the probability. For example, for a probability of 0.05, the odds are $0.05/(1 - 0.05) = 0.052$. This similarity does not exist when the value of a probability is large.

Probability and odds are different ways of expressing similar concepts. For example, when randomly selecting a card from a deck, the probability of selecting a spade is $13/52 = 25\%$. The odds of selecting a card with a spade are $25\%/75\% = 1:3$. Clinicians usually are interested in knowing probabilities, whereas gamblers think in terms of odds. Odds are useful when wagering because they represent fair payouts. If one were to bet $1 on selecting a spade from a deck of cards, a payout of $3 is necessary to have an even chance of winning your money back. From the gambler's perspective, a payout smaller than $3 is unfavorable and greater than $3 is favorable.

Differences between 2 different groups having a binary outcome such as mortality can be compared using odds ratios, the ratio of 2 odds. Differences also can be compared using probabilities by calculating the *relative risk ratio*, which is the ratio of 2 probabilities. Odds ratios commonly are used to express strength of associations from logistic regression to predict a binary outcome.[1]

WHY REPORT ODDS RATIOS FROM LOGISTIC REGRESSION?

Researchers often analyze a binary outcome using multivariable logistic regression. One potential limitation of logistic regression is that the results are not directly interpretable as either probabilities or relative risk ratios. However, the results from a logistic regression are converted easily into odds ratios because logistic regression estimates a parameter, known as the log odds, which is the natural logarithm of the odds ratio. For example, if a log odds estimated by logistic regression is 0.4 then the odds ratio can be derived by exponentiating the log odds (exp(0.4) = 1.5). It is the odds ratio that is usually reported in the medical literature. The odds ratio is always positive, although the estimated log odds can be positive or negative (log odds of −0.2 equals odds ratio of 0.82 = exp(−0.2)).

The odds ratio for a risk factor contributing to a clinical outcome can be interpreted as whether someone with the risk factor is more or less likely than someone without that risk factor to experience the outcome of interest. Logistic regression modeling allows the estimates for a risk factor of interest to be adjusted for other risk factors, such as age, smoking status, and diabetes. One feature of the logistic function is that an odds ratio for one covariate is constant for all values of the other covariates.

Another feature of odds ratios from a logistic regression is that it is easy to test the statistical strength of association. The standard test is whether the parameter (log odds) equals 0, which corresponds to a test of whether the odds ratio equals 1. Odds ratios typically are reported in a table with 95% CIs. If the 95% CI for an odds ratio does not include 1.0, then the odds ratio is considered to be statistically significant at the 5% level.

WHAT ARE THE LIMITATIONS OF ODDS RATIOS?

Several caveats must be considered when reporting results with odds ratios. First, the interpretation of odds ratios is framed in terms of odds, not in terms of probabilities. Odds ratios often are mistaken for relative risk ratios.[2,3] Although for rare outcomes odds ratios approximate relative risk ratios, when the outcomes are not rare, odds ratios always overestimate relative risk ratios, a problem that becomes more acute as the baseline prevalence of the outcome exceeds 10%. Odds ratios cannot be calculated directly from relative risk ratios. For example, an odds ratio for men of 2.0 could correspond to the situation in which the probability for some event is 1% for men and 0.5% for women. An odds ratio of 2.0 also could correspond to a probability of an event occurring 50% for men and 33% for women, or to a probability of 80% for men and 67% for women.

Second, and less well known, the magnitude of the odds ratio from a logistic regression is scaled by an arbitrary factor (equal to the square root of the variance of the unexplained part of binary outcome).[4] This arbitrary scaling factor changes when more or better explanatory variables are added to the logistic regression model because the added variables explain more of the total variation and reduce the unexplained variance. Therefore, adding more independent explanatory variables to the model will increase the odds ratio of the variable of interest (eg, treatment) due to dividing by a smaller scaling factor. In addition, the odds ratio also will change if the additional variables are not independent, but instead are correlated with the variable of interest; it is even possible for the odds ratio to decrease if the correlation is strong enough to outweigh the change due to the scaling factor.

Consequently, there is no unique odds ratio to be estimated, even from a single study. Different odds ratios from the same study cannot be compared when the statistical models that result in odds ratio estimates have different explanatory variables because each model has a different arbitrary scaling factor.[4-6] Nor can the magnitude of the odds ratio from one study be compared with the magnitude of the odds ratio from another study, because different samples and different model specifications will have different arbitrary scaling factors. A further implication is that the magnitudes of odds ratios of a given association in multiple studies cannot be synthesized in a meta-analysis.[4]

HOW DID THE AUTHORS USE ODDS RATIOS?

Tringale and colleagues[7] studied industry payments to physicians for consulting, ownership, royalties, and research as well as whether payments differed by physician specialty or sex. Industry payments were received by 50.8% of men across all specialties compared with 42.6% of women across all specialties. Converting these probabilities to odds, the odds that men receive industry payments is 1.03 (0.51/0.49), and the odds that women receive industry payments is 0.74 = (0.43/0.57).

The odds ratio for men compared with women is the ratio of the odds for men divided by the odds for women. In this case, the unadjusted odds ratio is 1.03/0.74 = 1.39. Therefore, the odds for men receiving industry payments are about 1.4 as large (40% higher) compared with women. Note that the ratio of the odds is different than the ratio of the probabilities because the probability is not close to 0. The unadjusted ratio of the probabilities for men and women (Tringale et al[7] report each probability, but not the ratio), the relative risk ratio, is 1.19 (0.51/0.43).

Greater odds that men may receive industry payments may be explained by their disproportionate representation in specialties more likely to receive industry payments. After controlling for specialty (and other factors), the estimated odds ratio was reduced from 1.39 to 1.28, with a 95% CI of 1.26 to 1.31, which did not include 1.0 and, therefore, is statistically significant.

The odds ratio probably declined after adjusting for more variables because they were correlated with physicians' sex.

HOW SHOULD THE FINDINGS BE INTERPRETED?

In exploring the association between physician sex and receiving industry payments, Tringale and colleagues[7] found that men are more likely to receive payments than women, even after controlling for confounders. The magnitude of the odds ratio, about 1.4, indicates the direction of the effect, but the magnitude of the number itself is hard to interpret. The estimated odds ratio is 1.4 when simultaneously accounting for specialty, spending region, sole proprietor status, sex, and the interaction between specialty and sex. A different odds ratio would be found if the model included a different set of explanatory variables. The 1.4 estimated odds ratio should not be compared with odds ratios estimated from other data sets with the same set of explanatory variables, or to odds ratios estimated from this same data set with a different set of explanatory variables.[4]

WHAT CAVEATS SHOULD THE READER CONSIDER?

Odds ratios are one way, but not the only way, to present an association when the main outcome is binary. Tringale et al[7] also report absolute rate differences. The reader should understand odds ratios in the context of other information, such as the underlying probability. When the probabilities are small, odds ratios and relative risk ratios are nearly identical, but they can diverge widely for large probabilities. The magnitude of the odds ratio is hard to interpret because of the arbitrary scaling factor and cannot be compared with odds ratios from other studies.

It is best to examine study results presented in several ways to better understand the true meaning of study findings.

Acknowledgment

The following disclosures were reported at the time this original article was first published in *JAMA*.

Conflict of Interest Disclosures: Dr Maciejewski reported receiving personal fees from the University of Alabama at Birmingham for a workshop presentation; receiving grants from NIDA and the Veterans Affairs; receiving a contract from NCQA to Duke University for research; being supported by a research career scientist award 10-391 from the Veterans Affairs Health Services Research and Development; and that his spouse owns stock in Amgen. No other disclosures were reported.

References

1. Meurer WJ, Tolles J. Logistic regression diagnostics: understanding how well a model predicts outcomes. *JAMA*. 2017;317(10):1068-1069. Medline:28291878 doi:10.1001/jama.2016.20441
2. Schwartz LM, Woloshin S, Welch HG. Misunderstandings about the effects of race and sex on physicians' referrals for cardiac catheterization. *N Engl J Med*. 1999;341(4):279-283. Medline:10413743 doi:10.1056/NEJM199907223410411
3. Holcomb WLJr, Chaiworapongsa T, Luke DA, Burgdorf KD. An odd measure of risk: use and misuse of the odds ratio. *Obstet Gynecol*. 2001;98(4):685-688. Medline:11576589
4. Norton EC, Dowd BE. Log odds and the interpretation of logit models. *Health Serv Res*. 2018;53(2):859-878. Medline:28560732 doi:10.1111/1475-6773.12712
5. Miettinen OS, Cook EF. Confounding: essence and detection. *Am J Epidemiol*. 1981;114(4):593-603. Medline:7304589 doi:10.1093/oxfordjournals.aje.a113225
6. Hauck WW, Neuhaus JM, Kalbfleisch JD, Anderson S. A consequence of omitted covariates when estimating odds ratios. *J Clin Epidemiol*. 1991;44(1):77-81. Medline:1986061 doi:10.1016/0895-4356(91)90203-L
7. Tringale KR, Marshall D, Mackey TK, Connor M, Murphy JD, Hattangadi-Gluth JA. Types and distribution of payments from industry to physicians in 2015. *JAMA*. 2017;317(17):1774-1784. Medline:28464140 doi:10.1001/jama.2017.3091

JAMAevidence
Using Evidence to Improve Care

Marginal Effects—Quantifying the Effect of Changes in Risk Factors in Logistic Regression Models

Edward C. Norton, PhD, Bryan E. Dowd, PhD, and Matthew L. Maciejewski, PhD

IN THIS CHAPTER

Use of Marginal Effects

Why Are Marginal Effects Used?

What Are Marginal Effects?

What Are the Limitations of Marginal Effects?

How Should the Marginal Effects Be Interpreted in Cummings et al?

This JAMA Guide to Statistics and Methods discusses the marginal effects approach to express the strength of the association between a risk factor and a binary outcome from a logistic regression.

Marginal effects can be used to express how the predicted probability of a binary outcome changes with a change in a risk factor. For example, how does 1-year mortality risk change with a 1-year increase in age or for a patient with diabetes compared with a patient without diabetes? This approach can make the results more easily understood. Marginal effects often are reported with logistic regression analyses to communicate and quantify the incremental risk associated with each factor.[1,2]

In an article published in *JAMA Psychiatry*, Cummings et al[3] studied factors that predicted access to US outpatient mental health facilities that accept Medicaid. Their main outcome had 3 categories, which were labeled "no access," "some access," and "good access." An ordered logistic regression model was developed and results were presented as the change in the probability of each outcome for a change in certain demographic factors.

USE OF MARGINAL EFFECTS

Why Are Marginal Effects Used?

There are several ways to express the strength of the association between a risk factor and a binary outcome from a logistic regression. One popular approach is the odds ratio (OR).[4] The odds are the ratio of the probability that an outcome occurs to the probability that the outcome does not occur. The ratio of the odds for 2 groups—the OR—is often used to quantify differences between 2 different groups; eg, treatment and control groups. Another approach is the risk ratio, which is the probability that the outcome occurs in the presence of the risk factor divided by the probability that the outcome occurs in the absence of the risk factor. Risk ratios are often easier to use in clinical practice than are ORs.[4,5]

A third alternative is the marginal effect, which is the change in the probability that the outcome occurs as the risk factor changes by 1 unit while holding all the other explanatory variables constant. When the risk factor is continuous (eg, age), the change in the probability that the outcome occurs that is associated with a 1-unit change in the risk factor has been called a *marginal* effect. When the risk factor is discrete (eg, presence or absence of diabetes), the change has been called an *incremental* effect. In this chapter, the term *marginal effect* represents this strength of association measure in both instances.

What Are Marginal Effects?

Of the 3 approaches, marginal effects are the most intuitive because they are expressed as the change in the predicted probability that the outcome occurs that is associated with a 1-unit change in the risk factor. Unlike ORs, it is easier to compare marginal effects across different studies because they are less sensitive to the statistical model conditions that influence the reported values of ORs.[6] Marginal effects depend on the values of the other explanatory variables and will not be the same for all members of a group.

For example, consider a linear regression analysis predicting body weight in pounds from a person's height measured in inches. If the regression coefficient is 5, it means that a 1-in increase in height is associated with a 5-lb increase in weight. In this instance, the marginal effect of the 1-unit change in the risk factor, height, is how it changes the predicted outcome, weight in pounds. This is true in linear regressions unless the predictors included in the model include higher powers of the risk factors (eg, age and age squared) or interactions among the explanatory variables (eg, 2 explanatory variables multiplied together). In a simple linear regression (eg, without interactions between predictors), this marginal effect is constant across all values of the risk factor. For instance, a change in height from 5 ft 8 in to 5 ft 9 in has the same predicted effect as does a change from 6 ft 3 in to 6 ft 4 in. The marginal effect is also constant across all values of the other explanatory variables, such as age or presence of diabetes.

In a nonlinear model like logistic regression, the marginal effect of the risk factor is an informative way to answer the research question—how does a change in a risk factor affect the probability that the outcome occurs? In logistic regression, neither the marginal effect nor the OR is the same as the regression coefficient. Instead, the marginal effect reflects the nonlinear function on which the logistic regression model is based. Logistic regression ensures that predicted probabilities lie between 0 and 1, even for extreme values of a continuous risk factor, by modeling the relationship as a curve that fits between 0 and 1. Thus, the marginal effect of a 1-unit increase in age is not constant. The marginal effect will be small when the probability of the outcome is close to 0 or 1 and relatively large when the probability is close to 0.5. Because the values of the other covariates change the predicted probabilities, the marginal effect of any covariate depends on the value of other covariates in the model. For example, the marginal effect of a 1-unit increase in age may depend on whether the study participant is a man or a woman, even without including an interaction term between sex and age.[7] The variability in marginal effects makes intuitive sense because it is expected that the effect of a risk factor on the outcome is heterogeneous; ie, different effects for different values of the risk factor and other explanatory variables.

In logistic regression, there is no single marginal effect for the entire sample of individuals, so analysts must choose how to present marginal effects. The most common way is to report the average marginal effect across all persons in the data set, knowing that it is larger for some individuals and smaller for others. A second way is to report the marginal effect calculated at the means of all covariates. This can lead to a challenging interpretation; for instance, an estimated marginal effect of a risk factor for a person who is 50% pregnant or 20% diabetic. A third way is to report the marginal effect for an individual with a specific set of characteristics; for example, the effect of an intervention on pregnant patients with diabetes.

An important advantage of marginal effects over ORs is that estimated marginal effects are less sensitive than ORs to inclusion of different sets of explanatory variables and estimation based on different samples of data.[4] The sensitivity of ORs and marginal effects to different model specifications and data sets was reviewed by Norton and Dowd.[6]

WHAT ARE THE LIMITATIONS OF MARGINAL EFFECTS?

Marginal effects vary across individuals, so it is important to present reported marginal effects in context by comparing the marginal effects with the magnitude of the baseline risk. For example, a change in probability of 1% may seem small if the baseline risk is 80% but may be large for a rare outcome (eg, baseline risk of 2%).

Care must be exercised when reporting marginal effects from case-control studies.[8] In this type of model, the sample proportions of the outcome values are not representative of the population.[5] Simple logistic models cannot provide either a meaningful marginal effect or a meaningful risk ratio from a case-control study, so ORs are the appropriate measures of association in this setting.

Until recently, it was challenging to compute marginal effects from logistic regressions and other nonlinear models such as ordered logistic, Poisson, negative binomial, and conditional logistic models. In recent years, standard statistical packages have added commands that make it easier to generate marginal effects, including the margins command in Stata and the margins package in R.

HOW SHOULD THE MARGINAL EFFECTS BE INTERPRETED IN CUMMINGS ET AL?

Cummings et al[3] described how changes in 4 county-level characteristics would change the predicted probability of either having no access or having good access to mental health outpatient treatment facilities that accept Medicaid (see Table 2 in the article[3]). For example, an increase of 31 percentage points in the fraction of the county population living in a rural community (the standard deviation of that variable) would on average increase the probability of no access to mental health care by 27.9 percentage points (baseline risk = 34.8%) but would also increase the probability of good access by 3.4 percentage points (baseline risk = 20.2%), holding the effect of other explanatory variables constant. Such a change in rural population therefore would decrease the probability of some access, the third possible outcome, by 31.3 percentage points (27.9 + 3.4).

Marginal effects are a useful way to describe the average effect of changes in explanatory variables on the change in the probability of outcomes in logistic regression and other nonlinear models. Marginal effects provide a direct and easily interpreted answer to the research question of interest.

Acknowledgment

The following disclosures were reported at the time this original article was first published in *JAMA*.

Conflict of Interest Disclosures: Dr Maciejewski reported being supported by research career scientist award 10-391 from the Veterans Affairs Health Services Research and Development and support from the Durham Veterans Affairs Health Services Research and Development Center of Innovation (CIN 13-410); receiving grants from the National Institute on Drug Abuse and the Department of Veterans Affairs; receiving a contract from the National Committee for Quality Assurance to Duke

University for research; and that his spouse owns stock in Amgen. No other disclosures were reported.

References

1. Meurer WJ, Tolles J. Logistic regression diagnostics: understanding how well a model predicts outcomes. *JAMA*. 2017;317(10):1068-1069. Medline:28291878 doi:10.1001/jama.2016.20441
2. Tolles J, Meurer WJ. Logistic regression: relating patient characteristics to outcomes. *JAMA*. 2016;316(5):533-534. Medline:27483067 doi:10.1001/jama.2016.7653
3. Cummings JR, Wen H, Ko M, Druss BG. Geography and the Medicaid mental health care infrastructure: implications for health care reform. *JAMA Psychiatry*. 2013;70(10):1084-1090. Medline:23965816 doi:10.1001/jamapsychiatry.2013.377
4. Norton EC, Dowd BE, Maciejewski ML. Odds ratios—current best practice and use. *JAMA*. 2018;320(1):84-85. Medline:29971384 doi:10.1001/jama.2018.6971
5. Sackett DL, Deeks JJ, Altman DG. Down with odds ratios! *BMJ Evid Based Med*. 1996;1(6):164-166. doi:10.1136/ebm.1996.1.164
6. Norton EC, Dowd BE. Log odds and the interpretation of logit models. *Health Serv Res*. 2018;53(2):859-878. Medline:28560732 doi:10.1111/1475-6773.12712
7. Karaca-Mandic P, Norton EC, Dowd B. Interaction terms in nonlinear models. *Health Serv Res*. 2012;47(1 pt 1):255-274. Medline:22091735 doi:10.1111/j.1475-6773.2011.01314.x
8. Irony TZ. Case-control studies: using "real-world" evidence to assess association. *JAMA*. 2018;320(10):1027-1028. Medline:30422270 doi:10.1001/jama.2018.12115

JAMAevidence
Using Evidence to Improve Care

Adjusting for Covariates: A Source of False Findings in Published Research Studies

Helena Chmura Kraemer, PhD

This JAMA Guide to Statistics and Methods discusses adjusting for covariates, a common cause of false findings in published research, by allowing variables to vary as they will but then using a mathematical model to assess their influence on the outcome.

Concern about erroneous conclusions of many published research findings has led to the conclusion that most published research findings are wrong.[1,2] What can be done about that? In what follows, I will focus on one common source of false findings: adjusting for covariates.

Here, *adjusting* means allowing variables to vary as they will but then using a mathematical model to assess their influence on the outcome. In contrast, *to control* means manipulation of variables by the researcher for a particular purpose (eg, in experimental design). Unfortunately, the terms *adjust* and *control* are often used as if they were synonymous. Adjusting often leads to false conclusions because the models used may not correspond to reality.

To illustrate this point, consider a randomized clinical trial (RCT) in which those sampled from the population of interest are randomly assigned to 2 treatment groups, T1 and T2. A valid test simply comparing the outcomes in the 2 groups tests the overall effect size (overall ES) that a randomly sampled patient from T1 has an outcome clinically preferable to that of a randomly sampled patient from T2.[3]

Often, the first table of an RCT report compares the baseline characteristics of the T1 vs T2 samples to assess the success of randomization, ignoring the fact that randomization (1) is a process, not an outcome, and (2) is meant to generate 2 random samples from the same population, not 2 matched samples. When a few baseline variables significantly differentiate the 2 groups at the 5% level, researchers often propose to adjust for those covariates in testing the treatment effect. This is post hoc testing (like offering to bet at prerace odds on a horse as it approaches the finish line), which frequently leads to false-positive results.

Any covariates to be used in adjusting should be specified a priori, listed in the RCT registration, and taken into consideration in the power analysis. Such adjustment changes the hypothesis to be tested from comparing all T1 patients vs all T2 patients (overall ES) to comparing T1 patients only with T2 patients matched in one way or another on the particular covariates proposed. Let's say that covariate ES is the ES for patients with one particular configuration of the covariates and typical ES is the ES specifically for patients who are at the mean of each such covariate (ie, for the typical patient). Overall ES, typical ES, and all possible covariate ES are the same only if the covariates are irrelevant to the treatment outcome. If the covariates are irrelevant, adjusting for those simply leads to a loss of power. If the covariates are not irrelevant, then estimation and testing of overall ES, typical ES, and covariate ES provide answers to different research questions.

The linear model used for covariate adjusting (eg, analysis of covariance [ANCOVA]) assumes, for all possible values of the covariates, that covariate ES is equal to typical ES; that is, that there is no interaction between the covariates and the treatment effect. If this assumption is violated, then the interactions that exist in the population (but are not included in the model) can bias the statistical tests and estimation of the treatment ES. Furthermore, not finding statistically significant interactions in the sample does not prove the null hypothesis that they do not exist in the population. Given these risks for bias, ANCOVA should not generally be used for such adjustment.

When treatment interactions are included in a linear model, how the variables are coded can impact the results.[4] The treatment effect refers to the treatment effect for patients having the zero value of all included covariates. Thus, if T1 and T2 were 2 treatments for Alzheimer disease, and the single covariate were chronological age at disease onset, the treatment effect would be the effect of the treatment for individuals with Alzheimer disease diagnosed as having the illness at age 0 years, which is a ludicrous result. Instead, age is better coded as deviations from the mean age at onset (centering at the mean). Then the treatment effect is typical ES and the interaction effect reflects the change in covariate ES as the covariate value changes. Examination of the covariate ES may well indicate to clinicians which patients will respond better to T1 or T2.[5] With multiple covariates, if each is centered at its mean,[4] the treatment effect tested is typical ES, the treatment effect for those at the mean of every covariate, which is sometimes a very small subpopulation.

There are still additional problems. For example, when multiple covariates are included, omitting interactions between them can introduce bias to the estimation of treatment ES. However, to include all interactions involving m covariates in a linear model requires estimation of 2^{m+1} parameters. To make matters even worse, the advantage of an RCT with random assignment is that, over replications, treatment choice and each covariate are uncorrelated. However, covariates may be correlated with each other (collinearity). Correlated variables share information. In fitting a model to the data, the computer is instructed to allocate the information shared between 2 variables to one variable or the other. The computer does this using information from within the sample. Because such information will change from one sample to another, the estimates of the adjusted treatment effects (typical ES and covariate ES) are unstable and difficult to replicate.

The bottom line is that covariates proposed a priori should always have strong rationale and justification and should be as few in number and as noncorrelated as possible. Often the best choice is to ignore covariates and to test and estimate overall ES and then to explore possible moderators of treatment response (ie, baseline variables for which covariate ES differs for different covariate values).[5] Subsequent hypothesis-testing studies can focus on those particular covariates that moderate treatment response.

Clearly, researchers bear the primary responsibility for the veracity of the findings they report. Post hoc hypothesis testing should not lead to conclusions. Instead, hypothesis-generating (exploratory) studies on the same data can provide rationale and justification for future hypothesis-testing studies. An interpretable ES and its confidence interval should be presented with each P value.[6,7] There should be no surprise when some statistically significant results (even with $P = 10^{-10}$) are of no clinical or practical significance. Tests that are not statistically significant should be regarded as indicative of poorly justified, designed, or executed hypothesis-testing studies, not as proof of the null hypothesis. Knowing and checking the assumptions made in any model is essential (eg, absence of interactions in ANCOVA models) and a clear interpretation of each parameter tested or estimated (such as overall ES vs typical ES vs covariate ES in an RCT) should be presented.

Journal editors and peer reviewers provide an additional level of protection against false findings in the literature. They should be sensitive to the problems of post hoc testing and refrain from suggesting post hoc hypotheses, such as inclusion of covariates or outcomes the researchers had not considered a priori. They should insist on ESs and confidence intervals that can be interpreted by the intended readers of the report. Finally, they should be alert to statistical errors justified by "But that's the way everyone does it." (eg, ANCOVA to adjust for multiple, interacting, and collinear variables).

We cannot eliminate false findings with such efforts; however, we can get the percentage of false findings closer to the conventional 5%.

Acknowledgment

The following disclosures were reported at the time this original article was first published.

Conflict of Interest Disclosures: None reported.

References

1. Ioannidis JPA. Contradicted and initially stronger effects in highly cited clinical research. *JAMA*. 2005;294(2):218-228. Medline:16014596

2. Ioannidis JPA. Why most published research findings are false. *PLoS Med.* 2005;2(8):e124. Medline:16060722

3. Kraemer HC, Kupfer DJ. Size of treatment effects and their importance to clinical research and practice. *Biol Psychiatry.* 2006;59(11):990-996. Medline:16368078

4. Kraemer HC, Blasey CM. Centring in regression analyses: a strategy to prevent errors in statistical inference. *Int J Methods Psychiatr Res.* 2004;13(3):141-151. Medline:15297898

5. Kraemer HC, Frank E, Kupfer DJ. Moderators of treatment outcomes: clinical, research, and policy importance. *JAMA.* 2006;296(10):1286-1289. Medline:16968853

6. Grissom RJ, Kim JJ. *Effect Sizes for Research: Univariate and Multivariate Applications.* New York, NY: Routledge; 2012.

7. Cumming G. *Understanding the New Statistics: Effect Sizes, Confidence Intervals, and Meta-analysis.* New York, NY: Routledge; 2012.

Treatment Effects in Multicenter Randomized Clinical Trials

Stephen J. Senn, PhD, and
Roger J. Lewis, MD, PhD

IN THIS CHAPTER

Estimating Treatment Effects in Multicenter Clinical Trials

Why Are Differences Between Centers Considered When Estimating Treatment Effects?

How Are Center Effects Incorporated into Estimates of Treatment Effects?

Limitations of Estimates of Treatment Effects From Multicenter Clinical Trials

How Were the Multicenter Data Analyzed in the Study by Dodick et al?

How Should the Results From This Study Be Interpreted?

This JAMA Guide to Statistics and Methods discusses analytical approaches to accounting for differences in treatment effect by study center when randomized trials enroll patients and administer interventions at multiple sites.

It is common for treatments to be evaluated in clinical trials that involve many sites or centers, primarily because one center rarely can enroll sufficient numbers of patients to complete the trial.[1] The use of multiple clinical sites introduces complexity because outcomes at different sites may be systematically different, eg, due to differences in patient populations, ancillary treatment practices, or other factors. Thus, appropriate statistical analyses of multicenter clinical trials consider these center effects to yield a better understanding of the overall mean treatment effect and the variability in treatment effects and patient outcomes among sites.[1]

In an article in *JAMA*, Dodick et al[2] published the results of a clinical trial that compared migraine prevention by 2 different dosing regimens of fremanezumab vs placebo. The number of migraine days were recorded during a 28-day baseline period and a 3-month treatment period. The primary outcome for the study was the change from baseline in the mean number of monthly migraine days during treatment. The 875 participating patients were recruited from 123 centers in 9 countries. Using a primary analysis that accounted for each patient's mean number of migraines during the baseline period,[2,3] treatment, country (US vs non-US), and other factors, the authors reported a difference with monthly dosing vs placebo of −1.5 days (95% CI, −2.01 to −0.93 days; $P < .001$) and with single higher dosing vs placebo of −1.3 days (95% CI, −1.79 to −0.72 days; $P < .001$). They also conducted a post hoc sensitivity analysis that accounted for effects of the specific country of enrollment.[2]

ESTIMATING TREATMENT EFFECTS IN MULTICENTER CLINICAL TRIALS

Why Are Differences Between Centers Considered When Estimating Treatment Effects?

The goals of the statistical analysis of a multicenter clinical trial include providing a valid estimate of the treatment effect (ie, the mean difference in outcomes between patients treated in the 2 groups) and understanding and quantifying the remaining uncertainty or precision in the estimated treatment effect.[1] Patients treated at different centers may differ in their overall prognoses but experience the same relative benefit of a treatment compared with standard care. Alternatively, patients at different centers may differ in both their overall prognoses and in the treatment effect. Only the first case is considered in this article.

The randomization of patients to treatments in multicenter trials is usually stratified by center to achieve balance in the numbers of patients receiving each treatment within each center and, in what follows, it is assumed this has been done.[4] Balance improves the statistical efficiency of the trial, increasing precision in the estimation of treatment effects given a particular sample size. It also reduces the risk in modestly sized trials that chance imbalance in treatment allocation at centers with smaller numbers of patients results in a bias if that center has better or worse outcomes on average than other centers.[1,4]

Center effects, including systematic differences in outcomes between patients enrolled in different centers, have the potential to affect the estimate of the treatment effect (eg, if patients vary in severity of illness from center to center, any imbalance in treatment allocation within centers could affect the estimate of the treatment effect). However, a potentially more important and less well-appreciated effect of differences between centers is on the uncertainty or the precision in the estimate of the treatment effect. Even when stratified randomization is used successfully to achieve balance between groups across centers,[4] the resulting confidence intervals (CIs) and P values can change substantially depending on whether the center effect is included in the statistical model used to estimate the treatment effect, potentially affecting the overall interpretation of the clinical trial result.[1]

The uncertainty in the estimate of the treatment effect is defined by the variability in the estimates that would be obtained, hypothetically, if equivalent multicenter clinical trials were independently repeated many times. There are two distinct ways that such repetition might be conducted. First, the same centers might be used but the random treatment allocation (eg, which treatment is assigned to each patient in sequence) would be changed from repetition to repetition, maintaining stratification to balance treatments within center each time. Second, different centers could also be used for each trial, selected from a larger pool of centers with similar characteristics. Only the first approach is considered here, which addresses the uncertainty in the treatment effect obtained from the original trial with those particular centers. The second type of repetition, with variation in the participating centers, would address a more general type of uncertainty—including uncertainty due to difference in the treatment effect among centers—that is beyond the scope of this discussion.

Suppose the same multicenter clinical trial results were analyzed using 2 different statistical models. First, a simple model is used that does not include a term for center effect, so all variability is assumed to arise only from the inherent variation among patients but without any systematic differences from center to center. Second, a more appropriate model is used that separates the variability arising from differences among patients within centers from the variability arising from differences among centers. The uncertainty in the treatment effect obtained from the 2 models, representing the variability in the mean treatment effect that would be seen in the repeated equivalent trials, and reflected in the width of the 95% CI around the estimated treatment effect, will be different. The first model, without the center effect, will overestimate the variability in the estimated mean treatment effect because it assumes that all variability is an inherent characteristic of the patient population. This will result in an overly wide CI and decreased statistical power (the overly wide CI will be more likely to include a zero or null treatment effect, equivalent to a nonstatistically significant P value). In contrast, the model incorporating the center effect will correctly recognize that some of the variability is a characteristic of patients within each center and some is a characteristic of differences in populations enrolled at different centers, and eliminate the latter. This will reduce the estimated variability for patients within each center, resulting in a narrower, more accurate CI and increased power.

How Are Center Effects Incorporated into Estimates of Treatment Effects?

Various statistical models can be used to account for center effects when estimating the treatment effect. The simplest way is to consider centers as fixed effects—each center is associated with its own effect on patient outcomes—in an appropriate model. This approach can be used in linear models, survival analysis, or logistic regression for dichotomous outcomes and, in each case, allows for the greater similarity among treatment outcomes within a center compared with across centers.[5]

LIMITATIONS OF ESTIMATES OF TREATMENT EFFECTS FROM MULTICENTER CLINICAL TRIALS

It is often stated that the purpose of enrolling patients at multiple centers is to increase the external generalizability of the trial results; however, centers are typically selected for factors (eg, academic affiliations, large patient volumes) intended to speed enrollment and that limits the generalizability of results to other clinical settings. Thus, even estimates from multicenter clinical trials may lack external validity when applied to qualitatively different practice settings.

Each of the models used to adjust for center effects has underlying assumptions regarding how the differences between centers affect patient outcomes or, similarly, how patients within centers are more similar on average than patients between centers. If these assumptions do not hold true, then the results of the analyses may be biased or estimates of uncertainty may be incorrect, affecting the statistical significance of results or the width of CIs.

HOW WERE THE MULTICENTER DATA ANALYZED IN THE STUDY BY DODICK ET AL?

The 875 participating patients were recruited in 123 centers in 9 countries and randomized in a 1:1:1 ratio to the 3 treatments.[2] Patient randomization was stratified by sex, country, and baseline preventive medication used. The primary analysis used analysis of covariance[3] to adjust for the influence of the 3 stratification factors, the number of episodes occurring in the baseline period, and the number of years since first onset of migraine. The effect of country was simplified by reducing this variable to only 2 groups: US vs non-US. To more completely evaluate the potential "country effect" (analogous to the "center effect" described above), the authors conducted a "post hoc sensitivity analysis using a mixed-effects model that included country instead of region as a random effect."[2] The results of this analysis are presented in eTable 4 in the article's Supplement 3, demonstrating a difference from placebo with monthly dosing of −1.5 (95% CI, −2.00 to −0.93) and a difference with the single higher dose of −1.3 (95% CI, −1.79 to −0.72).[2]

These results are almost identical to those of the primary analysis, suggesting that either there was little effect of country on the results or that all effect of the country was captured by simply distinguishing US sites from non-US sites.

HOW SHOULD THE RESULTS FROM THIS STUDY BE INTERPRETED?

The treatment effects estimated by Dodick et al,[2] and the associated CIs, were nearly identical regardless of whether the effect of location of enrollment was dichotomized as within or outside of the US, or captured as the country of enrollment, with 9 possibilities. The consistency suggests that the variability in outcomes associated with the location of enrollment is either small or captured similarly by both models. The results from the model adjusting for the country of enrollment is the preferred estimate, because there is no harm in the adjustment if the country-to-country variability is unimportant and the adjustment is critically important for correctly determining the uncertainty in the estimate of the mean treatment effect if the country-to-country variability turns out to be substantial. In both the primary and post hoc sensitivity analyses, the models partitioned the variability in patient outcomes between that associated with the location of enrollment (US vs non-US or by country) and that associated with differences between patients, resulting in more accurate CIs than would have obtained had these effects not been included.

Acknowledgment

The following disclosures were reported at the time this original article was first published in *JAMA*.

Conflict of Interest Disclosures: Dr Senn reported serving as a consultant to the pharmaceutical industry.

References

1. Senn S. Some controversies in planning and analysing multi-centre trials. *Stat Med.* 1998;17(15-16):1753-1765. Medline:9749445 doi:10.1002/(SICI)1097-0258(19980815/30)17:15/16<1753::AID-SIM977>3.0.CO;2-X
2. Dodick DW, Silberstein SD, Bigal ME, et al. Effect of fremanezumab compared with placebo for prevention of episodic migraine: a randomized clinical trial. *JAMA.* 2018;319(19):1999-2008. Medline:29800211 doi:10.1001/jama.2018.4853
3. Vickers AJ, Altman DG. Statistics notes: analysing controlled trials with baseline and follow up measurements. *BMJ.* 2001;323(7321):1123-1124. Medline:11701584 doi:10.1136/bmj.323.7321.1123
4. Broglio K. Randomization in clinical trials: permuted blocks and stratification. *JAMA.* 2018;319(21):2223-2224. Medline:29872845 doi:10.1001/jama.2018.6360
5. Meurer WJ, Lewis RJ. Cluster randomized trials: evaluating treatments applied to groups. *JAMA.* 2015;313(20):2068-2069. Medline:26010636 doi:10.1001/jama.2015.5199

The Propensity Score

Jason S. Haukoos, MD, MSc, and
Roger J. Lewis, MD, PhD

IN THIS CHAPTER

Use of the Method

Why Were Propensity Methods Used?

What Are the Limitations of Propensity Score Methods?

Why Did the Authors Use Propensity Methods?

How Should the Findings Be Interpreted?

What Caveats Should the Reader Consider When Assessing the Results of Propensity Analyses?

This JAMA Guide to Statistics and Methods discusses the use of propensity scores as a way to reduce bias in estimates of treatment effect when randomized trials are not feasible.

Many observational studies analyze data to estimate the effect of a treatment on patient outcomes. For example, in a study by Rozé et al,[1] a large observational data set was analyzed to estimate the relationship between early echocardiographic screening for patent ductus arteriosus and mortality among preterm infants. The authors compared mortality rates of 847 infants who were screened for patent ductus arteriosus and 666 who were not. The 2 infant groups were dissimilar; infants who were screened were younger, more likely female, and less likely to have received corticosteroids. The authors used propensity score matching to create 605 matched infant pairs from the original cohort to adjust for these differences. In another study by Huybrechts et al,[2] the Medicaid Analytic eXtract data set was analyzed to estimate the association between antidepressant use during pregnancy and persistent pulmonary hypertension of the newborn. The authors included 3 789 330 women, of which 128 950 had used antidepressants. Women who used antidepressants were different from those who had not, with differences in age, race/ethnicity, chronic illnesses, obesity, tobacco use, and health care use. The authors adjusted for these differences using, in part, the technique of propensity score stratification.

USE OF THE METHOD

Why Were Propensity Methods Used?

Many considerations influence the selection of one therapy over another. In many settings, more than one therapeutic approach is commonly used. In routine clinical practice, patients receiving one treatment will tend to be different from those receiving another, eg, if one treatment is thought to be better tolerated by elderly patients or more effective for patients who are more seriously ill. This results in a correlation—or confounding—between patient characteristics that affect outcomes and the choice of therapy (often called "confounding by indication"). If observational data obtained from routine clinical practice are examined to compare the outcomes of patients treated with different therapies, the observed difference will be the result of both differing patient characteristics and treatment choice, making it difficult to delineate the true effect of one treatment vs another.

The effect of an intervention is best assessed by randomizing treatment assignments so that, on average, the patients are similar in the 2 treatment groups. This allows a direct assessment of the effect of the intervention on outcome. In observational studies, randomization is not possible, so investigators must adjust for differences between groups to obtain valid estimates of the associations between the treatments being compared and the outcomes of interest.[3] Multivariable statistical methods are often used to estimate this association while adjusting for confounding.

Propensity score methods are used to reduce the bias in estimating treatment effects and allow investigators to reduce the likelihood of confounding when analyzing nonrandomized, observational data. The propensity score is the probability that a patient would receive the treatment of interest, based on characteristics of the patient, treating clinician, and clinical environment.[4] Such probabilities can be estimated using multivariable statistical methods (eg, logistic regression), in which case the treatment of interest is the dependent variable and the characteristics of the patient, prescribing clinician, and clinical setting are the predictors. Investigators estimate these probabilities, ranging from 0 to 1, for each patient in the study population. These probabilities—the propensity scores—are then used to adjust for differences between groups. In biomedical studies, propensity scores are often used to compare treatments, but they can also be used to estimate the relationship between any nonrandomized factor, such as the exposure to a toxin or infectious agent and the outcome of interest.

There are 4 general ways propensity scores are used. The most common is *propensity score matching*, which involves assembling 2 groups of study participants, one group that received the treatment of interest and the other that did not, while matching individuals with similar or identical propensity scores.[1] The analysis of a propensity score–matched sample can then approximate that of a randomized trial by directly comparing outcomes between individuals who received the treatment of interest and those who did not, using methods that account for the paired nature of the data.[5]

The second approach is *stratification* on the propensity score.[4] This technique involves separating study participants into distinct groups or strata based on their propensity scores. Five strata are commonly used, although increasing the number can reduce the likelihood of bias. The association between the treatment of interest and the outcome of interest is estimated within each stratum or pooled across strata to provide an overall estimate of the relationship between treatment and outcome. This technique relies on the notion that individuals within each stratum are more similar to each other than individuals in general; thus, their outcomes can be directly compared.

The third approach is *covariate adjustment* using the propensity score. For this approach, a separate multivariable model is developed, after the propensity score model, in which the study outcome serves as the dependent variable and the treatment group and propensity score serve as predictor variables. This allows the investigator to estimate the outcome associated with the treatment of interest while adjusting for the probability of receiving that treatment, thus reducing confounding.

The fourth approach is *inverse probability of treatment weighting* using the propensity score.[6] In this instance, propensity scores are used to calculate statistical weights for each individual to create a sample in which the distribution of potential confounding factors is independent of exposure, allowing an unbiased estimate of the relationship between treatment and outcome.[7]

Alternative strategies—other than use of propensity scores—for adjusting for baseline differences between groups in observational studies include matching on baseline characteristics, performing stratified analyses, or using multivariable statistical methods to adjust for confounders. Propensity score methods are often more practical or statistically more efficient than these methods, in part because propensity score methods can substantially limit the number of predictor variables used in the final analysis. Propensity score methods generally allow many more variables to be included in the propensity score model, which increases the ability of these approaches to effectively adjust for confounding, than could be incorporated directly into a multivariable analysis of the study outcome.

What Are the Limitations of Propensity Score Methods?

The propensity score for each study participant is based on the available measured patient characteristics, and unadjusted confounding may still exist if unmeasured factors influenced treatment selection. Therefore, using fewer variables in the propensity score model reduces the likelihood of effectively adjusting for confounding.

Although propensity score matching may be used to assemble comparable study groups, the quality of matching depends on the quality of the propensity score model, which in turn depends on the quality and size of the available data and how the model was built. Conventional modeling methods (eg, variable selection, use of interactions, regression diagnostics, etc) are not typically recommended for the development of propensity score models. For example, propensity score models may optimally include a larger number of predictor variables.

Why Did the Authors Use Propensity Methods?

In the reports by Rozé et al[1] and Huybrechts et al,[2] both of whom used propensity score methods because their data were observational, the treatments of interest (ie, screening by echocardiography and use of antidepressants in pregnancy) were not randomly allocated, and important characteristics differed between groups. Direct comparisons of the outcomes between treated and untreated groups would have likely resulted in significantly biased estimates. Instead, use of propensity score matching and stratification enabled the investigators to create study groups that were similar to one another and more accurately measure the relationship between treatment and outcome.

How Should the Findings Be Interpreted?

Given the observational nature of these studies, the fact that individuals in the treated and untreated groups were dissimilar, and the goal of accurately estimating the association between treatment and outcome, the investigators had to adjust for differences in the treatment groups. Use of propensity score methods, whether by matching or stratification, resulted in less biased estimates than if such methods were not used. Even though observational data cannot definitely establish causal relationships or determine treatment effects as rigorously as a randomized clinical trial, assuming propensity score methods are properly used and the sample size is sufficiently large, these methods may provide a useful approximation of the likely effect of a treatment. This approach is particularly valuable for clinical situations in which randomized trials are not feasible or are unlikely to be conducted.

WHAT CAVEATS SHOULD THE READER CONSIDER WHEN ASSESSING THE RESULTS OF PROPENSITY ANALYSES?

The studies by Rozé et al[1] and Huybrechts et al[2] used propensity score matching and propensity score stratification, respectively. Although both methods are more valid in terms of balancing study groups than simple matching or stratification based on baseline characteristics, they vary in their ability to minimize bias. In general, propensity score matching minimizes bias to a greater extent than propensity score stratification. Assessment of balance between the groups, after use of propensity score methods, is important to allow readers to assess the comparability of patient groups.

Although no single standard approach exists to assess balance, comparing characteristics between treated and untreated patients typically begins with comparing summary statistics (eg, means or proportions) and the entire distributions of observed characteristics. For propensity score—matched samples, standardized differences (ie, differences divided by pooled standard deviations) are often used and, although no threshold is universally accepted, a standard difference less than 0.1 is often considered negligible. Assessing for balance provides a general sense for how well matching or stratification occurred and thus the extent to which the results are likely to be valid. Unfortunately, balance can only be demonstrated for patient characteristics that were measured in the study. Differences could still exist between patient groups that were not measured, resulting in biased results.

Acknowledgment

The following disclosures were reported at the time this original article was first published in *JAMA*.

Conflict of Interest Disclosures: None reported.

Funding/Support: Dr Haukoos is supported, in part, by grants R01AI106057 from the National Institute of Allergy and Infectious Diseases (NIAID) and R01HS021749 from the Agency for Healthcare Research and Quality (AHRQ).

Disclaimer: The views expressed herein are those of the authors and do not necessarily represent the views of NIAID, the National Institutes of Health, or AHRQ.

References

1. Rozé JC, Cambonie G, Marchand-Martin L, et al. Hemodynamic EPIPAGE 2 Study Group. Association between early screening for patent ductus arteriosus and in-hospital mortality among extremely preterm infants. *JAMA*. 2015;313(24):2441-2448. Medline:26103028

2. Huybrechts KF, Bateman BT, Palmsten K, et al. Antidepressant use late in pregnancy and risk of persistent pulmonary hypertension of the newborn. *JAMA*. 2015;313(21):2142-2151. Medline:26034955

3. Greenland S, Pearl J, Robins JM. Causal diagrams for epidemiologic research. *Epidemiology*. 1999;10(1):37-48. Medline:9888278

4. Rosenbaum PR, Rubin DB. The central role of the propensity score in observational studies for causal effects. *Biometrika*. 1983;70:41-55.

5. Austin PC. An introduction to propensity score methods for reducing the effects of confounding in observational studies. *Multivariate Behav Res*. 2011;46(3):399-424. Medline:21818162

6. Schaffer JM, Singh SK, Reitz BA, Zamanian RT, Mallidi HR. Single- vs double-lung transplantation in patients with chronic obstructive pulmonary disease and idiopathic pulmonary fibrosis since the implementation of lung allocation based on medical need. *JAMA*. 2015;313(9):936-948. Medline:25734735

7. Robins JM, Hernán MA, Brumback B. Marginal structural models and causal inference in epidemiology. *Epidemiology*. 2000;11(5):550-560. Medline: 10955408

Using Free-Response Receiver Operating Characteristic Curves to Assess the Accuracy of Machine Diagnosis of Cancer

Chaya S. Moskowitz, PhD

IN THIS CHAPTER

Why Are FROC Curves Used?

How Are FROC Curves Constructed?

What Are the Limitations of FROC Curves?

How Should the FROC Curves Be Interpreted in This Study?

Caveats to Consider When Looking at FROC Curves

This JAMA Guide to Statistics and Methods discusses the use of free-response receiver operating characteristic curves to test the accuracy of computer algorithms to detect the localization of disease on pathology slide images.

In a machine learning study, Ehteshami Bejnordi et al[1] evaluated and compared the ability of 32 computer algorithms to identify the presence and location of metastatic lesions on pathology slide images of sentinel axillary lymph nodes from women with breast cancer. The authors used free-response receiver operating characteristic (FROC) curve analysis to assess diagnostic and localization accuracy. They found that the best algorithm performed similarly to a pathologist working without a time constraint (Figure 11).

Free-response operating characteristic analysis assesses the ability of a medical test to identify abnormalities on an image. Examples include identifying tumors in radiographs or foci of malignancy on histological slides. There are similarities between FROC analysis and the more commonly used receiver operating characteristic (ROC) curve analysis.[2,3] Conventional ROC curves, however, evaluate the accuracy of a test for detecting the presence or absence of disease but do not evaluate whether a test correctly identifies the location.

WHY ARE FROC CURVES USED?

When trying to characterize how well a test determines the location of disease and decide if one test is better than another at this task, it is necessary to account for variations in the appearances of the lesions and the fact that lesions may be located anywhere on an image. One approach that can be used for this purpose is called free-response analysis, meaning that a person or machine reading the image assesses the entire image, marks the portions of the image that look abnormal and may be diseased, and makes a determination regarding the probability that

FIGURE 11

FROC Curves of the Top 5 Performing Algorithms vs Pathologist WOTC for the Metastases Identification Task (Task 1) From the CAMELYON16 Competition

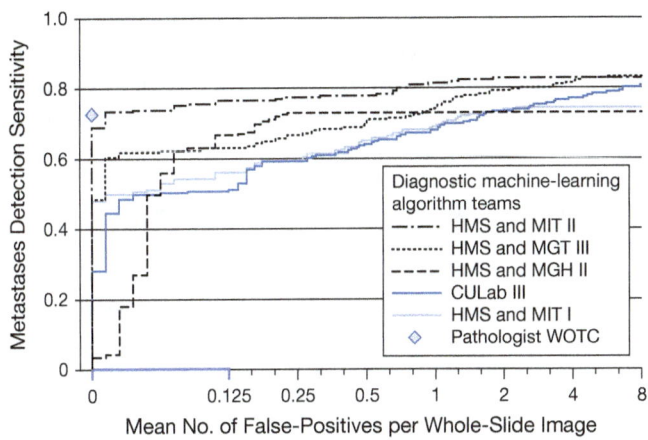

CAMELYON16 indicates Cancer Metastases in Lymph Nodes Challenge 2016; CULab, Chinese University Lab; FROC, free-response receiver operator characteristic; HMS, Harvard Medical School; MGH, Massachusetts General Hospital; MIT, Massachusetts Institute of Technology; WOTC, without time constraint. The range on the x-axis is linear between 0 and 0.125 (blue) and base 2 logarithmic scale between 0.125 and 8. Teams were those organized in the CAMELYON16 competition. Task 1 was measured on the 129 whole-slide images in the test data set, of which 49 contained metastatic regions. The pathologist did not produce any false-positives and achieved a true-positive fraction of 0.724 for detecting and localizing metastatic regions.

the marked areas represent disease. A single image may have several locations with the disease entity.

When performing this sort of analysis, a rating (either continuous or ordinal) is given regarding the likelihood that there is disease in any marked spot. Lesions identified as pathological by the person or machine assessing the image may or may not correspond to truly diseased areas previously identified by some reference standard. Areas that raters mark that have disease are considered true positives and areas they mark in which disease is not present are considered false positives. The marked locations do not need to overlie the true diseased locations but they must be reasonably close using a proximity criterion defined by the investigators. False negatives occur when a rater fails to mark a lesion.

Because the number of lesions is known, the true-positive fraction (TPF) can be calculated by dividing the number of areas identified (ie, marked) by the rater as having disease by the total number of areas on the images known to have disease. This is equivalent to the sensitivity of the test. The number of false-positive marks is counted but there is no true negative equivalent in this analysis precluding the calculation of a false-positive fraction. Consequently, the false-positive rate (FPR) is calculated as the mean number of false-positive locations per image.

HOW ARE FROC CURVES CONSTRUCTED?

Ehteshami Bejnordi et al[1] constructed FROC curves by requiring the algorithms to mark areas suspected of having disease and to assign ratings between 0 and 1 to these marked areas. Marked areas were first classified as true positives or false positives depending on whether the identified locations were within 75 μm of lesions outlined on the reference standard created by 2 expert pathologists using immunohistochemistry. The ratings were then compared with various thresholds to characterize the accuracy of the ratings relative to the thresholds. For any given threshold, c, the FPR at this threshold, FPR(c), was defined as the total number of false-positive locations rated higher than c divided by the number of slides without lesions. It has been recommended that the FPR only be estimated among images without disease because the tendencies of raters to incorrectly mark nondiseased areas on images containing disease may be very different than their tendencies to incorrectly identify nondiseased areas on images in which no disease is present.

The distribution of the ratings assigned to the locations is likely to be different as well.[4] The TPF at c, TPF(c), was defined as the total number of true-positive locations with ratings higher than c divided by the total number of lesions on all the slides. c was varied across the values of the rating scale, and the resultant FROC curve plotted the pairs of FPR(c) and TPF(c) for all values of c. The points were connected by straight lines.

WHAT ARE THE LIMITATIONS OF FROC CURVES?

In ROC curve analysis, the diagonal 45° line characterizes a test that cannot distinguish between diseased and nondiseased states. The line serves as a benchmark for judging how well a test works. There is no analogous, simply defined line for FROC curves. Thus, it can be more difficult to infer from FROC curves how well a test is performing. Moreover, because the FPR is not a fraction and can take values greater than 1, the FROC curve may extend endlessly along the horizontal axis.

An integral component in calculating an FROC curve is the proximity criterion. Choosing a different distance for this criterion may result in a different FROC curve.[4,5] Furthermore, the decision regarding how to handle multiple findings close to a single lesion affects the FROC curve.[6] In addition, analysis of FROC data can be complicated because there are many sources of variability, and appropriately accounting for these may be difficult.[4,6]

HOW SHOULD THE FROC CURVES BE INTERPRETED IN THIS STUDY?

The FROC curves in Figure 1 and eFigure 4 in the study by Ehteshami Bejnordi et al facilitate visualization of how well the automated computer algorithms performed across the spectrum of the rating scale when compared with the criterion standard. One algorithm performed better than the others at all thresholds. At each average FPR per slide, the TPF was greater for the HMS-MIT II team (Harvard Medical School and Massachusetts Institute of Technology) than for other algorithms. In addition to looking at the entire FROC curve, the operating characteristics can be explored at particular points of interest. Examining certain TPFs at specific FPRs allows readers to judge if the algorithms performed well enough to be useful in clinical practice. For instance, if an average of at most 1 false positive per slide was determined to be acceptable, team HMS-MIT II had a TPF of approximately 0.81 (see eTable 4 in the article's supplement). At the operating point of having 1 false positive per slide, the TPF of 0.81 means that team HMS-MIT II identified 81% of all metastases and failed to identify 19% of them.

CAVEATS TO CONSIDER WHEN LOOKING AT FROC CURVES

FROC curves depend on the sample chosen and do not necessarily generalize to other populations or sets of cases with different distributions of disease locations.[5] While several numerical indices have been proposed for summarizing FROC curve results as a simple number,[5,7] none of them have been universally accepted as has the area under the curve used to summarize an ROC curve. Ehteshami Bejnordi et al identified specific FPRs of interest and took the mean value of TPFs at those FPRs as a summary measure.

Acknowledgment

The following disclosures were reported at the time this original article was first published in *JAMA*.

Conflict of Interest Disclosures: None reported.

Funding/Support: This work was supported by core grant P30 CA008748 to Memorial Sloan Kettering Cancer Center from the National Cancer Institute.

Role of the Funder/Sponsor: The National Cancer Institute had no role in the preparation, review, or approval of the manuscript; and decision to submit the manuscript for publication.

References

1. Ehteshami Bejnordi B, Veta M, van Diest PJ, et al. CAMELYON16 Consortium. Diagnostic assessment of deep learning algorithms for detection of lymph nodes metastases in women with breast cancer. *JAMA*. 2017;318(22): 2199-2210. doi:10.1001/jama.2017.14585
2. Alba AC, Agoritsas T, Walsh M, et al. Discrimination and calibration of clinical prediction models: Users' Guides to the Medical Literature. *JAMA*. 2017;318(14):1377-1384. Medline:29049590
3. Hanley JA. Receiver operating characteristic (ROC) methodology: the state of the art. *Crit Rev Diagn Imaging*. 1989;29(3):307-335. Medline:2667567
4. Chakraborty DP. A brief history of free-response receiver operating characteristic paradigm data analysis. *Acad Radiol*. 2013;20(7):915-919. Medline:23583665
5. Zou KH, Liu A, Bandos AI, Ohno-Machado L, Rockette HE. *Statistical Evaluation of Diagnostic Performance: Topics in ROC Analysis*. Boca Raton, FL: Chapman & Hall; 2012.
6. Gur D, Rockette HE. Performance assessments of diagnostic systems under the FROC paradigm: experimental, analytical, and results interpretation issues. *Acad Radiol*. 2008;15(10):1312-1315. Medline:18790403
7. Bandos AI, Rockette HE, Song T, Gur D. Area under the free-response ROC curve (FROC) and a related summary index. *Biometrics*. 2009;65(1):247-256. Medline:18479482

# Random-Effects Meta-analysis: Summarizing Evidence With Caveats

Stylianos Serghiou, MD, and
Steven N. Goodman, MD, PhD

IN THIS CHAPTER

Why Is Random-Effects Meta-analysis Used?

Description of Random-Effects Meta-analysis

Why Did the Authors Use Random-Effects Meta-analysis?

What Are Limitations of a Random-Effects Meta-analysis?

Caveats to Consider When Assessing the Results of a Random-Effects Meta-analysis

How Should the Results of a Random-Effects Meta-analysis Be Interpreted in This Particular Study?

This JAMA Guide to Statistics and Methods explains the difference between fixed and random effects in treatment effect estimates, and the rationale for using random-effects meta-analysis to determine treatment effects across randomized trials conducted in heterogeneous patients and settings.

Questions involving medical therapies are often studied more than once. For example, numerous clinical trials have been conducted comparing opioids with placebos or nonopioid analgesics in the treatment of chronic pain. In a study published in *JAMA*, Busse et al[1] evaluated the evidence on opioid efficacy from 96 randomized clinical trials and, as part of that work, used random-effects meta-analysis to synthesize results from 42 randomized clinical trials on the difference in pain reduction among patients taking opioids vs placebo using a 10-cm visual analog scale (Figure 2 in Busse et al[1]). Meta-analysis is the process of quantitatively combining study results into a single summary estimate and is a foundational tool for evidence-based medicine. Random-effects meta-analysis is the most common approach.

WHY IS RANDOM-EFFECTS META-ANALYSIS USED?

Each study evaluating the effect of a treatment provides its own answer in terms of an observed or estimated effect size. Opioids reduced pain by 0.54 cm more than placebo on a visual analog scale in 1 study[2]; this was the observed effect size and represents the best estimate from that study of the true opioid effect. The true effect is the underlying benefit of opioid treatment if it could be measured perfectly, and is a single value that cannot directly be known.

If a particular study was replicated with new patients in the same setting multiple times, the observed treatment effects would vary by chance even though the true effects would be the same in each. The belief that the true effect was the same in each study is called the fixed-effect assumption, whereby the fixed effect is the common, unknown true effect underlying each replication. A meta-analysis making the fixed-effect assumption is called a fixed-effect meta-analysis. The corresponding fixed-effect estimate of the treatment effect is a weighted average of the individual study estimates and is always more precise (ie, it has a narrower confidence interval [CI] than that of any individual study, making the estimate appear closer to the true value than any individual study).

However, medical studies addressing the same question are typically not exact replications and they can use different types of medication or interventions for different amounts of time, at different intensities, within different populations, and have differently measured outcomes.[3] Differences in study characteristics reduce the confidence that each study is actually estimating the same true effect. The alternative assumption is that the true effects being estimated are different from each other or heterogeneous. In statistical jargon, this is called the random-effects assumption. The plural in effects implies there is more than 1 true effect and random implies that the reasons the true effects differ are unknown.

A random-effects assumption is less restrictive than a fixed-effect assumption and reflects the variation or heterogeneity in the true effects estimated by each trial. This usually results in a more realistic estimate of the uncertainty in the overall treatment effect with larger CIs than would be obtained if a fixed effect was assumed. A random-effects model can also be used to provide differing, study-specific estimates of the treatment effect in each trial, something that cannot be done under the fixed-effect assumption.

DESCRIPTION OF RANDOM-EFFECTS META-ANALYSIS

In a random-effects meta-analysis, the statistical model estimates multiple parameters. First, the model estimates a separate treatment effect for each trial, representing the estimate of the true effect for the trial. The assumption that the true effects can vary from trial to trial is the foundation for a random-effects meta-analysis. Second, the model estimates an overall treatment effect, representing an average of the true effects over the group of studies included. Third, the model estimates the variability or degree of heterogeneity in the true treatment effects across trials. Compared with a fixed-effect estimate, the random-effects estimate for the overall effect is more influenced by smaller studies and has a wider CI, reflecting not just the chance variation that is reflected in a fixed-effect estimate, but also the variation among the true effects.[4] In the report by Busse et al,[1] the random-effects average opioid benefit was −0.69 cm (95% CI, −0.82 to −0.56 cm).

Whether the variability observed in the estimates of treatment effect is consistent with chance variation alone is reflected in statistical measures of heterogeneity, often expressed as an I^2, the percentage of total variation in the random-effects estimate due to heterogeneity in the true underlying treatment effects. An I^2 value greater than 50% to 75% is considered large.[5] Busse et al[1] report an I^2 of 70.4%, reflecting the marked variation among studies, which is also demonstrated by nonoverlapping CIs around some individual treatment estimates.

A more natural heterogeneity measure is the standard deviation of the true effects, often denoted as τ. A τ of 0.35 cm can be derived from the data in Figure 2 in the article by Busse et al.[1] Given the overall random-effects estimate of −0.69 cm, this means that the true effects in individual studies could vary over the range of −0.69 cm $\pm 2\tau$ or −1.39 cm to 0.01 cm, namely a true benefit in some studies roughly twice as large as the average and no benefit in some others. This reflects the display provided in the study by Busse et al[1] in which 10 of 42 studies estimated a benefit larger than 1 cm, which was the minimum clinically important difference. Quantifying the variability in treatment effects among studies helps readers decide whether combining these results makes sense. Like the proverbial person said to be at normal average temperature with 1 foot in ice and the other in boiling water, the estimated average effect can be nonsensical if the true individual study effects are too variable.

WHY DID THE AUTHORS USE RANDOM-EFFECTS META-ANALYSIS?

Meta-analyses incorporate some uncertainties that mathematical summaries cannot reflect. A sensible approach is to use the statistical method least likely to overstate certainty almost regardless of perceptions or philosophy about true effects being fixed or random, which is why random-effects models are a frequent choice in meta-analyses.

The studies in the report by Busse et al[1] demonstrate substantial variability, being both qualitatively and quantitatively different. Tominaga et al[6] examined the effect of tapentadol extended release tablets in Japanese patients with either chronic osteoarthritic knee pain or lower back pain, whereas Simpson and Wlodarczyk[7] examined the effect of transdermal buprenorphine in Australian patients with diabetic peripheral neuropathic pain. These studies used different opioids to treat different sources of pain in culturally different populations that may assess pain differently; indeed, the variability in observed effects between the 2 studies suggests that the differences seen are probably beyond chance variation.

Taken together, these features provide substantial evidence that these studies are not examining the same effect, consistent with the random-effects assumption. Thus, a fixed effect is not plausible and a random-effects meta-analysis is the appropriate method.

WHAT ARE LIMITATIONS OF A RANDOM-EFFECTS META-ANALYSIS?

First, the random-effects model does not explain heterogeneity, it merely incorporates it. The standard recommendation is that researchers should attempt to reduce heterogeneity[8,9] by using subgroups of studies or a meta-regression; however, such methods represent exploratory data-dependent exercises and their results must be interpreted accordingly.

Second, there are many approaches to calculating the random-effects estimates. Although most produce similar estimates, the DerSimonian-Laird method is the most widely used and it produces CIs that are too narrow and P values that are too small when there are few studies (<10-15) and sizable heterogeneity; accordingly, this approach is not optimal in the setting of few studies and high heterogeneity and often may be contraindicated.[10]

Third, small studies more strongly influence estimates from random-effects than from fixed-effect models; in fact, the larger the heterogeneity, the larger their relative influence. If smaller studies are judged as more likely to be biased, this can be a substantial concern.

CAVEATS TO CONSIDER WHEN ASSESSING THE RESULTS OF A RANDOM-EFFECTS META-ANALYSIS

The overall summary effect of a random-effects meta-analysis is representative of the study-specific true effects without the estimate representing a true effect (ie, there may be no population of patients or interventions for which this summary value is true). This is why a random-effects meta-analysis should be interpreted with consideration of the qualitative and quantitative heterogeneity, particularly the range of effects calculated using $\pm 2 \times \tau$. If the range is too broad, or if I^2 exceeds 50% to 75%, the meta-analytic estimate might be too unrepresentative of the underlying effects, potentially obscuring important differences. Busse et al[1] assessed qualitative heterogeneity partly through their assessment of directness and judged it to be minimal, although that may not capture every dimension of importance.

Other caveats apply to all meta-analyses and include whether the analyses include all relevant studies, whether the studies are representative of the population of interest, whether study exclusions are justified, and whether study quality was adequately assessed. Sometimes heterogeneity reflects a mixture of diverse biases, with few of the studies properly estimating even their own true effects. Busse et al[1] addressed this by using a risk-of-bias assessment.

HOW SHOULD THE RESULTS OF A RANDOM-EFFECTS META-ANALYSIS BE INTERPRETED IN THIS PARTICULAR STUDY?

Three of 8 meta-analyses reported in Busse et al[1] (using 7 different outcome measures) have an I^2 of 50% or greater, and the meta-analysis we have been discussing that used the outcome of pain has an I^2 of 70.4%, reflecting conflict or a high degree of variability among studies. The meta-analysis by Busse et al[1] provided evidence against opioids increasing pain and suggested that opioids are generally likely to reduce chronic noncancer pain by a modest 0.69 cm more than placebo (less than the 1 cm minimum clinically important difference). However, in view of the amount of heterogeneity, it is possible that in some settings and patients, the benefit of opioids could be lesser or greater than this random-effects estimate. As such, physicians should consider this summary result with caution, and in conjunction with the effect from the subset of studies most relevant to the patients they need to treat.

Acknowledgment

The following disclosures were reported at the time this original article was first published in *JAMA*.

Conflict of Interest Disclosures: None reported.

References

1. Busse JW, Wang L, Kamaleldin M, et al. Opioids for chronic noncancer pain: a systematic review and meta-analysis. *JAMA*. 2018;320(23):2448-2460. doi:10.1001/jama.2018.18472

2. Wen W, Sitar S, Lynch SY, et al. A multicenter, randomized, double-blind, placebo-controlled trial to assess the efficacy and safety of single-entity, once-daily hydrocodone tablets in patients with uncontrolled moderate to severe chronic low back pain. *Expert Opin Pharmacother*. 2015;16(11): 1593-1606. Medline:26111544

3. Serghiou S, Patel CJ, Tan YY, et al. Field-wide meta-analyses of observational associations can map selective availability of risk factors and the impact of model specifications. *J Clin Epidemiol*. 2016;71:58-67. Medline:26415577

4. Nikolakopoulou A, Mavridis D, Salanti G. Demystifying fixed and random effects meta-analysis. *Evid Based Ment Health*. 2014;17(2):53-57. Medline:24692250

5. Higgins JP, Thompson SG, Deeks JJ, Altman DG. Measuring inconsistency in meta-analyses. *BMJ*. 2003;327(7414):557-560. Medline:12958120

6. Tominaga Y, Koga H, Uchida N, et al. Methodological issues in conducting pilot trials in chronic pain as randomized, double-blind, placebo-controlled studies. *Drug Res (Stuttg)*. 2016;66(7):363-370. Medline:27224908 doi:10.1055/s-0042-107669

7. Simpson RW, Wlodarczyk JH. Transdermal buprenorphine relieves neuropathic pain. *Diabetes Care*. 2016;39(9):1493-1500. Medline:27311495 doi:10.2337/dc16-0123

8. Thompson SG, Sharp SJ. Explaining heterogeneity in meta-analysis. *Stat Med*. 1999;18(20):2693-2708. Medline:10521860

9. Riley RD, Higgins JP, Deeks JJ. Interpretation of random effects meta-analyses. *BMJ*. 2011;342:d549. Medline:21310794

10. Cornell JE, Mulrow CD, Localio R, et al. Random-effects meta-analysis of inconsistent effects. *Ann Intern Med*. 2014;160(4):267-270. Medline: 24727843

Bayesian Hierarchical Models

Anna E. McGlothlin, PhD, and Kert Viele, PhD

IN THIS CHAPTER

Why Is a BHM Used?

What Are the Limitations of BHMs?

How Were BHMs Used in This Case?

How Should BHMs Be Interpreted?

This JAMA Guide to Statistics and Methods discusses the use, limitations, and interpretation of Bayesian hierarchical modeling, a statistical procedure that integrates information across multiple levels and uses prior information about likely treatment effects and their variability to estimate true vs random treatment effects.

Treatment effects will differ from one study to another evaluating similar therapies, both because of random variation between individual patients and owing to true differences that exist because of other differences, including inclusion criteria and temporal trends. The sources of variability have many levels; one level involves the random differences between individual patients, and another level involves the systematic differences that exist between studies. This multilevel or hierarchical information occurs in many research settings, such as in cluster-randomized trials and meta-analyses.[1,2] Sources of variation can be better understood and quantified if treatment effect estimates from each individual study are examined in relation to the totality of information available in all the studies.

Bayesian analysis differs from the usual frequentist approach (eg, use of P values or confidence intervals). Rather than focusing on the probability of different patterns in outcomes assuming specific treatment effects, Bayesian analysis relies on the use of prior information in combination with data from a study to calculate the probabilities of a treatment effect.[3] Readers may be familiar with Bayesian analysis when used in randomized clinical trials.[4,5] In this type of Bayesian analysis, patients are considered largely equivalent except with respect to the assigned treatment, and the goal is to estimate the probability of an overall treatment effect in the population.

In contrast, a Bayesian hierarchical model (BHM) is a statistical procedure that integrates information across many levels, so multiple quantities are estimated simultaneously, and explicitly separates the observed variability into parts attributable to random differences and true differences.[6] The model has

2 key characteristics. First, there is a hierarchical or multilevel structure. For example, if multiple studies were conducted to evaluate diabetes management strategies, the first-level data may be improvements in hemoglobin A_{1C} values in individual patients, the second-level data may be the mean improvements for patients within each trial, and the third-level data may be the average improvements in trials grouped according to the type of disease management strategy. Second, prior information is used to reflect available information, even if vague, regarding the likely values and variability at each level of the hierarchy (eg, the variability of improvements in patients in a single trial, the variability of average treatment effects between trials using similar disease management strategies, and the variability of treatment effects among groups of trials that use different disease management strategies). Using Bayes theorem, prior information, and the data, the BHM yields estimates of the true effects at each level of the hierarchy.[3,6] Estimates of true treatment effects may be derived for individual patients, patient subgroups, individual trials, or groups of trials. Each of these estimates are informed by the entire data set included in the statistical model.[6]

Stunnenberg and colleagues[8] reported the results of a trial that used a BHM to integrate data from a series of N-of-1 crossover trials[7] comparing mexiletine with placebo in the treatment of patients with nondystrophic myotonia. An N-of-1 trial uses a patient as his or her own control by repeatedly exposing the patient to a treatment or placebo and measuring the effect of the intervention. Each N-of-1 trial exposes the patient to between 1 and 4 treatment pairs or sets, with each set randomizing the order of mexiletine and placebo, with a 1-week washout period between therapies. After each treatment set, prespecified rules were used to determine whether the patient should continue to the next treatment set or discontinue, either for evidence of benefit of mexiletine, evidence of no benefit, or for reaching the maximum allowed number of treatment sets. A BHM was used to integrate data from all available N-of-1 trials performed in all the patients to produce estimates of treatment effects for each patient individually and also for 2 genetic subtypes of the disease.

WHY IS A BHM USED?

Multilevel data have an underlying hierarchical structure. In the report by Stunnenberg et al,[8] each trial had data from a single patient, and patients were grouped into genetic subtypes. Properly integrating this information required acknowledging the commonalities, eg, data from 2 patients having the same genetic subtype are more likely to be similar than data from 2 patients having different genetic subtypes. Heterogeneity between genetic subtypes and patient-to-patient variability are simultaneously accounted for in the BHM. A pooled analysis, ie, simply combining data from all patients, would not account for systematic patient-to-patient differences. At the other extreme, analyzing each individual patient's trial separately would not account for the information available across all the trials. This could result in underpowered analyses.

By considering the results across all trials, BHMs allow for more accurate estimates of the treatment effects for each individual trial because of a fundamental fact about multilevel data—namely, that regardless of the true systematic differences between the true treatment effects estimated by each trial, random variability is more likely to amplify these differences than diminish them. For example, suppose 4 single-intervention group trials of 100 patients each are conducted to estimate a common rate of a particular patient outcome, which is, hypothetically, 60% for all of the trials. Because of random variability in 100 patients, it is likely that one of the studies will produce an observed rate less than 60%, while another will produce an observed rate greater than 60%. Even though the studies all have exactly equal true underlying rates, numerical simulation demonstrates that the lowest observed value will average 54.9% and the highest will average 65.0%. Even though no true heterogeneity exists, when actual observations are made the results will appear heterogeneous because of random variation. Consider a different scenario in which the 4 trials are truly different, with true underlying rates of 54%, 58%, 62%, and 66%. Although the true rates range from 54% to 66%, the observed rates on average will range from 52.5% to 67.4% because of the additional random variation seen in a trial with a finite sample size. Here again, the observed values tend to be farther apart than the true values. The lowest observed value in a group is likely lower than its true value, and the highest observed value in a group is likely higher than its true value.

Knowing that observed values tend to be farther apart than the true values, the best estimates of the true values are closer together than the observed values. These estimates (which are more accurate than if each estimate were based only on the results from the individual trial) can be obtained using "shrinkage estimation."[6,9] The term "shrinkage" refers to the reduction in the observed differences between the trials. The purpose of the BHM is to determine the proper amount to move the observed treatment differences closer together to obtain the shrinkage estimates. The model estimates the proportion of total variability attributable to random (within-trial) variability and the amount attributable to systematic differences. By eliminating random noise, the resulting estimates are, on average, closer to the underlying truth.[6]

If the observed heterogeneity is consistent entirely with random variation, the resulting estimates for each group will be close to each other. In contrast, if the observed heterogeneity far exceeds what may be explained by random variation, the heterogeneity will be attributed to true differences that exist between the groups, and the treatment effect estimates will not shift much from the observed rates.

Estimates from a BHM typically have reduced variability compared with those from independent analyses, in which each trial is analyzed separately. This results in tighter interval estimates of treatment effects and may result in statistical hypothesis tests with greater power and lower type I error. For these reasons, BHMs are especially promising for studies of rare diseases for which large sample sizes are not feasible.

WHAT ARE THE LIMITATIONS OF BHMS?

All statistical models are predicated on assumptions that should be understood before applying the method. Bayesian hierarchical models rely on various assumptions (eg, the number of levels and the prior probability distributions used as the basis for Bayesian estimation of treatment effects) to estimate and separate within- and across-group variability.[6] Additionally, most BHMs assume a certain type of distribution for the across-group variability—for example, a bell-shaped curve. This assumption may fail if there is an outlying group inconsistent with a bell shape, potentially resulting in biased estimates for that outlying group.[10] It is important to consider sensitivity analyses that verify the robustness of the conclusions to changes in the choices of prior distributions.

HOW WERE BHMS USED IN THIS CASE?

In the study by Stunnenberg et al,[8] information from 27 N-of-1 trials was integrated to produce estimates of the treatment effect of mexiletine relative to placebo for 2 genetic subgroups and for the overall population. The outcome was a reduction in self-reported muscular stiffness on a 1-to-9 scale using a validated questionnaire. The mean reduction in stiffness was 3.84 (95% CI, 2.52 to 5.16) for the *CLNC1* genotype and 1.94 (95% CI, 0.35 to 3.53) for the *SCN4A* genotype. The mean reduction across all subgroups was 3.06 (95% CI, 1.96 to 4.15). Bayesian hierarchical models were used to successfully and rigorously integrate information with a complex underlying structure: a variable number of treatment sets per patient, with patients grouped into 2 genotype subgroups.

The BHM allows analysis at different levels of aggregation. In the study by Stunnenberg et al,[8] the aggregation occurred at 3 levels. First, data from each patient were aggregated across multiple treatment sets to estimate a single treatment effect for each patient. At the second level of the hierarchy, data were aggregated to estimate the treatment effect within 2 genotype subgroups. The third level described the distribution across subgroups.

HOW SHOULD BHMS BE INTERPRETED?

A BHM provides estimates of treatment effects, or other relevant clinical metrics, at each level of the hierarchy, based on all data included in the model. Because of the inclusion of a greater amount of information, these estimates are generally more accurate than if analyses were conducted on subgroups separately, increasing the power of statistical comparisons. For example, in a 3-level model with multiple measurements for each patient, multiple patient subtypes (eg, genetic subtypes), and an overall treatment effect for all patients, the hierarchical model provides estimates for each patient individually, for each patient subtype, and across all subtypes.

Acknowledgment

The following disclosures were reported at the time this original article was first published in *JAMA*.

Conflict of Interest Disclosures: Drs McGlothlin and Viele are employees of Berry Consultants LLC, a private consulting firm specializing in Bayesian adaptive clinical trial design, implementation, and analysis.

References

1. Meurer WJ, Lewis RJ. Cluster randomized trials. *JAMA*. 2015;313(20):2068-2069. Medline:26010636 doi:10.1001/jama.2015.5199

2. Whitehead A. *Meta-analysis of Controlled Clinical Trials*. Sussex, United Kingdom: Wiley West; 2002. doi:10.1002/0470854200

3. Quintana M, Viele K, Lewis RJ. Bayesian analysis: using prior information to interpret the results of clinical trials. *JAMA*. 2017;318(16):1605-1606. Medline:29067406 doi:10.1001/jama.2017.15574

4. Goligher EC, Tomlinson G, Hajage D, et al. Extracorporeal membrane oxygenation for severe acute respiratory distress syndrome and posterior probability of mortality benefit in a post hoc Bayesian analysis of a randomized clinical trial [published online October 22, 2018]. *JAMA*. Medline:30347031 doi:10.1001/jama.2018.14276

5. Lewis RJ, Angus DC. Time for clinicians to embrace their inner Bayesian? reanalysis of results of a clinical trial of extracorporeal membrane oxygenation [published online October 22, 2018]. *JAMA*. doi:10.1001/jama.2018.16916

6. Gelman A, Stern HS, Carlin JB, Dunson DB, Vehtari A, Rubin DB. *Bayesian Data Analysis*. 3rd ed. Boca Raton, FL: CRC Press; 2013.

7. Zucker DR, Schmid CH, McIntosh MW, et al. Combining single patient (N-of-1) trials to estimate population treatment effects and to evaluate individual patient responses to treatment. *J Clin Epidemiol*. 1997;50(4):401-410. Medline:9179098 doi:10.1016/S0895-4356(96)00429-5

8. Stunnenberg BC, Raaphorst J, Groenewoud HM, et al. Effect of mexiletine on muscle stiffness in patients with nondystrophic myotonia evaluated using aggregated N-of-1 trials [published December 11, 2018]. *JAMA*. doi:10.1001/jama.2018.18020

9. Lipsky AM, Gausche-Hill M, Vienna M, Lewis RJ. The importance of "shrinkage" in subgroup analyses. *Ann Emerg Med*. 2010;55(6):544-552. Medline:20138396 doi:10.1016/j.annemergmed.2010.01.002

10. Neuenschwander B, Wandel S, Roychoudhury S, Bailey S. Robust exchangeability designs for early phase clinical trials with multiple strata. *Pharm Stat*. 2016;15(2):123-134. Medline:26685103 doi:10.1002/pst.1730

Evaluating Discrimination of Risk Prediction Models: The C Statistic

Michael J. Pencina, PhD, and
Ralph B. D'Agostino Sr, PhD

IN THIS CHAPTER

Use of the Method

Why Are C Statistics Used?

What Are the Limitations of the C Statistic?

Why Did the Authors Use C Statistics in Their Study?

How Should the Findings Be Interpreted?

Caveats to Consider When Using C Statistics to Assess Predictive Model Performance

This JAMA Guide to Statistics and Methods characterizes the strengths and limitations of the C statistic as a measure of a risk prediction model's ability to discriminate between and predict future events.

Risk prediction models help clinicians develop personalized treatments for patients. The models generally use variables measured at one time point to estimate the probability of an outcome occurring within a given time in the future. It is essential to assess the performance of a risk prediction model in the setting in which it will be used. This is done by evaluating the model's discrimination and calibration. *Discrimination* refers to the ability of the model to separate individuals who develop events from those who do not. In time-to-event settings, discrimination is the ability of the model to predict who will develop an event earlier and who will develop an event later or not at all. *Calibration* measures how accurately the model's predictions match overall observed event rates.

In a prospective cohort study, Melgaard et al[1] used the C statistic, a global measure of model discrimination, to assess the ability of the CHA_2DS_2-VASc model to predict ischemic stroke, thromboembolism, or death in patients with heart failure and to do so separately for patients who had or did not have atrial fibrillation (AF).

USE OF THE METHOD

Why Are C Statistics Used?

The C statistic is the probability that, given 2 individuals (one who experiences the outcome of interest and the other who does not or who experiences it later), the model will yield a higher risk for the first patient than for the second. It is a measure of concordance (hence, the name "C statistic") between model-based risk estimates and observed events. C statistics measure the ability of a model to rank patients from high to low risk but do not assess the ability of a model to assign accurate probabilities of an event occurring (that is measured by the model's calibration). C statistics generally range from 0.5 (random concordance) to 1 (perfect concordance).

C statistics can also be thought of as being the area under the plot of sensitivity (proportion of people with events for whom the model predicts are high risk) vs 1 minus specificity (proportion of people without events for whom the model predicts are high risk) for all possible classification thresholds. This plot is called the receiver operating characteristic (ROC) curve, and the C statistic is equal to the area under this curve.[2] For example, in the study by Melgaard et al,[1] CHA_2DS_2-VASc scores ranged from a low of 0 (heart failure only) to a high of 5 or higher, depending on the number of comorbidities a patient had. One point on the ROC curve would be when high risk is defined as a CHA_2DS_2-VASc score of 1 or higher and low risk as a CHA_2DS_2-VASc score of 0. Another point on the curve would be when high risk is defined as a CHA_2DS_2-VASc score of 2 or higher and low risk as a CHA_2DS_2-VASc score of lower than 2, etc. Each cut point is associated with a different sensitivity and specificity.

It is useful to quantify the performance and clinical value of predictive models using the positive predictive value (PPV; the proportion of patients in whom the model predicts an event will occur who actually have an event) and the negative predictive value (NPV; the proportion of patients whom the model predicts will not have an event who actually do not experience the event). An important measure of a model's misclassification of events is 1 minus NPV, or the proportion of patients the model predicts will not have an event who actually have the event. The PPV and 1 minus NPV can be more informative for individual patients than the sensitivity and specificity because they answer the question "What are this patient's chances of having an event when the model predicts they will or will not have one?" If the event rate is known, then the PPV and NPV can be estimated based on sensitivity and specificity and, hence, the C statistic can be viewed as a summary for both sets of measures.

What Are the Limitations of the C Statistic?

The C statistic has several limitations. As a single number, it summarizes the discrimination of a model but does not communicate all the information ROC plots contain and lacks direct clinical application. The NPV, PPV, sensitivity, and specificity have more clinical relevance, especially when presented as plots across all meaningful classification thresholds (as is done with ROCs). A weighted sum of sensitivity and specificity (known as the standardized net benefit) can be plotted to assign different penalties to the 2 misclassification errors (predicting an individual who ultimately experiences an event to be at low risk; predicting an individual who does not experience an event to be at high risk) according to the principles of decision analysis.[3,4] In contrast, the C statistic does not effectively balance misclassification errors.[5] In addition, the C statistic is only a measure of discrimination, not calibration, so it provides no information regarding whether the overall magnitude of risk is predicted accurately.

Why Did the Authors Use C Statistics in Their Study?

Melgaard et al[1] sought to determine if the CHA_2DS_2-VASc score could predict occurrences of ischemic stroke, thromboembolism, or death among patients who have heart failure with and without AF. The authors used the C statistic to determine how well the model could distinguish between patients who would or would not develop each of the 3 end points they studied. The C statistic yielded the probability that a randomly selected patient who had an event had a risk score that was higher than a randomly selected patient who did not have an event.

How Should the Findings Be Interpreted?

The value of the C statistic depends not only on the model under investigation (ie, CHA_2DS_2-VASc score) but also on the distribution of risk factors in the sample to which it is applied. For example, if age is an important risk factor, the same model can appear to perform much better when applied to a sample with a wide age range compared with a sample with a narrow age range.

The C statistics reported by Melgaard et al[1] range from 0.62 to 0.71 and do not appear impressive (considering that a C statistic of 0.5 represents random concordance). This might be due to limitations of the model; eg, if there were an insufficient number of predictors or the predictors had been dichotomized for simplicity. The nationwide nature of the data used by Melgaard et al suggests that the unimpressive values of the C statistic cannot be attributed to narrow ranges of risk factors in the analyzed cohort. Rather, it might suggest inherent limitations in the ability to discriminate between patients with heart failure who will and will not die or develop ischemic stroke or thromboembolism.

The C statistic analysis suggested that the CHA_2DS_2-VASc model performed similarly among heart failure patients with and without AF (C statistics between 0.62 and 0.71 among patients with AF and 0.63 to 0.69 among patients without AF). An additional insight emerges from NPV analysis looking at misclassification of events occurring at 5 years, however. Between 19% and 27% of patients without AF who were predicted to be at low risk actually had 1 of the 3 events and thus were misclassified, yielding an NPV of 73% to 82%. Between 24% and 39% of patients with AF whom the model classified as low risk had major events, yielding an NPV of 61% to 76%. Because there was less misclassification among patients without AF who were predicted to be at low risk, a CHA_2DS_2-VASc score of 0 is a better determinant of long-term low risk among patients without AF than patients with AF. This aspect of the model performance is not apparent when looking at C statistics alone.

CAVEATS TO CONSIDER WHEN USING C STATISTICS TO ASSESS PREDICTIVE MODEL PERFORMANCE

Special extensions of the C statistic need to be used when applying it to time-to-event data[6] and competing-risk settings.[7] Furthermore, there exist several appealing single-number alternatives to the C statistic. They include the discrimination slope, the Brier score, or the difference between sensitivity and 1 minus specificity evaluated at the event rate.[3]

The C statistic provides an important but limited assessment of the performance of a predictive model and is most useful as a familiar first-glance summary. The evaluation of the discriminating value of a risk model should be supplemented with other statistical and clinical measures. Graphical summaries of model calibration and clinical consequences of adopted decisions are particularly useful.[8]

Acknowledgment

The following disclosures were reported at the time this original article was first published in *JAMA*.

Conflict of Interest Disclosures: None reported.

References

1. Melgaard L, Gorst-Rasmussen A, Lane DA, Rasmussen LH, Larsen TB, Lip GYH. Assessment of the CHA_2DS_2-VASc score in predicting ischemic stroke, thromboembolism, and death in patients with heart failure with and without atrial fibrillation. *JAMA*. 2015;314(10):1030-1038. doi:10.1001/jama.2015.10725.

2. Hanley JA, McNeil BJ. The meaning and use of the area under a receiver operating characteristic (ROC) curve. *Radiology*. 1982;143(1):29-36. Medline:7063747

3. Pepe MS, Janes H. Methods for evaluating prediction performance of biomarkers and tests. In: Lee M-LT, Gail M, Pfeiffer R, Satten G, Cai T, Gandy A, eds. *Risk Assessment and Evaluation of Predictions*. New York, NY: Springer; 2013:107-142.

4. Vickers AJ, Elkin EB. Decision curve analysis: a novel method for evaluating prediction models. *Med Decis Making*. 2006;26(6):565-574. Medline:17099194

5. Hand DJ. Measuring classifier performance: a coherent alternative to the area under the ROC curve. *Mach Learn*. 2009;77:103-123.

6. Pencina MJ, D'Agostino RB. Overall C as a measure of discrimination in survival analysis: model specific population value and confidence interval estimation. *Stat Med*. 2004;23(13):2109-2123. Medline:15211606

7. Blanche P, Dartigues JF, Jacqmin-Gadda H. Estimating and comparing time-dependent areas under receiver operating characteristic curves for censored event times with competing risks. *Stat Med*. 2013;32(30): 5381-5397. Medline:24027076

8. Moons KGM, Altman DG, Reitsma JB, et al. Transparent reporting of a multivariable prediction model for individual prognosis or diagnosis (TRIPOD): explanation and elaboration. *Ann Intern Med*. 2015;162(1):W1-W73. Medline:25560730

Overview of Cost-effectiveness Analysis

Gillian D. Sanders, PhD,
Matthew L. Maciejewski, PhD, and
Anirban Basu, PhD

IN THIS CHAPTER

The Use of Cost-effectiveness Analysis

Description of Cost-effectiveness Analysis

Limitation in the Use of Cost-effectiveness Analysis

How Was the Cost-effectiveness Analysis Performed in This Study?

How Should the Cost-effectiveness Analysis Be Interpreted in This Study?

This JAMA Guide to Statistics and Methods reviews the use of cost-effectiveness analysis to quantify the tradeoffs in costs, harms, and benefits of new health care interventions compared with existing interventions.

Health care decision makers, including patients, clinicians, hospitals, private health systems, and public payers (eg, Medicare), are often challenged with choosing among several new or existing interventions or programs to commit their limited resources to. This choice is ideally based on a comparison of health benefits, harms, and costs associated with each alternative. How best to determine the optimal intervention is a challenging task because benefits, harms, and costs must be weighed for a given option and compared with alternatives.

One way to inform such decisions is to perform a cost-effectiveness analysis. A cost-effectiveness analysis is an analytic method for quantifying the relative benefits and costs among 2 or more alternative interventions in a consistent framework. In a study published in *JAMA Oncology*, Moss et al[1] examined the cost-effectiveness of multimodal ovarian cancer screening with serum cancer antigen 125 compared with no screening in the United States, based on findings from the large United Kingdom Collaborative Trial of Ovarian Cancer Screening (UKCTOCS). The UKCTOCS evaluated the effect of screening on ovarian cancer mortality[2] and demonstrated that multimodal screening reduced mortality among women without prevalent ovarian cancer.

THE USE OF COST-EFFECTIVENESS ANALYSIS

Choosing among alternative treatments or programs is complicated because benefits, harms, and costs vary in the following ways: (1) benefits may be reflected in varying patterns of reduced morbidity or mortality in patients; (2) interventions vary in price and also in costs of acquiring or providing them (eg, time costs); and (3) benefits and costs accrue differently to different constituents (patients, caregivers, clinicians, health systems, and society). A cost-effectiveness analysis is designed to allow decision makers to clearly understand the tradeoffs of costs, harms, and benefits between alternative treatments and to combine those considerations into a single metric, the incremental cost-effectiveness ratio (ICER), that can be used to inform decision making when limited resources are available.

DESCRIPTION OF COST-EFFECTIVENESS ANALYSIS

Cost-effectiveness analysis is an analytic tool in which the costs and harms and benefits of an intervention (intervention A) and at least 1 alternative (intervention B) are calculated and presented as a ratio of the incremental cost (cost of intervention A − cost of intervention B) and the incremental effect (effectiveness of intervention A − effectiveness of intervention B). This ratio is known as the ICER.

The incremental cost in the numerator represents the additional resources (eg, medical care costs, costs from productivity changes) incurred from the use of intervention A over intervention B. The incremental effect in the denominator of the ICER represents the additional health outcomes (eg, the number of cases of a disease prevented or the quality-adjusted life-years [QALYs] gained) through the use of intervention A over intervention B.[3]

QALYs are the most commonly used benefit measure in cost-effectiveness analyses, in which the length of life is left unchanged or adjusted downward to reflect the health-related quality of life. Specifically, a quality weight of 1 indicates optimal health, 0 indicates the equivalent of death, and weights between 0 and 1 indicate less-than-optimal health. The weight for each period is multiplied by the length of the period to yield the QALYs for that period.

A primary rationale for using QALYs as a standard effectiveness outcome in cost-effectiveness analyses is the ability for policy makers to compare ICERs for various interventions across different diseases when allocating scarce resources to the intervention(s) that provide the greatest value for money. ICER values that are low suggest that intervention A improves health at a small additional cost per unit of health, assuming that A is both more costly and effective than B. If the ICER is negative, interpretation is more complex because negative ICERs can result from negative incremental costs (ie, the new treatment is less costly than the existing treatment) or from negative incremental benefits (ie, the new treatment is less effective than the existing treatment). A new treatment is said to be "dominant" if it is lower in cost and more effective than the comparator and is clearly of better value for money. However, the new treatment is said to be "dominated" if it is higher in cost and less effective than the comparator and is not of good value for money.

LIMITATION IN THE USE OF COST-EFFECTIVENESS ANALYSIS

There are important qualifications to consider when reviewing a cost-effectiveness analysis. What is considered cost-effective depends on comparing the ICER to the threshold value (eg, $50 000 or $100 000 per additional QALY) of the decision maker, which represents the willingness to pay for a unit of increased effectiveness (eg, 1 QALY). The threshold helps to determine which interventions merit investment. This willingness to pay is often represented by the largest ICER among all the interventions that were adopted before current resources were exhausted, because adoption of any new intervention would require removal of an existing intervention to free up resources. There is no fixed threshold for cost per QALY to determine what is cost-effective. Most decision makers do not rely on a single threshold to determine investment decisions.

Cost-effectiveness analyses have numerous limitations, including that available data may be drawn from heterogeneous populations, data on important outcomes may be unavailable, and that only short-term outcomes may be available and long-term outcomes must be extrapolated. Further, simplifying assumptions often must be made about how to represent the health states associated with the disease being studied that may not accurately represent the nuance and complexities of the clinical setting.

In 2016, the Second Panel on Cost-Effectiveness in Health and Medicine[4] recommended that all cost-effectiveness analyses should include a discussion of relevant limitations and efforts to compensate for the shortcomings of cost-effectiveness analyses. The Second Panel also recommended that all cost-effectiveness analyses should provide their findings from a health care sector perspective, which would incorporate the costs, benefits, and harms that are incurred by a payer, and from a societal perspective, which would incorporate all costs and health effects regardless of who incurs the costs or experiences the effects. To ensure that all consequences to patients, caregivers, social services, and others outside the health care sector are considered, the Second Panel recommended use of an "Impact Inventory" that lists the health and non–health-related effects of an intervention. This tool allows analysts to evaluate categories of effects that may be most important to diverse stakeholders. Checklists for the various items that should be included when reporting cost-effectiveness analysis results were provided by the Second Panel.[4]

HOW WAS THE COST-EFFECTIVENESS ANALYSIS PERFORMED IN THIS STUDY?

Moss et al evaluated the cost-effectiveness of a multimodal screening (MMS) program for ovarian cancer in the United States from a health care sector perspective (eg, Medicare).[1] In a health care sector perspective, only costs, health benefits, and harms that were observed by the health care sector are considered, and other costs, benefits, and harms that may affect patients or their caregivers are ignored.[4]

The authors developed a Markov simulation model using data from the UKCTOCS to compare MMS with no screening for women beginning at 50 years of age in the general population. The model, which involved a mathematical simulation that evaluated the benefits of the screening strategies in hypothetical cohorts of patients as they moved from one health state to the next, according to transition probabilities, demonstrated that MMS was both more expensive and more effective in reducing ovarian cancer mortality than no screening.

Clinical effectiveness was estimated from the UKCTOCS trial estimates of the effects of MMS on ovarian cancer mortality, with extrapolation of the long-term effects beyond the 11-year follow-up period. Direct medical costs were estimated based on Medicare claims data. Quality of life–related weights were included for the health states of being cancer free, undergoing MMS screening, and having ovarian cancer (incorporating lower weights for the chemotherapy and cancer stage).

HOW SHOULD THE COST-EFFECTIVENESS ANALYSIS BE INTERPRETED IN THIS STUDY?

In the main, base-case analysis, MMS screening with a risk algorithm cost estimate of $100 reduced ovarian cancer mortality by 15%, resulting in an incremental cost-effectiveness ratio of $106 187 per QALY gained (95% CI, $97 496-$127 793). The authors explored the uncertainty in the underlying parameters and found that screening women starting at 50 years of age with MMS was cost-effective in 70% of the simulations at a willingness to pay of $150 000 per QALY. If the willingness to pay were $100 000 per QALY, then screening was cost-effective 47% of the time.

A cost-effectiveness analysis does not make the decision for patients, clinicians, health care systems, or policy makers, but rather provides information that they can use to facilitate decision making. A cost-effectiveness analysis is also not designed for cost containment. These analyses do not set the level of resources to be spent on health care, but rather they provide information that can be used to ensure that those resources, whatever the level available, are used as effectively as possible to improve health. When reviewing cost-effectiveness analyses, readers should examine the study and use the recommendations from the Second Panel on Cost-Effectiveness in Health and Medicine[4] to help understand the implications of cost-effectiveness analysis research.

Acknowledgment

The following disclosures were reported at the time this original article was first published in *JAMA*.

Conflict of Interest Disclosures: Dr Maciejewski reported receiving research and center funding (CIN 13-410) from the VA Health Services Research and Development Service, receiving a contract for research from the National Committee for Quality Assurance, receiving research funding from the National Institute on Drug Abuse (RCS 10-391), and that his spouse owns stock in Amgen. Dr Basu reported consulting for Merck, Pfizer, GlaxoSmithKline, Janssen, and AstraZeneca as an expert on issues related to cost-effectiveness analysis. No other disclosures were reported.

References

1. Moss HA, Berchuck A, Neely ML, Myers ER, Havrilesky LJ. Estimating cost-effectiveness of a multimodal ovarian cancer screening program in the United States: secondary analysis of the UK Collaborative Trial of Ovarian Cancer Screening (UKCTOCS). *JAMA Oncol*. 2018;4(2):190-195. Medline:29222541 doi:10.1001/jamaoncol.2017.4211

2. Jacobs IJ, Menon U, Ryan A, et al. Ovarian cancer screening and mortality in the UK Collaborative Trial of Ovarian Cancer Screening (UKCTOCS): a randomised controlled trial. *Lancet*. 2016;387(10022):945-956. Medline:26707054 doi:10.1016/S0140-6736(15)01224-6

3. Neumann PJ, Cohen JT. QALYs in 2018—advantages and concerns. *JAMA*. 2018;319(24):2473-2474. Medline:29800152 doi:10.1001/jama.2018.6072

4. Sanders GD, Neumann PJ, Basu A, et al. Recommendations for conduct, methodological practices, and reporting of cost-effectiveness analyses: Second Panel on Cost-effectiveness in Health and Medicine. *JAMA*. 2016;316(10):1093-1103. Medline:27623463 doi:10.1001/jama.2016.12195

JAMAevidence
Using Evidence to Improve Care

Choosing a Time Horizon in Cost and Cost-effectiveness Analyses

Anirban Basu, PhD, and
Matthew L. Maciejewski, PhD

IN THIS CHAPTER

The Use of Time Horizon in a Cost-effectiveness Analysis

Limitations Regarding Selection of Time Horizons

How Was Time Horizon Defined and Used in the Study?

How Does the Time Horizon Selected by Wittenborn et al Affect the Interpretation of the Study?

This JAMA Guide to Statistics and Methods reviews considerations that go into investigators' choice of time over which to define and measure the benefits and costs of interventions in risk-benefit and cost-effectiveness analyses.

When designing a comparative outcomes or a cost-effectiveness analysis, the time horizon defining the duration of time for outcomes assessment must be carefully considered. The time horizon must be long enough to capture the intended and unintended benefits and harms of the intervention(s).[1,2] In some instances, the time horizon should extend beyond the duration of a clinical trial when a specific end point is measured, whereas in other instances modeling outcomes over a longer period is unnecessary. Using a longer time horizon than is necessary may add unnecessary cost and complexity to the cost-effectiveness analysis model.

In a study published in *JAMA Ophthalmology,* Wittenborn et al[3] examined costs and effectiveness of home-based macular degeneration monitoring systems using a lifetime horizon in a cost-effectiveness analysis and a 10-year horizon in a budget impact analysis. The rationale for selection of time horizons and their implications for interpreting the research is reviewed in this JAMA Guide to Statistics and Methods article.

THE USE OF TIME HORIZON IN A COST-EFFECTIVENESS ANALYSIS

For cost-effectiveness, the time horizon is the time over which the costs and effects are measured.[1,2] Cost-effectiveness analyses should consider time horizons that capture all intended and unintended consequences of the interventions being evaluated, irrespective of when they occur. When a cost-effectiveness analysis is performed as part of a clinical trial, the time in which the data are collected may be limited to the duration of the trial itself. This is called a within-trial horizon.[4] For example, cost-effectiveness of antibiotics used to treat acute sinusitis can use a within-trial time horizon because the disease and its treatment occur over a very short period and extrapolation of benefits over a long period is not required.

If benefits and harms of an intervention can occur over the entirety of a patient's life, then a lifetime horizon is appropriate. For example, cost-effectiveness for the use of a low vs a high dose of aspirin may affect the primary end point of cardiovascular events within the trial period, but the effects are likely to continue throughout the patients' lifetime. In such cases, within-trial analyses based on the primary end point are incomplete and potentially misleading because the long-term population effects on health and costs and results would not be captured.[5] In some instances, the appropriate time horizon can be somewhere between the duration of the trial and the lifetime of patients; eg, when a cost-effectiveness analysis is conducted from a payer's perspective. However, choice of time horizon can have substantial influence on cost-effectiveness analysis results in such cases.[6]

LIMITATIONS REGARDING SELECTION OF TIME HORIZONS

Studies using long time horizons can be difficult and expensive to complete. Consequently, 2 types of information external to the trial are generally needed because few trials collect patient information for their entire lives. If the trial studied the effect of an intervention on an intermediate outcome such as cholesterol level, it must have a plausible epidemiological link between the intermediate outcome and more comprehensive outcomes such as survival. When the epidemiological links are weak, assumptions about the comprehensive outcome cannot reliably be made from observations of intermediate outcomes. Second, the treatment effect found within the trial must persist in time beyond the trial follow-up. For example, if a trial of aspirin demonstrates an annual reduction of stroke by a risk ratio of 0.8 over 3 years, would this effect be expected to continue beyond 3 years? Extrapolations regarding long-term treatment effects depend on both clinical assumptions such as the known efficacy of an intervention and behavioral assumptions such as long-term adherence to treatment. These assumptions are commonly based on empirical evidence arising from other research studies such as information describing aspirin treatment adherence from real-world data. In the absence of prior information to fulfill these 2 conditions, the assumptions should be explicitly stated and alternate analyses that vary the scenarios and assumptions should be conducted to understand how the results are influenced by these assumptions.

Choosing the time horizon for a cost-effectiveness study depends on what perspective is selected to study. The perspective (eg, patient, private or public payer, society) defines whose costs are included and thus the types of resource use to be considered in a cost-effectiveness analysis. A private payer's perspective may require a relatively short time horizon such as for 1 to 2 years so may not capture an intervention's full benefits and harms that occur with time. In this scenario, benefits and harms determined from a payer perspective may differ from societal perspective that will be longer and will also include the effect of an intervention on patients, caregivers, and other sectors of the society. The Second Panel on Cost-effectiveness in Health and Medicine recommends using health care sector and a societal perspectives for cost-effectiveness analysis.[2] These 2 perspectives should be prioritized in selecting the appropriate time horizon and may involve selection of the same time horizon.

When designing studies with long time horizons, investigators must anticipate how outcomes for the treatment and control groups might change over time. For example, will the control group's outcome trend change linearly over time, such as a slow, linear gain until a certain age, then slow linear decline until death? Will the treatment group's outcome change in a non-linear fashion in the short-term and then stabilize into a fairly linear trend after a number of years? How may survival curves be extrapolated over time? These time-dependent changes in outcomes can be very difficult to anticipate.

HOW WAS TIME HORIZON DEFINED AND USED IN THE STUDY?

Wittenborn et al[3] compared costs and effectiveness of patients randomized to supplementing usual care with home-based macular degeneration monitoring systems or randomized to usual care. A lifetime horizon was used for the cost-effectiveness analysis from a societal perspective and a 10-year horizon for a budget impact analysis from a public payer (Medicare) perspective. It considered costs that would be incurred by patients, clinicians and health care systems necessary for monitoring, and medical costs. It also examined costs incurred by patients and employers such as productivity costs due to the time employees were unable to do their usual activities such as work. The incremental cost-effectiveness ratio, which summarizes the benefits (eg, effectiveness) and costs of the 2 alternatives in a single metric, attributable to monitoring based on a social perspective with a lifetime horizon was $35 663 (95% CI, cost-saving to $235 613) per quality-adjusted life-year gained. In the budget impact analysis that estimated the cumulative cost for covering monitoring in the initial 10 years found that Medicare would be projected to spend $1312 (95% CI: $222-$2848) per patient. Taken together, these analyses demonstrated that coverage of home telemonitoring would require additional Medicare expenditures over the first 10 years but could be a good value for money when the time horizon was expanded from 10 years to patient lifetimes and when the set of relevant benefits and costs were broadened from a public payer perspective (Medicare) to a social perspective.

HOW DOES THE TIME HORIZON SELECTED BY WITTENBORN ET AL AFFECT THE INTERPRETATION OF THE STUDY?

The lifetime analysis was warranted because the natural history of age-related macular degeneration continues over patients' lifetimes. However, the challenges faced by the authors were to extrapolate the HOME trial results of 1.4 years mean duration to a lifetime horizon.[3] The trial end point of best-corrected visual acuity scores at the detection of age-related macular degeneration–associated choroidal neovascularization (CNV) had to be extrapolated to lifetime quality-adjusted life-years; and the acuity score at time of CNV diagnosis and the false-positive rates of CNV diagnosis observed in the trial had to be extrapolated beyond the duration of the trial. The authors relied on extensive epidemiological studies to estimate these parameters, and found that their results were relatively insensitive to variation in the input value of one parameter at a time over a range. However, to what extent continuous monitoring would lead to additional behavioral changes (prevention of scheduled eye examination or fidelity to monitoring recommendations) beyond the duration of the HOME trial remains uncertain and were not captured by the model parameters. The authors studied some of these considerations by changing underlying assumptions of the model to reflect slightly higher benefits of monitoring and found that the monitoring interventions became cost-saving when modeled using a lifetime horizon.

Acknowledgment

The following disclosures were reported at the time this original article was first published in *JAMA*.

Conflict of Interest Disclosures: Dr Basu reports receiving fees from Salutis Consulting LLC. Dr Maciejewski reports owning stock through spouse's employment at Amgen; grants and other support from the Veterans Affairs Health Services Research and Development and the National Committee for Quality Assurance; and grants from the National Institute on Drug Abuse.

References

1. Gold MR, Siegel JE, Russell LB, Weinstein MC, eds. *Cost-Effectiveness in Health and Medicine*. New York, NY: Oxford University Press; 1996.
2. Sanders GD, Neumann PJ, Basu A, et al. Recommendations for conduct, methodological practices, and reporting of cost-effectiveness analyses: Second Panel on Cost-effectiveness in Health and Medicine. *JAMA*. 2016;316(10):1093-1103. Medline:27623463 doi:10.1001/jama.2016.12195
3. Wittenborn JS, Clemons T, Regillo C, Rayess N, Liffmann Kruger D, Rein D. Economic evaluation of a home-based age-related macular degeneration monitoring system. *JAMA Ophthalmol*. 2017;135(5):452-459. Medline:28358948 doi:10.1001/jamaophthalmol.2017.0255
4. Hlatky MA, Owens DK, Sanders GD. Cost-effectiveness as an outcome in randomized clinical trials. *Clin Trials*. 2006;3(6):543-551. Medline:17170039 doi:10.1177/1740774506073105
5. Sculpher MJ, Claxton K, Drummond M, McCabe C. Whither trial-based economic evaluation for health care decision making? *Health Econ*. 2006;15(7):677-687. Medline:16491461 doi:10.1002/hec.1093
6. Kim DD, Wilkinson CL, Pope EF, Chambers JD, Cohen JT, Neumann PJ. The influence of time horizon on results of cost-effectiveness analyses. *Expert Rev Pharmacoecon Outcomes Res*. 2017;17(6):615-623. Medline:28504026 doi:10.1080/14737167.2017.1331432

JAMAevidence
Using Evidence to Improve Care

On Deep Learning for Medical Image Analysis

Lawrence Carin, PhD, and
Michael J. Pencina, PhD

IN THIS CHAPTER

Opening the Deep Learning Black Box

What Are the Limitations of Deep Learning Methods?

This JAMA Guide to Statistics and Methods explains the basic concepts underlying convolutional neural networks (CNNs), a type of machine learning being used to automate the reading of medical images.

Neural networks, a subclass of methods in the broader field of machine learning, are highly effective in enabling computer systems to analyze data, facilitating the work of clinicians. Neural networks have been used since the 1980s, with convolutional neural networks (CNNs) applied to images beginning in the 1990s.[1-3] Examples include identifying natural images of everyday life,[4] classifying retinal pathology,[5] selecting cellular elements on pathological slides,[6] and correctly identifying the spatial orientation of chest radiographs.[7] Successful neural networks for such tasks are typically composed of multiple analysis layers; the term *deep learning* is also (synonymously) used to describe this class of neural networks.

OPENING THE DEEP LEARNING BLACK BOX

One way to understand how CNNs work is to use an analogy of written language. Ideas are communicated in written articles that are composed of a series of paragraphs that are, in turn, made of sentences, sentences of words, and words from collections of letters. Understanding text comes after assessing the relationships of the letters to one another in increasing layers of complexity (a "deep" hierarchical representation: from letters, to words, to sentences, to paragraphs). Images are analyzed by computers via motifs, instead of letters. A motif is a collection of pixels that form a basic unit of analysis, the simplest of which represent the most basic pattern for communicating visual information, just as a letter does for language. After the computer learns the form of these motifs, they are detected in images using a filter that is matched to the motif's structure.

VIDEO

Understanding How Machine Learning Works

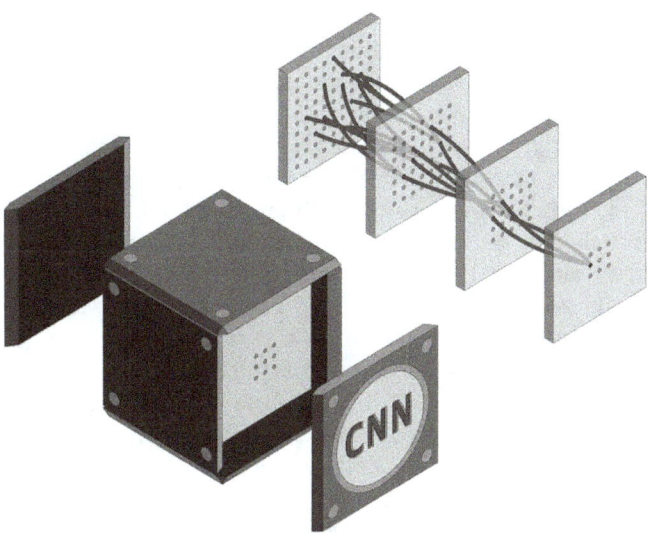

This video at https://edhub.ama-assn.org/jn-learning/video-player/16845576 illustrates how a convolutional neural network works, a type of machine learning being used to automate the reading of medical images.

Consider the image in the accompanying Video corresponding to a collection of words. An image may be considered as a map, with the location-dependent pixel value reflecting the signal strength at a given point; the collection of pixels yields an image, and in this example the image forms a set of words.

The most primitive building blocks that make up the images are on the first layer of the CNN model; these building blocks correspond to the motifs. The CNN detects these motifs by applying filters to the images. Each filter is a set of pixels that are of similar form as the respective motif. In this example, the first layer filters correspond to the letters of the alphabet. Each filter is shifted sequentially to each location in the image and measures the degree to which the local properties of the image match the filter at each location, a process called *convolution*. The result of this convolution process is projected to another array (or new image) called a feature map. Feature maps quantify the degree of match between the filter and each local region in the original image. If there are N first layer filters, there are N 2D feature maps created by the convolutional process.

The N feature maps output from layer 1 are now aligned spatially and "stacked" atop each other; this is the input to layer 2 of the model. At layer 2, another set of filters is used to process the image. Each layer 2 filter has N motifs associated with each filter, matched to the N components (layers) of the input "image" at layer 2. If there are M second-layer filters, there are M feature maps output from layer 2. These M feature maps are again spatially aligned and "stacked" and correspond to the input to layer 3, and the process repeats again. A sequential analysis of this form is repeated for a desired number of layers, and the final set of feature maps at the top (last layer) are used to make a classification decision. This decision may correspond to determining if a sentence being searched for is in the image (as in the video), or a lesion is present in a photograph, as was the case for recent work identifying pathology from retinal photographs.[5]

The Video illustrates how a CNN works. Consider the word "Ada" from the name Ada Lovelace. Each first layer filter corresponds to one of the letters in the alphabet. For simplicity, all letters are assumed to be uppercase. Consider "ADA" located within the original image being analyzed. When the *A* motif overlies the letter *A* in the original image, the convolution output generates a strong signal that is mapped to the corresponding feature map. This map has weak signals everywhere *A* is absent, including in the space where the *D* in ADA is present. On the feature map corresponding to the letter/filter *D*, a strong signal is situated spatially where all *D*s are located, including at the location between the 2 *A*s in ADA. The N feature maps (where N is the number of motifs or letters assessed) output from first layer of the model detect the presence and location of each of the N building-block motifs/letters. The second layer filters simultaneously analyze all N feature maps output from layer one, looking for combinations of letters.

For the example shown in the accompanying Video, each second layer filter is designed to detect a short sequence of letters, for example, the sequence ADA. Each second layer filter has N components, corresponding to the N feature maps output from the first layer. The N-component filter that is seeking to detect the sequence ADA will have zero amplitude on N-2 of its components (associated with the N-2 letters other than *A* and *D*). The component of the filter corresponding to the letter *A* will seek 2 nearby strong signals (corresponding to *A* "space" *A*), and the filter component corresponding to the letter *D* will have a single strong amplitude, situated between where the *A*'s reside. After the N components of the ADA filter are convolved with the N first layer output feature maps, and then summed, a strong signal will be manifested at the location of the word ADA.

Each of the M feature maps output from layer 2 corresponds to a different short collections of letters. Moving to layer 3, larger words and groups of words are detected. Moving to layer 4, sequences of words and sentences are detected. Finally, at layers 5 and above paragraphs are detected. At each layer the same process is used: convolutions with filters, with the number of filter components matched to the number feature maps from the layer below. There are a few additional details of the CNN omitted here for simplicity, but this captures the essence of the model.

What is the advantage of this hierarchy? Why not directly learn filters for sequences like ADA? The hierarchy facilitates a more complete ability to share data (termed *sharing strength* in statistics). The words ADA, ADAPT, ADAM, and MADAM all have the sequence ADA, and the presence of all these words may be shared in learning the sequence ADA. By learning a hierarchical representation (rather than directly learn separate filters for each word) the model is able to more fully utilize all data (the model is able to learn what the word ADA may look like, by leveraging experience with ADAPT, ADAM, etc). Similar concepts exist for analysis of medical images: images of different states of health may be distinct at one level of granularity (scale), but at a finer scale they may share substructural characteristics (hence, at that finer scale the model can learn motifs that are shared between different states of health/disease).

WHAT ARE THE LIMITATIONS OF DEEP LEARNING METHODS?

The deep network has a specified number of layers, and at each layer there are a specified number of filters to learn. There are currently no means of defining the appropriate number of layers and filters. For example, the model in eFigure 1 of the article by Ting et al[5] was not designed for medical images, but rather was originally specified for analysis of natural imagery.[8] This suggests that the already excellent performance can be further improved, by refinement/tuning of the model structure for medical images.

Because numerous parameters must be tuned in the learning process (number of layers, number of kernels at each layer, form of the classifier, etc), it is essential that the test data set be completely separate from all data used for training and for evaluating model performance. If one examines the results on the test data set, then goes back and adjusts the model structure, and then retrains the model, effectively all the data are being used in the training process (the "test" data set becomes part of the training process and is not independent). This separation is necessary so that deep learning results are not overly optimistic and will generalize to medical settings outside those used for model development.

Acknowledgment

The following disclosures were reported at the time this original article was first published in *JAMA*.

Conflict of Interest Disclosures: Dr Pencina reported that his institution received grant support from Bristol-Myers Squibb and Regeneron/Sanofi. Dr Carin reported no disclosures.

References

1. LeCun Y, Boser BE, Denker JS, et al. Handwritten digit recognition with a back-propagation network. *Adv Neural Inf Process Syst*. 1990:396-404. https://www.cs.rit.edu/~mpv/course/ai/lecun-90c.pdf.
2. Hinton G. Deep learning—a technology with the potential to transform health care [published online August 30, 2018]. *JAMA*. doi:10.1001/jama.2018.11100
3. Naylor CD. On the prospects for a (deep) learning health care system [published online August 30, 2018]. *JAMA*. doi:10.1001/jama.2018.11103
4. Krizhevsky A, Sutskever I, Hinton GE. ImageNet classification with deep convolutional neural networks. Presented at: NIPS 12 Proceedings of the 25th International Conference on Neural Information Processing Systems. December 2012.
5. Ting DSW, Cheung CY, Lim G, et al. Development and validation of a deep learning system for diabetic retinopathy and related eye diseases using retinal images from multiethnic populations with diabetes. *JAMA*. 2017;318(22):2211-2223. Medline:29234807 doi:10.1001/jama.2017.18152
6. Kraus OZ, Ba JL, Frey BJ. Classifying and segmenting microscopy images with deep multiple instance learning. *Bioinformatics*. 2016;32(12):i52-i59. Medline:27307644 doi:10.1093/bioinformatics/btw252
7. Rajkomar A, Lingam S, Taylor AG, Blum M, Mongan J. High-throughput classification of radiographs using deep convolutional neural networks. *J Digit Imaging*. 2017;30(1):95-101. Medline:27730417 doi:10.1007/s10278-016-9914-9
8. Simonyan K, Zisserman A. Very deep convolutional networks for large-scale image recognition. arXiv:1409.1556v6. Last updated April 2015.

A Checklist to Elevate the Science of Surgical Database Research

Adil H. Haider, MD, MPH,
Karl Y. Bilimoria, MD, MS, and
Melina R. Kibbe, MD

This JAMA Guide to Statistics and Methods provides an overview of the 11 most widely used surgical data sets, as well as a 10-item checklist that authors can use to improve the quality of their analyses.

Each year, *JAMA Surgery* receives hundreds of submissions that retrospectively analyze large surgical databases. Although many of these attempt to shed light on new and important questions, most do not get published. A majority of submissions are not even sent out for peer review because they have clear flaws in the data analytic techniques or they attempt to address a research question that cannot be adequately answered with the proposed data set. Of those that are sent out for peer review, many are recommended to be rejected by expert peer reviewers as they find major methodological flaws in the use of these otherwise powerful data sets. Articles that are published frequently come from a select group of investigators who have developed a mastery of specific data sets and the analytic techniques required to truly harness their potential.

This series is aimed at providing short, practical guides for investigators in the use of the most widely available surgical data sets that can be used across the research continuum, from conceptualization to peer-reviewed publication. To achieve this, *JAMA Surgery* partnered with the Surgical Outcomes Club (http://www.surgicaloutcomesclub.com).

The following chapters provide succinct overviews of the 11 most widely used data sets[1-11] (Box 1), their specific features, strengths, limitations, and some important statistical considerations. In addition, we present a 10-item checklist (Box 2) that authors can use to ensure that they have covered what is "at minimum" expected from a manuscript that uses 1 of these databases. Finally, our biostatistician colleagues provide more in-depth information on statistical methodologies mentioned in the practical guides as well as potential pitfalls that need to be avoided.[12]

To help authors improve the quality of their analyses of large surgical databases, we have developed a 10-item checklist

> **BOX 1**
>
> ### Databases Covered in This Series
>
> Agency for Healthcare Research and Quality Healthcare Cost and Utilization Project databases: National Inpatient Sample, State Inpatient Databases, and Kids' Inpatient Database[1]
>
> Surveillance, Epidemiology, and End Results Program[2]
>
> Medicare Claims Data[3]
>
> Military Health System Tricare Encounter Data[4]
>
> Veterans Affairs Surgical Quality Improvement Program[5]
>
> National Surgical Quality Improvement Program[6]
>
> Metabolic and Bariatric Surgery Accreditation and Quality Improvement Program[7]
>
> National Cancer Database[8]
>
> National Trauma Data Bank[9]
>
> Society for Vascular Surgery Vascular Quality Initiative[10]
>
> The Society of Thoracic Surgeons National Database[11]

(Box 2). The first item in our checklist encourages authors to pursue hypothesis-driven science. Defining a solid research question is key to translating a problem into an operational hypothesis. The FINER (Feasible, Interesting, Novel, Ethical, Relevant) criteria or the PICO (Patient, Population, or Problem; Intervention, Prognostic Factor, or Exposure; Comparison or Intervention; Outcome) format can help develop a meaningful research question.[13,14] Adequately defining the population of interest lays a solid groundwork for the interpretation, applicability, and generalizability of the research findings. We understand that in many cases, authors may be using these large databases for "hypothesis-generating" research. That is of course acceptable, but one must start with a solid research question to conduct a meaningful research project that will generate important hypotheses from the large data sets that can then be

BOX 2

Checklist to Elevate the Science of Surgical Database Research

1. Have a solid research question and clear hypothesis. Consider using the FINER (Feasible, Interesting, Novel, Ethical, Relevant) or PICO (Patient, Population, or Problem; Intervention, Prognostic Factor, or Exposure; Comparison or Intervention; Outcome) criteria to develop these.
2. Ensure compliance with the institutional review board and data use agreements.
3. Conduct a thorough literature review. Use a reference management program for ease in manuscript development.
4. Make sure this is the best data set available and that it has the appropriate variables to answer your research question.
5. Clearly define the inclusion criteria, exclusion criteria, and outcome variables. Use a flow diagram to describe final patient selection.
6. Identify potential confounders and use risk adjustment to minimize bias. Consider using a directed acyclic graph to represent potential associations. Avoid use of causal language in reporting results of these observational studies.
7. Ensure that the data variables have not changed over time. If so, account for this.
8. Ensure that competing risks are identified and addressed.
9. Ensure that data issues, such as missing data, are discussed and that any sensitivity analyses or imputations performed are reported in a clear and cohesive way.
10. Ensure that your article has a clear take-home message that addresses how your research advances current knowledge and has important policy or clinical implications.

further studied with translational or prospective approaches. Some authors ask if it is acceptable to try and see what they can find in a data set that they may have access to without a real research question. This is never acceptable.

Second, we remind authors to seek approval or an exemption from an institutional review board and to properly document and comply with applicable data use agreements. These are often overlooked, but compliance with applicable rules is necessary for patient privacy and a variety of important reasons. Third, a thorough literature review will assist in making sure the best database is selected to answer research questions and to make sure the research question has not been previously answered. Fourth, we encourage authors to invest enough time early on to get to know the database, confirm that it has the appropriate variables, and understand methodological considerations to make sure this is the best data set available for the study. Fifth, a clear definition of the inclusion and exclusion criteria, as well as outcome variables, is necessary for reviewers and readers to understand the population under study. This also helps facilitate data query and extraction of a complete and useful data set.

Sixth, another important aspect of working with databases is the need to identify potential confounders or covariates and use risk adjustment to minimize bias. Given the observational nature of data in these surgical registries, 1 approach to do this is to create a directed acyclic graph,[15] which will allow a visual depiction of the potential association being explored along with the covariates and confounders that need to be kept in mind or accounted for while studying the association. Please refer to the chapter, Tips for Analyzing Large Data Sets From the JAMA Surgery Statistical Editors, for further details. Authors should also avoid use of causal language when describing the results of these observational studies. Seventh, authors must account for any updates or significant changes to the variables of interest over time as this might jeopardize comparison between and across years (for example, in the National Cancer Database, the definition of sentinel lymph node biopsy for breast and melanoma has changed during the last 10 years, and this must be accounted for). Eighth, authors are encouraged to identify if competing risks exist in outcomes.[16] For example, if authors are studying complication rates 30 days after surgery, one must account for patients who may have already died and are not at risk for developing these complications. Ninth, authors must ensure that any data issues, such as missing data, are openly discussed in a clear, cohesive, and replicable way. Authors must lay out any data limitations, how they were addressed, and measures taken to reduce their impact (eg, sensitivity analyses, multiple imputation[17] for missing data). Finally, as our last item in the checklist, we encourage authors to clearly state a take-home message. It is best to communicate how the study advances the science, addresses gaps in knowledge, highlights further research opportunities, and discusses important policy or clinical implications of the work.

We recommend that authors use this checklist, the practical guide for their chosen data set, and the statistical tips for analyzing data sets as a 3-part series to consult before submission of their manuscript. We hope that by following these simple guides, authors can benefit from the collective wisdom of so many colleagues who have successfully completed similar analyses in the past.

Acknowledgment

The following disclosures were reported at the time this original article was first published.

Conflict of Interest Disclosures: Dr Haider reports receiving grants from the Henry M. Jackson Foundation of the Department of Defense, the Orthopaedic Research and Education Foundation, and the National Institutes of Health, and nonfinancial research supports from the Centers for Medicare and Medicaid Services Office of Minority Health. Dr Bilimoria was the president of the Surgical Outcomes Club from 2016 to 2017. No other disclosures were reported.

Funding/Support: This work is supported by the Henry M. Jackson Foundation for the Advancement of Military Medicine of the Department of Defense (Dr Haider).

Role of the Funder/Sponsor: The funder had no role in the preparation, review, or approval of the manuscript and decision to submit the manuscript for publication.

References

1. Stulberg JJ, Haut ER. AHRQ Healthcare Cost and Utilization Project Databases: National Inpatient Sample (NIS) [published online April 4, 2018]. *JAMA Surg*. doi:10.1001/jamasurg.2018.0542.

2. Doll KM, Rademaker A, Sosa JA. Longitudinal outcomes reporting using the Surveillance, Epidemiology, and End Results (SEER) Database [published online April 4, 2018]. *JAMA Surg*. doi:10.1001/jamasurg.2018.0501.

3. Ghaferi AA, Dimick JB. Longitudinal outcomes reporting using Medicare claims [published online April 4, 2018]. *JAMA Surg*. doi:10.1001/jamasurg.2018.0489.

4. Schoenfeld AJ, Kaji AH, Haider AH. Outcomes reporting using Tricare claims [published online April 4, 2018]. *JAMA Surg*. doi:10.1001/jamasurg.2018.0480.

5. Massarweh NM, Kaji AH, Itani KMF. Veterans Affairs Surgical Quality Improvement Program [published online April 4, 2018]. *JAMA Surg*. doi:10.1001/jamasurg.2018.0504.

6. Raval MV, Pawlik TM. National Surgical Quality Improvement Program (NSQIP) and pediatric NSQIP [published online April 4, 2018]. *JAMA Surg*. doi:10.1001/jamasurg.2018.0486.

7. Telem DA, Dimick JB. Metabolic and Bariatric Surgery Accreditation and Quality Program (MBSAQIP) [published online April 4, 2018]. *JAMA Surg*. doi:10.1001/jamasurg.2018.0495.

8. Merkow RP, Rademaker AW, Bilimoria KY. National Cancer Database [published online April 4, 2018]. *JAMA Surg*. doi:10.1001/jamasurg.2018.0492.

9. Hashmi ZG, Kaji AH, Nathens AB. National Trauma Data Bank [published online April 4, 2018]. *JAMA Surg*. doi:10.1001/jamasurg.2018.0483.

10. Desai SS, Kaji AH, Upchurch G. Society for Vascular Surgery Vascular Quality Improvement Program [published online April 4, 2018]. *JAMA Surg*. doi:10.1001/jamasurg.2018.0498.

11. Farjah F, Kaji AH, Chu D. Society of Thoracic Surgery (STS) Dataset [published online April 4, 2018]. *JAMA Surg*. doi:10.1001/jamasurg.2018.0545.

12. Kaji AH, Rademaker AW, Hyslop T. Tips for analyzing large data sets from the JAMA Surgery statistical editors [published online April 4, 2018]. *JAMA Surg*. doi:10.1001/jamasurg.2018.0647.

13. Cummings SR, Browners WS, Hulley SB. Conceiving the research question and developing the study plan. In: Hulley SB, Cummings SR, Browner WS, Grady DG, Newman TB, eds. *Designing Clinical Research*. 3rd ed. Philadelphia, PA: Lippincott Williams & Wilkins; 2007:19-22.

14. Brian Haynes R. Forming research questions. *J Clin Epidemiol*. 2006;59(9):881-886. Medline:16895808.

15. Shrier I, Platt RW. Reducing bias through directed acyclic graphs. *BMC Med Res Methodol*. 2008;8:70. Medline:18973665.

16. Sun M, Choueiri TK, Hamnvik OP, et al. Comparison of gonadotropin-releasing hormone agonists and orchiectomy: effects of androgen-deprivation therapy. *JAMA Oncol*. 2016;2(4):500-507. Medline:26720632.

17. Oyetunji TA, Crompton JG, Ehanire ID, et al. Multiple imputation in trauma disparity research. *J Surg Res*. 2011;165(1):e37-e41. Medline:21067775.

Tips for Analyzing Large Data Sets From the *JAMA Surgery* Statistical Editors

Amy H. Kaji, MD, PhD,
Alfred W. Rademaker, PhD, and
Terry Hyslop, PhD

IN THIS CHAPTER

Study Population Considerations

Methodological and Sample Size Considerations

Data Elements and Presentation

Analytic and Statistical Considerations

Conclusions

This JAMA Guide to Statistics and Methods offers tips for handling big data, including important considerations regarding study population, methodology and sample size, data elements and presentation, and analysis and statistics.

With the advent of administrative databases and patient registries, big data is increasingly accessible to researchers. The large sample size of these data sets makes the study of rare outcomes easier and provides the potential to determine national estimates and regional variations. However, no database is completely free of bias and measurement error. With bigger data, random signals may denote statistical significance, and precision may be incorrectly inferred because of narrow confidence intervals. While many principles apply to all studies, the importance of these methodological issues is amplified in large, complex data sets.

STUDY POPULATION CONSIDERATIONS

It is important for the reader to understand how the investigator arrived at the study population. Usually, it is drawn from a larger source population to which inclusion criteria have been applied. A flowchart of the included and excluded participants, with the number excluded and reasons why, should be clearly delineated. Similarly, if the study is longitudinal, loss to follow-up should be reported. This will help readers understand any selection bias present.

METHODOLOGICAL AND SAMPLE SIZE CONSIDERATIONS

The objective and outcome(s) of the study should have been defined prior to data collection and analysis. If an author is looking for a difference in some variable between 2 cohorts, this difference and its confidence intervals should also be preplanned. The difference in the effect estimate should be reported as a patient-centered, clinically meaningful, and interpretable difference[1] in addition to the statistical result (eg, regression coefficient, *P* value). Unfortunately, mining large data sets without preplanning can lead to unintentional, often mistaken conclusions. Statistical significance is related to sample size, and with a large enough sample, statistical significance between groups may occur with very small differences that are not clinically meaningful.

When reporting the results of observational studies, authors should consider following the Strengthening the Reporting of Observational Studies in Epidemiology (STROBE) reporting guidelines.[2] The study design should be clearly described and be consistent with how the data were collected and analyzed, and the study results should be presented in a concise yet complete manner. There should be some statement that the study was performed after institutional review board approval or exemption was obtained. Authors should also describe whether any interim analyses were performed and if there were any protocol violations. Limitations should be reported to promote scientific integrity and validity of conclusions, which should be fully supported by the data analysis. Interpretations of observational studies should only lead to descriptions of associations between variables, not to conclusions of causality.

Although insufficient power would not seem to be a problem with large databases, this is simply not true. Study samples may be inadequate to answer questions about rare outcomes. Thus, regardless of the size of the database, the sample size and power analysis should have been calculated a priori. A power analysis is particularly helpful in interpreting the study findings when statistically significant effects are not found.[3] If a post hoc subgroup or power analysis is performed, then this should be stated in the Methods section of the resulting article. Consideration should also be given to adjusting for multiple comparisons and/or multiple testing, especially if these were not preplanned. If there are more than 20 tests performed, then by chance, one will be statistically significant. One strategy is to employ methods of correction (eg, Bonferroni correction, Hochberg sequential procedure) when the number of tests or comparisons exceeds 20.[4]

DATA ELEMENTS AND PRESENTATION

Authors should present their data with sufficient detail that a reader could calculate and reproduce the results. Rather than simply reporting summary data or proportions, it is preferred that the authors present granular, raw data. The proportion of missing data for the variables and outcomes of interest should be clearly described.[5] When there is a large proportion of missing data (>30%), the author should describe the pattern of missingness in the data, and there should be consideration for using techniques such as multiple imputation. In addition to reduced power, performing analyses in which only participants with complete data are included will result in bias. For example, if income data are more likely to be missing for those who do not have insurance and are considered sicker, there will potentially be problems analyzing the effect of socioeconomic status on surgical outcomes.

Given the observational nature of registry data, one consideration is to create a directed acyclic graph,[6] which will allow the reader to understand the role of potential confounders and intermediates. When there are a large number of tables, ancillary to the primary study objective, submitting online supplementary files should be considered. If the data can be depicted in a table or figure, there is no need to describe the results in the manuscript text. Pie charts and bar graphs add very little to what is already stated in the text, unless there are multiple, complex bins. If bar graphs are to be used, the 95% CI bars (sometimes called whiskers) should also be denoted.

If medical record abstraction was used, the methods for medical record review should be detailed, such as describing who the abstractors were, their background, how they were trained, and whether there was a standardized data collection instrument.[7] Ideally, medical record abstractors should be blinded to the study hypothesis and objectives, and there should be at least 2 independent medical record abstractors. The inter-rater reliability (eg, κ) of the abstractors should also be described.

ANALYTIC AND STATISTICAL CONSIDERATIONS

Since studies based on secondary analyses of large data sets are by definition observational, it would be preferred if there were less emphasis placed on statistical hypothesis testing and the reporting of P values. As per the American Statistical Association,[8] a description of effect estimates (odds ratios, risk ratios, etc.) and the 95% CI is more informative than reporting P values. If 2 cohorts are being compared for a continuous variable (eg, duration of operation, length of hospital stay), then the mean difference (or median, if the data are not normally distributed) and its 95% CI should be reported.

When presenting a multivariable model, the theoretical basis of the model should be described. The type of model (eg, logistic, linear, Poisson) and the assumptions on which it is based should be clear (eg, the model assumed linearity or normality of the distribution of the data). The authors should demonstrate that model assumptions were not violated, thereby supporting the validity of the model. Additionally, a description of why certain predictor variables and which variables were chosen for the model should be clearly stated. Ideally, a model with its predictors will not be selected simply using criteria for statistical significance. Rather, the predictor variables should be chosen based on background literature and/or biological and clinical plausibility. If model selection is performed purely based on statistical significance, then the model should be presented as hypothesis-generating, rather than conclusive.[9] For the purposes of sample size calculation for multivariable logistic regression analysis, for each additional included predictor, there should be at least 10 to 15 participants with the outcome of interest. Thus, if there are 20 deaths in a study sample, it would only be possible to assess 2 variables as predictors at most, such as age and diabetes in a multivariable model.

One other consideration in multivariable modeling is the potential for correlations within a cluster of participants. As an example, if one is assessing regional differences in postoperative wound infections after hernia repair, one would expect correlations of outcomes by surgeon. In this case, a cluster analysis using generalized estimating equations should be used. Similarly, if a study is evaluating repeated measures of a variable over time in the same patient (eg, quality of life scores at 3 months and 9 months after surgery), then a mixed model approach should be used.[10] Finally, in presenting the model, authors should describe how they assessed for model fit, multicollinearity, and effect modification.[11]

CONCLUSIONS

Large data sets have many unique strengths, including broad representation, efficient sampling design, and often consistency in data structure. However, large data sets are not free from bias and measurement error, and it is important to respect and acknowledge the limitations of the data. The challenge with big data is that it requires a carefully thought-out research question and a transparent analytic strategy. The resulting article should have sufficient information demonstrating that appropriate design and statistical methods were used. Yet there needs to be a balance between the amount of information provided and journal space limits; thus, relevant methodologic information can be placed in a supplement if needed. For additional information, see the chapter, A Checklist to Elevate the Science of Surgical Database Research.

Acknowledgment

The following disclosures were reported at the time this original article was first published.
   Conflict of Interest Disclosures: None reported.

References

1. McGlothin AE, Lewis RJ. Minimally clinically important difference: defining what really matters to patients. *JAMA*. 2014;312(13):1342-1343. Medline:25268441.
2. Strengthening the Reporting of Observational Studies in Epidemiology Group. Strengthening the Reporting of Observational Studies in Epidemiology (STROBE) statement. https://www.strobe-statement.org/index.php?id=strobe-home. Published 2009. Accessed March 7, 2018.
3. Stokes L. Sample size calculation for a hypothesis test. *JAMA*. 2014;312(2):180-181. Medline:25005655.
4. Cao J, Zhang S. Multiple comparison procedures. *JAMA*. 2014;312(5):543-544. Medline:25096694.
5. Newgard CD, Lewis RJ. Missing data: how to best account for what is not known. *JAMA*. 2015;314(9):940-941. Medline:26325562.
6. Shrier I, Platt RW. Reducing bias through directed acyclic graphs. *BMC Med Res Methodol*. 2008;8:70. Medline:18973665.
7. Kaji AH, Schriger D, Green S. Looking through the retrospectoscope: reducing bias in emergency medicine chart review studies. *Ann Emerg Med*. 2014;64(3):292-298. Medline:24746846.
8. American Statistical Association. The ASA's statement on P values: context, process and purpose. *Am Stat*. 2016;70:129-133.
9. Meurer WJ, Tolles J. Logistic regression diagnostics: understanding how well a model predicts outcomes. *JAMA*. 2017;317(10):1068-1069. Medline:28291878.
10. Detry MA, Ma Y. Analyzing repeated measurements using mixed models. *JAMA*. 2016;315(4):407-408. Medline:26813213.
11. Tolles J, Meurer WJ. Logistic regression: relating patient characteristics to outcomes. *JAMA*. 2016;316(5):533-534. Medline:27483067.

Practical Guide to Surgical Data Sets: Healthcare Cost and Utilization Project National Inpatient Sample (NIS)

Jonah J. Stulberg, MD, PhD, MPH, and Elliott R. Haut, MD, PhD

IN THIS CHAPTER

Introduction to the Healthcare Cost and Utilization Project

Strengths of Administrative Data

Limitations of Administrative Data and the HCUP Databases

   Administrative Data Limitations

   NIS Limitations

Critical Methodologic Considerations

Unique Capabilities of HCUP

This JAMA Guide to Statistics and Methods summarizes the key characteristics, strengths, and limitations of the National Inpatient Sample, a data set within AHRQ's Healthcare Cost and Utilization Project (HCUP) data set collection, for use in surgical health services research.

INTRODUCTION TO THE HEALTHCARE COST AND UTILIZATION PROJECT

Managed by the Agency for Healthcare Research and Quality, the Healthcare Cost and Utilization Project (HCUP, pronounced *H-Cup*) is a collection of data sets that represent the largest collection of administrative, longitudinal health care data in the United States. The data represent all-payer encounter-level information beginning in 1988 and is a collaborative effort between state data organizations, hospital associations, private data organizations, and the federal government. The stated objective of the project is to "conduct and translate research to inform decision making and improve health care delivery." Because an extensive description of all HCUP data sets is beyond the scope of this review, we will focus on the National Inpatient Sample (NIS, formerly *Nationwide Inpatient Sample*) as it relates to surgical research. This guide is an introduction; interested readers can explore the resources available on the HCUP website (http://www.hcup-us.ahrq.gov/). Many of the ideas we discuss will be applicable to the entire HCUP suite (Table 2).

STRENGTHS OF ADMINISTRATIVE DATA

The HCUP databases are considered administrative data sets because they capture the administrative components (eg, diagnosis codes, procedure codes, and costs) of a hospital encounter and not the clinical components (eg, vital signs and laboratory values).

TABLE 2

Available Healthcare Cost and Utilization Project Data Resources

Full Name	Acronym	Year Begun	New Records/y	Key Strengths	Key Limitations	Ideal Use
National Data						
National Inpatient Sample (formerly *Nationwide Inpatient Sample*)	NIS	1988	7 Million	Large size, long history, and inclusion of all inpatient hospital encounters	Lack of longitudinal data	Researching national prevalence/incidence, changes over time, and associations between diagnoses, procedures, and outcomes
Kids' Inpatient Database	KID	1997	2 Million–3 million	Large size and use of national estimates	Lack of state-specific granularity	Researching national prevalence/incidence, changes over time, and associations between diagnoses, procedures, and outcomes in the pediatric population

(*Continued*)

TABLE 2

Available Healthcare Cost and Utilization Project Data Resources (*Continued*)

Full Name	Acronym	Year Begun	New Records/y	Key Strengths	Key Limitations	Ideal Use
Nationwide Emergency Department Sample	NEDS	2006	30 Million	Large size and focus on emergency care	Inability to observe patients through system of care	Understanding patient use of emergency department services
Nationwide Readmissions Database	NRD	2013	15 Million	Readmissions and longitudinal data	Unsuitability for regional, state, or hospital-specific analysis	Studying readmissions following surgical procedures
State Data						
State Inpatient Database	SID	1995	Varies by state	All-payer state-specific data	Inconsistency of state participation over time	Studying state-level policy on surgical services

(*Continued*)

TABLE 2

Available Healthcare Cost and Utilization Project Data Resources (*Continued*)

Full Name	Acronym	Year Begun	New Records/y	Key Strengths	Key Limitations	Ideal Use
State Ambulatory Surgery and Services Databases	SASD	1997	Varies by state	All-payer ambulatory facility data	Inclusion of only 20 states	Understanding state-specific trends in inpatient vs ambulatory surgery
State Emergency Department Databases	SEDD	1999	Varies by state	All-payer emergency care data	Inability to observe patients through system of care	Understanding state-specific emergency surgery

They differ from clinical registries (eg, the National Surgical Quality Improvement Project) because they represent an aggregation of existing claims files rather than data prospectively collected by trained data abstractors for research or quality improvement. Although they are not clinical data sets, these administrative databases have been used to help shape policy decisions, assess the effectiveness of surgical techniques, examine disparities in surgical care, perform comparative effectiveness research, and drive quality-improvement efforts.[1-3]

The NIS is a 20% representative sampling of all inpatient hospital encounters in the United States. It is designed to be representative of health care use overall, making it ideal for performing basic descriptive studies, deriving national estimates, studying costs, studying rare disease, and understanding trends over time.

LIMITATIONS OF ADMINISTRATIVE DATA AND THE HCUP DATABASES

Regardless of what data source a researcher chooses to use for a given project, the data will have important limitations that could potentially affect the conclusions reached. Researchers should be transparent, acknowledge the limitations inherent in the data they are using, and discuss how the limitations may affect their findings. Researchers must always carefully select a data set that will allow them to reliably answer their research question or test their research hypothesis with a minimal amount of limitations.

Administrative Data Limitations

Although the size and scope of the HCUP databases affords wonderful research latitude, the data were originally collected for billing purposes and therefore have inherent limitations.[4] The most obvious limitation is the lack of clinical data. Additionally, the *International Classification of Diseases, Ninth Revision, Clinical Modification* (*ICD-9-CM*) system changes over time. As of October 2015, hospitals in the United States converted to using *International Statistical Classification of Diseases, Tenth Revision, Clinical Modification* codes, which will have consequences for those attempting longitudinal trend analyses. The specification of diagnoses is also limited by the inherent limitations of the coding system used. For example, in trauma research, the Injury Severity Score is not directly available. Instead, the International Classification of Diseases Programs for Injury Categorization can be used to estimate the Injury Severity Score based on *ICD-9-CM* codes. Another important limitation is surveillance bias, the phenomenon of "the more you look, the more you find," which may make examination of certain diagnoses or complications (eg, venous thromboembolism) invalid.[5] Finally, the systematic undercoding of certain low-cost diagnostic procedures can lead to inaccurate estimations of procedural use.

NIS Limitations

The most significant limitations involve the redesign (and associated renaming) of the NIS in 2012. There were several changes, including removing long-term acute care hospitals and using state hospital identifiers rather than the American Hospital Association hospital identifiers. The most dramatic change was the switch from using all discharges from a sample of hospitals to using a sample of discharges from all hospitals. These changes have important implications for researchers interested in studying trends over time, and anyone performing this type of analysis should refer to the NIS redesign report (http://www.hcup-us.ahrq.gov/reports/methods/methods.jsp) for further details.

CRITICAL METHODOLOGIC CONSIDERATIONS

With sample sizes in the millions, P values for statistical significance frequently far exceed the typical cutoff of less than .05. Therefore, we urge caution when interpreting P values from

> **BOX 3**
>
> ### Best Practices When Using the National Inpatient Sample for Research
>
> 1. Ensure the National Inpatient Sample is the appropriate data set to address the question of interest.
> 2. Consult the HCUP website (http://www.hcup-us.ahrq.gov) to guide the project through the nuances and common pitfalls of the data set.
> 3. Map out variables of interest to your research question and write out the benefits and disadvantages of that variable generated from administrative records. Assure these do not undermine your primary hypothesis.
> 4. Focus the research question on the strengths of the HCUP data sets (Table 2).
> 5. Review the HCUP website to determine which code sets and downloadable files pertain to your research.

NIS studies and recommend considering clinical significance in the context of statistical significance. By starting with a clearly thought-out research question and understanding the limitations of asking this question using the data available, findings can be appropriately interpreted to improve surgical practice. These data should not be used for causal inference; instead, they are best suited for hypothesis generation or evaluation of trends. Recent articles note the lack of rigor in published manuscripts using the NIS and make suggestions for best practices in research using the NIS (Box 3).[6,7]

UNIQUE CAPABILITIES OF HCUP

The HCUP is working to develop solutions for known limitations within their suite of databases. One shining example is the development of variables that track an individual over time (eg, VisitLink and DaysToEvent). All HCUP databases are deidentified, making the study of an individual patient over time impossible. The solution: developing a linking variable that would allow researchers to track an individual over time within the data without compromising the individual's identity by exposing protected health information. The combination of these variables allows researchers to track an individual from an initial visit, eg, a surgical encounter, over time, which will allow studies of readmissions, cancer recurrence, and others.

The HCUP also provides user support features, such as downloadable statistical programming codes that help with risk adjustment using Elixhauser comorbidities, clinical classifications software tools, and chronic condition indicators. With improved computing power and a well-established base of surgeon-researchers capable of using these resources, the HCUP suite will be increasingly valuable.

Acknowledgment

The following disclosures were reported at the time this original article was first published.

Conflict of Interest Disclosures: None reported.

References

1. Stulberg JJ, Delaney CP, Neuhauser DV, Aron DC, Fu P, Koroukian SM. Adherence to surgical care improvement project measures and the association with postoperative infections. *JAMA*. 2010;303(24):2479-2485. Medline:20571014.
2. Schwartz DA, Hui X, Schneider EB, et al. Worse outcomes among uninsured general surgery patients. *Surgery*. 2014;156(2):345-351. Medline:24953267.
3. Zafar SN, Shah AA, Hashmi ZG, et al. Outcomes after emergency general surgery at teaching versus nonteaching hospitals. *J Trauma Acute Care Surg*. 2015;78(1):69-76, 76-77. Medline:25539205.
4. Haut ER, Pronovost PJ, Schneider EB. Limitations of administrative databases. *JAMA*. 2012;307(24):2589. Medline:22735421.
5. Haut ER, Pronovost PJ. Surveillance bias in outcomes reporting. *JAMA*. 2011;305(23):2462-2463. Medline:21673300.

6. Khera R, Angraal S, Couch T, et al. Adherence to methodological standards in research using the national inpatient sample. *JAMA*. 2017;318(20):2011-2018. Medline:29183077.

7. Khera R, Krumholz HM. With great power comes great responsibility. *Circ Cardiovasc Qual Outcomes*. 2017;10(7):e003846. Medline:28705865.

JAMAevidence
Using Evidence to Improve Care

Practical Guide to Surgical Data Sets: Surveillance, Epidemiology, and End Results (SEER) Database

Kemi M. Doll, MD, MSCR,
Alfred Rademaker, PhD, and Julie A. Sosa, MD

IN THIS CHAPTER

Introduction

Data Considerations
  Data Sources
  Time Trend Data
  Cancer Data
  Treatment Data

Statistical Considerations

Conclusions

This JAMA Guide to Statistics and Methods summarizes the Surveillance, Epidemiology, and End Results (SEER) data sets, including longitudinal details, included and excluded data, and uses in surgical research.

INTRODUCTION

The Surveillance, Epidemiology, and End Results (SEER) database is a publicly available, federally funded cancer reporting system that represents a collaboration between the US Centers for Disease Control and Prevention, the National Cancer Institute, and regional and state cancer registries.[1] SEER data are national, with information from 18 states that represent all regions of the country. In contrast to other commonly used data sets (eg, the National Cancer Data Base), SEER is population-based, because local registries report information for all cancer cases within a specific region and/or defined racial/ethnic population. Given that SEER data is both a cancer reporting system and a research tool, we aim to present salient aspects of these data, strengths and limitations for analyses, and important statistical considerations.

DATA CONSIDERATIONS

Data Sources

SEER data are gathered at the local level. Trained registrars collect data from all clinical settings that diagnose or treat cancer and include patients of all ages, regardless of insurance status. Dates and causes of death come from death certificates, and mortality statistics are calculated using data from the US Census Bureau (Table 3). SEER data captures 28% of the US population; because of its targeted sampling strategy, it includes a high

TABLE 3

Overview of the Surveillance, Epidemiology, and End Results Database

Type	Included in SEER	Not Included in SEER
Sociodemographic factors	Age at diagnosis, year of birth, race/ethnicity, sex, census tract education, census tract income, marital status, place of birth	Individual income, family income
Geographic variables	County and state of residence, originating SEER registry, urban/rural designation	Zip codes, site of treatment
Clinical factors	Prior cancer history	Comorbidity, functional status, medications
Cancer specific factors	Site, laterality, stage,[a] grade, lymph node status, extent of disease,[b] tumor markers[b]	Depending on the cancer site, information may be missing to varying degrees.
Pathologic variables	Lymphovascular invasion, perineural invasion, margin status	Pathologic variables collected vary by cancer site.
Treatment factors	Method of diagnostic confirmation, receipt of surgery, extent of surgery,[b] receipt of radiation, order of treatment	Clinician information, surgical approach, radiation dose, chemotherapy, hormonal therapy, immunotherapy

(Continued)

TABLE 3

Overview of the Surveillance, Epidemiology, and End Results Database (*Continued*)

Type	Included in SEER	Not Included in SEER
Outcomes	Date of death, cause of death	Cancer recurrence

Abbreviation: SEER, Surveillance, Epidemiology, and End Results.
[a] These data points are SEER summary stages; American Joint Committee on Cancer Tumor, Nodes, and Metastases classification system was put in place starting in 2004.
[b] These data points are specific to certain cancer sites.

proportion of racial/ethnic minorities, foreign-born individuals, and those with income below the federal poverty line.

Time Trend Data

The SEER program originated in 1974, so it can be used to study trends in cancer incidence, prevalence, and survival in the United States over time. The addition of SEER registries since 1974 has resulted in numbered cohorts (eg, SEER-9 from 1974, SEER-13 from 1992, and SEER-18 from 2000). Trend studies should be restricted to a consistent SEER cohort for all years of the analysis to avoid shifts in base populations that create erroneous findings.

Cancer Data

Stage and histologic details are reported for all cancers, allowing for specific subpopulations and rare cancers to be studied. Unique to SEER is a variable termed *Summary Stage*, defined for each cancer site (local, regional, distant, and unknown) in manuals published online. Given the longevity of SEER data collection, shifts in stage classifications over time should be accounted for in time trend studies, using stratification or manually recoding for consistency. American Joint Committee on Cancer stage is available, usually for patients with summary stages reported. The *Collaborative Stage* variables (Box 4) for each cancer are site-specific factors that range from serum tumor markers (eg, cancer antigen 19-9) to diagnostic details (eg, number of prostate biopsy cores). Missingness, quality, and the time when each variable was introduced into the data set vary. (For example, in breast cancer, although HER2 laboratory test results are available for 76% of patients since 2010, they are often inconsistent with the HER2 status variable and therefore should not be used in analysis.[2]) Multiple imputation is a recommended method of accounting for variables with a high proportion of missing values, such as estrogen receptor status in breast cancer over time.[3]

BOX 4

Details of SEER Data

1. SEER is a nationally representative, population-based cancer reporting system that includes all cancer cases within specific US geographic regions.

2. Longitudinal trends in cancer diagnosis, treatment, and survival can be analyzed starting from 1974 to the present.

3. The SEER data are particularly well suited for longitudinal studies on specific subpopulations and rare or indolent cancer types.

4. The Collaborative Stage Data Collection system can be used to gather additional site-specific prognostic and treatment details for individual cancer sites.

5. Care should be taken to document and account for changes in staging classifications over time.

6. Comparative effectiveness analyses are limited by lack of information on comorbidity, recurrence, and chemotherapy.

Abbreviation: SEER, Surveillance, Epidemiology, and End Results.

Treatment Data

SEER data report receipt of surgery and radiation, and treatment sequence is captured such that analysis of treatment trends by specific histologic indications can be performed. For example, Ko et al[4] measured the use of adjuvant radiation therapy for high-to-intermediate–risk endometrial cancer after 2 national clinical trials. It is more difficult to study treatment outcomes and perform comparative effectiveness research in SEER. Important details, such as comorbidity, intent of surgery (cure vs palliation), surgical route (minimally invasive vs open approaches), radiation dosing, and other treatments (eg, chemotherapy, hormonal therapy, or immunotherapy) are absent. The inability to address the influence of these missing variables on outcomes makes comparative effectiveness analyses prone to unmeasured confounding. Using the SEER-Medicare linked database can address this, but largely in adults 65 years and older.

STATISTICAL CONSIDERATIONS

SEER data are available in 2 ways: (1) a binary format for which SEER*Stat software can be used to perform common but limited analyses; or (2) as text data that can be directly imported into external statistical software for more complex projects.[1] For incidence and mortality rates, results should be age-adjusted and reported as cases per 100 000 person-years. A trend analysis evaluates how rates change over time by comparing the annual percent change in rates using standard t or rank sum tests. A modeling strategy (eg, log-linear regression) can then be used to calculate the rate of change and generate illustrative graphics. The addition of joinpoint regression[5] can pinpoint years that demonstrate the most dramatic changes, as in a study by Lim et al[6] for thyroid cancer rates from 1974 through 2013.

Population-level survival statistics can be reported as relative survival (the ratio of overall survival of patients with the disease to the expected survival in a comparable cohort of the general population) or cancer-specific survival (the proportion of patients alive with a specific disease). Which to use depends on how best to limit bias for the population in question. Relative survival, which is based on the overall survival of patients with the disease, is less accurate for cancers for which patients commonly have other serious comorbidities (eg, lung cancer) because the competing mortality risks from these comorbidities are not taken into account. Cancer-specific survival is less reliable in cases of multiple primary cancers because of difficulty in identifying accurate causes of death from death certificates.[7] Cox proportional hazard models can be used to calculate how demographic factors and prognostic differences influence individual mortality. Overall, missing clinical data mean that comparative effectiveness research using SEER data alone should be undertaken with caution, given the limited ability to account for important clinical differences between treatment groups.

CONCLUSIONS

SEER is a long-established resource that allows for population-based surveillance and analysis of all cancers in the United States. Excellent uses of SEER include epidemiologic studies of incidence, prevalence, and mortality rates over time, shifting treatment patterns between surgery and radiation, and quantifying diagnostic and treatment patterns by geographic and demographic factors.

Acknowledgment

The following disclosures were reported at the time this original article was first published.

Conflict of Interest Disclosures: Dr Doll receives research support from the National Comprehensive Cancer Network Foundation through a grant supported by Pfizer. Dr Sosa is a member of the data monitoring committee of the Medullary Thyroid Cancer Consortium Registry, which is supported by NovoNordisk, GlaxoSmithKline, AstraZeneca, and Eli Lilly. No other disclosures are reported.

References

1. National Cancer Institute. Surveillance, Epidemiology, and End Results program website. http://www.seer.cancer.gov. Published 2018. Accessed February 26, 2018.
2. Howlader N, Chen VW, Ries LA, et al. Overview of breast cancer collaborative stage data items—their definitions, quality, usage, and clinical implications: a review of SEER data for 2004-2010. *Cancer*. 2014;120(suppl 23):3771-3780. Medline:25412389.
3. Krieger N, Jahn JL, Waterman PD. Jim Crow and estrogen-receptor-negative breast cancer: US-born black and white non-Hispanic women, 1992-2012. *Cancer Causes Control*. 2017;28(1):49-59. Medline:27988896.
4. Ko EM, Funk MJ, Clark LH, Brewster WR. Did GOG99 and PORTEC1 change clinical practice in the United States? *Gynecol Oncol*. 2013;129(1):12-17. Medline:23376807.
5. Dehkordi ZF, Tazhibi M, Babazade S. Application of joinpoint regression in determining breast cancer incidence rate change points by age and tumor characteristics in women aged 30-69 (years) and in Isfahan city from 2001 to 2010. *J Educ Health Promot*. 2014;3:115. Medline:25540788.
6. Lim H, Devesa SS, Sosa JA, Check D, Kitahara CM. Trends in thyroid cancer incidence and mortality in the United States, 1974-2013. *JAMA*. 2017;317(13):1338-1348. Medline:28362912.
7. Sarfati D, Blakely T, Pearce N. Measuring cancer survival in populations: relative survival vs cancer-specific survival. *Int J Epidemiol*. 2010;39(2):598-610. Medline:20142331.

Practical Guide to Surgical Data Sets: Medicare Claims Data

Amir A. Ghaferi, MD, MS, and
Justin B. Dimick, MD, MPH

IN THIS CHAPTER

Introduction

Pros and Cons of Medicare Data

Potential Avenues of Research
   Comparative Effectiveness Research
   Health Policy Evaluation
   Understanding Variation

Where to Find More Information

This JAMA Guide to Statistics and Methods describes the Medicare claims data available from the Centers for Medicare and Medicaid Services and its use in comparative effectiveness research and health policy analysis.

INTRODUCTION

The Centers for Medicare and Medicaid Services (CMS) administers Medicare, the primary US health insurance program for people aged 65 years and older and people who qualify for Social Security Administration disability benefits (Box 5). Medicare includes Part A, which is hospital insurance; Part B,

---

BOX 5

Attributes of Medicare Claim Data

1. Medicare data are an excellent national representation of a large proportion of the older adult population.
2. While a cost-effective way of evaluating a large population, securing independent funding to purchase the data is highly recommended.
3. The data sets available from the Centers for Medicare and Medicaid Services are suitable for linkages to several existing data sets (ie, American Heart Association, US Census, and others).
4. Data can be tracked longitudinally across episodes of care, making this a uniquely positioned data set to study long-term outcomes in surgical patients.
5. Several advanced statistical methods can increase the robustness of inferences made using this data; inclusion of experienced methodologists in research is highly recommended.

medical insurance; Part C, Medicare Advantage (private health insurance approved by the CMS and paid on a per-capita basis); and Part D, prescription drug coverage. The CMS maintains and makes several data files available for purchase (https://www.cms.gov/Research-Statistics-Data-and-Systems/Files-for-Order/FilesForOrderGenInfo/index.html). Because the Medicare Advantage data are administered by private insurance, these claims are unavailable. However, national fee-for-service Medicare files are available and represent approximately 70% of beneficiaries.

Medicare data represent claims submitted to the CMS for reimbursement of services rendered. The Medicare data set has very little missing data because accurate claims are necessary for hospital and physician payments.

PROS AND CONS OF MEDICARE DATA

Several features make this data set a useful research tool. First, specific demographic data are included (eg, age, birthdate, sex, race/ethnicity, and place of residence). Second, these data can be linked to other CMS data sets on health care utilization, insurance enrollment, and clinician characteristics. Third, the data cover nearly 70% of adults aged 65 years and older, making fee-for-service Medicare data a rich source of utilization and outcomes data and allowing for subgroup analyses without decreased statistical power. Fourth, the data can be linked to non-CMS data, such as the US Census, cancer registries (eg, the Surveillance, Epidemiology, and End Results Program; Medicare), other government insurance programs (eg, Medicaid), the Social Security death index, and clinician information (ie, American Hospital Association data). Fifth, patients can be tracked across episodes of care, which permits longitudinal evaluations of outcomes and health care utilization. Finally, Medicare data files are a cost-effective way to assess a large patient population across multiple health care settings.

However, there are important limitations when using Medicare data for research. First, it only includes a diagnosis documented via the *International Classification of Diseases, Ninth Revision (ICD-9)* or *ICD-10* codes (ie, hypertension, depression, diabetes). This can prove difficult when assessing surgical complications. Iezzoni et al[1] identified the most appropriate *ICD* codes to measure comorbidities and complications, but these are imperfect. Second, there is no physiological or biochemical patient information, such as vital signs, laboratory test results, and pathology results. Third, there are no timestamps during a hospital stay. This can limit the study of how care progresses or when events and complications occur during a hospitalization. Fourth, evaluation of outpatient utilization patterns can be limited by the lack of data on uncovered services or benefits and managed care enrollee information. Finally, derivation from billing data limits reliability. This is especially important in patients undergoing surgery, for whom comorbidity and severity of illness may be inconsistently documented.

POTENTIAL AVENUES OF RESEARCH

Medicare data can provide valuable insights to several topical areas of surgical research. Three commonly studied categories are health policy evaluation, comparative effectiveness research, and outcome variations. Table 4 summarizes these 3 themes and methodologies.

Comparative Effectiveness Research

Comparative effectiveness research is the direct comparison of health care interventions to determine which works best, for whom, and in what circumstances. Although randomized clinical trials are excellent at identifying the efficacy of a procedure or treatment, these studies are limited by strict inclusion criteria and short-term follow-up. Large claims databases

TABLE 4

Common Research Uses for Medicare Data and Statistical Approaches for Addressing Common Methodological Problems

Major Research Theme	Methodological Problem	Statistical Methods
Comparative effectiveness research	Adjusting for selection bias (eg, differences in characteristics between treated and control groups)	Multivariate regression, instrumental variable analysis, and propensity score analysis
Health policy evaluation	Adjusting for background time trends (eg, improvements in outcomes over time)	Difference-in-differences analysis
Understanding variation across clinicians	Risk adjustment (eg, accounting for differences in patient characteristics across clinicians); accounting for clustering within clinicians and adjusting for reliability	Multivariate regression and hierarchical modeling

facilitate assessments in real-world settings with broader groups of patients and clinicians. For example, after 2 large national trials demonstrated the efficacy of carotid endarterectomy, a classic comparative effectiveness study[2] evaluated the real-world effectiveness of the procedure outside the confines of a clinical trial. Using multivariate logistic regression, Wennberg et al[2] found perioperative mortality after carotid endarterectomy in patients receiving Medicare to be markedly higher than in a control group. This raised concerns about translating randomized clinical trials' efficacy into effectiveness in everyday practice. Researchers interested in using Medicare data to study comparative effectiveness should develop expertise or seek collaborators experienced in using advanced methods for causal inference, such as instrumental variable analysis[3] and propensity score matching.[4]

Health Policy Evaluation

Health policy shapes many aspects of our environment, including payment, performance measurement, and training. However, to our knowledge, there is little evidence that policies have the desired effect of improving outcomes or reducing costs. Medicare data provide the use of rigorous methods on a large cohort of patients and clinicians to examine broad policy implications, intended and some unintended. Dimick et al[5] evaluated the implications of a CMS national coverage decision restricting bariatric surgery to centers of excellence. However, studies supporting this well-intentioned policy lacked control groups. Using longitudinal Medicare claims data and sophisticated statistical methods, this study identified no difference in outcomes before and after policy implementation, leading to a reconsideration and ultimately a reversal of that coverage decision. The specific method used was difference-in-differences, an econometric technique that accounts for background trends in outcomes and is common in health care policy evaluations.

Understanding Variation

Developing a better understanding of the magnitude of variation and its associations with measurable characteristics is a valuable way to gain insight into surgical practice and levers for change. These evaluations lend themselves to new policies to reduce variation in surgical care. Ghaferi et al[6] examined drivers of variation in mortality rates with high-risk surgery in patients receiving Medicare benefits. Mortality rates varied significantly, with a nearly 2.5-fold difference between the best and worst hospitals. Most interestingly, complication rates were similar across hospitals, but the rate at which patients were rescued from complications were much higher at hospitals with low mortality. These findings helped guide surgical quality improvement efforts toward reducing failure to rescue rates by focusing on timely and effective management of postoperative complications. The statistical methods used in this study included multivariate logistic regression to adjust for confounding patient variables and reliability adjustment to account for random chance as a driver of outcomes.[7]

WHERE TO FIND MORE INFORMATION

Medicare data are useful for studying comparative effectiveness of procedures, health care policy, and outcome variations. However, it is important to frame questions carefully and use appropriate methods to ensure scientific rigor, as each of the cited studies have done.

Acknowledgment

The following disclosures were reported at the time this original article was first published.

Conflict of Interest Disclosures: Dr Dimick reports receiving personal fees and holding equity interest in ArborMetrix, Inc. No other conflicts of interest were disclosed.

Funding/Support: This work is supported by grants from the Agency for Healthcare Research and Quality (grants 5K08HS02362 and P30HS024403, Dr Ghaferi) and a Patient Centered Outcomes Research Institute Award (grant CE-1304-6596, Dr Ghaferi).

Role of the Funder/Sponsor: The funders had no role in the design and conduct of the study; collection, management, analysis, and interpretation of the data; preparation, review, or approval of the manuscript; and decision to submit the manuscript for publication.

References

1. Iezzoni LI, Daley J, Heeren T, et al. Identifying complications of care using administrative data. *Med Care*. 1994;32(7):700-715. Medline:8028405.
2. Wennberg DE, Lucas FL, Birkmeyer JD, Bredenberg CE, Fisher ES. Variation in carotid endarterectomy mortality in the Medicare population: trial hospitals, volume, and patient characteristics. *JAMA*. 1998;279(16):1278-1281. Medline:9565008.
3. Tan HJ, Norton EC, Ye Z, Hafez KS, Gore JL, Miller DC. Long-term survival following partial vs radical nephrectomy among older patients with early-stage kidney cancer. *JAMA*. 2012;307(15):1629-1635. Medline:22511691.
4. Haukoos JS, Lewis RJ. The Propensity Score. *JAMA*. 2015;314(15):1637-1638. Medline:26501539.
5. Dimick JB, Nicholas LH, Ryan AM, Thumma JR, Birkmeyer JD. Bariatric surgery complications before vs after implementation of a national policy restricting coverage to centers of excellence. *JAMA*. 2013;309(8):792-799. Medline:23443442.
6. Ghaferi AA, Birkmeyer JD, Dimick JB. Complications, failure to rescue, and mortality with major inpatient surgery in Medicare patients. *Ann Surg*. 2009;250(6):1029-1034. Medline:19953723.
7. Dimick JB, Ghaferi AA, Osborne NH, Ko CY, Hall BL. Reliability adjustment for reporting hospital outcomes with surgery. *Ann Surg*. 2012;255(4):703-707. Medline:22388108.

JAMAevidence
Using Evidence to Improve Care

Practical Guide to Surgical Data Sets: Military Health System Tricare Encounter Data

Andrew J. Schoenfeld, MD, MSc,
Amy H. Kaji, MD, PhD, and
Adil H. Haider, MD, MPH

IN THIS CHAPTER

Introduction

Use of the Data

Salient and Unique Features of the Data Set

How Are Data Compiled?

What Are Common Outcomes That Can Be Studied?

What Are the Limitations With This Data Set?

Statistical Considerations

Where to Find More Information

This JAMA Guide to Statistics and Methods describes the use of Tricare insurance claims data from the US Department of Defense to assess health care needs, utilization, and outcomes in active, retired, and disabled military service members.

INTRODUCTION

Tricare (often styled TRICARE) is the insurance product owned and operated by the US Department of Defense (DoD); it covers more than 9 million beneficiaries nationwide (Box 6).[1-3] Tricare

---

BOX 6

Attributes of Tricare Claims Data

1. Tricare claims have been used to study health care utilization, prescription drug use, provider-induced demand, and the potential impact of universal insurance to reduce disparities in surgical care.
2. The demographic, educational, and vocational diversity of the population covered through Tricare likely renders data generalizable to the average American individual under age 65 years.
3. Tricare data has many of the limitations inherent to administrative claims data sets.
4. Reweighted estimating equations or multiple imputation may be used to adjust for the percentage of the population with missing data.
5. Analyses employing Tricare data should account for the environment of care (eg, Direct vs Purchased Care) in some fashion.

claims data are maintained by the Military Health System Data Repository (MDR).[1-5] Research is performed using administrative insurance claims prepared by the MDR.

USE OF THE DATA

Salient and Unique Features of the Data Set

Tricare insurance is available to active duty service members, retirees, and individuals who are separated from service with certain disabilities, as well as their dependents.[1] At present, only 20% of the covered population consists of active military personnel, with the remaining 80% composed of civilians.[1-5] Eligible beneficiaries can maintain Tricare coverage through age 65 years, when transition to Medicare coverage typically occurs. The diverse sociodemographic, vocational, educational, and occupational characteristics of the population insured through Tricare have been found to be representative of the general US population up to age 64 years.[1,5,6] Tricare insurance is not used to cover services administered in combat zones or health care provided through the Veterans Administration (VA). Individuals with both VA benefits and Tricare may choose to receive some or all aspects of their care at VA hospitals.

How Are Data Compiled?

Tricare beneficiaries may receive care at DoD-administered health care facilities (termed *direct care*) or at civilian hospitals and clinics that accept Tricare (termed *purchased care*).[1,3,5,6] Direct Care centers include 60 inpatient acute care hospitals, 385 stand-alone medical clinics, and 350 dental clinics. Irrespective of the site of service or the environment of care (eg, DoD vs civilian centers), all claims filed through Tricare (including inpatient and outpatient facility and physician fees, dental services, prescription medications, and durable medical equipment) are captured by the MDR.[2,5,6] Claims are verified using standard administrative practices for the purposes of providing payment. Data for the individual subscriber are linked over time, allowing for longitudinal analysis of care.

Clinician information is recorded in the MDR using National Provider Identifiers (NPI) and system-specific designations. The MDR also maintains a variety of demographic information for its beneficiaries, including age, race/ethnicity (if or as reported by the sponsor), marital status, census region of residence, and sponsor rank, a unique feature of this data which can be used as a proxy measure for socioeconomic status.[1,3,6] The MDR may be used to calculate Charlson comorbidity indices for beneficiaries via the *International Statistical Classification of Diseases and Related Health Problems, Ninth Revision (ICD-9)* or *ICD-10* diagnosis codes, develop Injury Severity Scores, and determine duration of hospital admissions. The MDR can be queried using *ICD-9* procedure or diagnosis codes. TRICARE claims data are deidentified before disbursal to data users. Access to Tricare requires application and approval from the DoD.

What Are Common Outcomes That Can Be Studied?

Tricare claims have frequently been used to study postsurgical morbidity, mortality, health care utilization, prescription drug use, and quality of care.[1-5] A unique advantage rests in the fact that retirees, disabled individuals, and their dependents can remain insured through Tricare until age 65 years. Thus, there is an enhanced potential for long-term observation, compared with private payer data sets that include individuals who may lose coverage or switch carriers. The substantial demographic, socio-ethnic, educational, occupational, and vocational diversity of the population covered through Tricare likely renders this data more generalizable to the US population than that of data derived from Medicare, private payer claims, or institutional registries.[1-6] Given the attributes inherent to the covered population, as well as the means through which care is provided, Tricare data has also been used to model the effects of universal health insurance in the United States.[5] The capacity to evaluate differences in health care provided to similar patients insured through Tricare but treated in a fee-for-service setting (Purchased Care) or salaried health care setting (Direct Care) has potentiated investigations of procedural inducement and provider induced demand.[4]

What Are the Limitations With This Data Set?

Similar to other administrative claims data sets, Tricare data are not clinically granular, and perioperative or trauma-specific measures (such as estimated blood loss, the extent or invasiveness of a surgical intervention, Glasgow Coma Scale scores, vital signs, and radiographic results) are typically unavailable. Likewise, Tricare claims may be prone to medication exposure misclassification if medications are purchased without using the insurance benefit.[1,3] Low-cost generic drug programs offered at major chain pharmacies can be a source of misclassification because these initiatives can incentivize individuals to purchase medications out of pocket. As a result, a pharmacy claim may never be submitted. Also, the means by which Tricare pays for services in the Direct Care setting, in which lump sum payments are allocated over a fiscal period in a manner that cannot be correlated with fee-for-service, makes it difficult to accurately determine the costs of specific surgical episodes.

STATISTICAL CONSIDERATIONS

Most studies conducted using TRICARE data have used traditional statistical approaches (eg, logistic regression and Cox proportional hazards regression).[1,5] Causal inference techniques, including propensity score matching, have been used as well. In all settings, it is important to adjust for the environment of care (eg, direct care or purchased care), and this has been performed in prior studies with hierarchical modeling.

Data on patient race/ethnicity are purely based on reports by the Tricare sponsor, and sponsors can decline to answer this question. As a result, missing data on patient race/ethnicity has been found to be as high as 31% in studies relying on Tricare.[5] This has been addressed in prior work by using reweighted estimating equations.[1,5,7] The limitation with this method is that this is a complete case analysis, and this analysis will be biased if the data are not missing at random. Thus, other statistical techniques, such as multiple imputation (which allows individuals with incomplete data to be included in analyses), could also be used. Limiting analyses to individuals with complete information or using missing data indicators may result in confounding. As a result, sensitivity analyses should be performed to examine the effect of different assumptions (missing completely at random, missing at random, or missing not at random) on the missing data mechanism.

WHERE TO FIND MORE INFORMATION

In a recent investigation, Chaudhary et al[1] used a multivariable logistic regression model to evaluate demographic and clinical factors associated with opioid prescription at discharge after trauma. In this study, incidence of an opioid prescription at discharge was closely aligned with reported prevalence of moderate or severe pain in patients who had experienced trauma. Older age and higher Injury Severity Score were associated with a greater likelihood of opioid prescription at discharge.

In a separate study of Tricare data collected between 2006 and 2010, Schoenfeld et al[5] modeled the association of universal insurance on disparities with outcomes of major surgical interventions among African American patients, including joint replacement, coronary artery bypass graft surgery, radical cystectomy, and appendectomy. Differences in outcomes between African American and white Tricare recipients were compared with individuals treated with identical surgeries in California during a similar period. Multivariable hierarchical logistic regression analysis was used to adjust for differences in case mix (age, sex, medical comorbidities, and socioeconomic status), hospital cluster effects, and the type of surgical intervention. The authors reported that while disparities in California were readily apparent for African American patients, especially those without private health insurance, they were absent in the Tricare setting.

Acknowledgment

The following disclosures were reported at the time this original article was first published.

Conflict of Interest Disclosures: Dr Schoenfeld reports receiving grants from the Henry M. Jackson Foundation of the Department of Defense, the Orthopaedic Research and Education Foundation, and the National Institutes of Health, and non-financial research supports from the Centers for Medicare and Medicaid Services Office of Minority Health and royalties from Wolters-Kluwer Health and Springer Publishers. Dr Haider reports receiving grants from the Henry M. Jackson Foundation of the Department of Defense, the Orthopaedic Research and Education Foundation, and the National Institutes of Health, and non-financial research supports from the Centers for Medicare and Medicaid Services Office of Minority Health. No other disclosures were reported.

Funding/Support: This work is supported by the Henry M. Jackson Foundation for the Advancement of Military Medicine of the Department of Defense (Drs Schoenfeld and Haider).

Role of the Funder/Sponsor: The funder had no role in the design and conduct of the study; collection, management, analysis, and interpretation of the data; preparation, review, or approval of the manuscript; and decision to submit the manuscript for publication.

References

1. Chaudhary MA, Schoenfeld AJ, Harlow AF, et al. Incidence and predictors of opioid prescription at discharge after traumatic injury. *JAMA Surg.* 2017;152(10):930-936. Medline:28636707.

2. Schoenfeld AJ, Jiang W, Chaudhary MA, Scully RE, Koehlmoos T, Haider AH. Sustained prescription opioid use among previously opioid-naive patients insured through TRICARE (2006-2014). *JAMA Surg.* 2017;152(12):1175-1176; E-pub ahead of print. Medline:28813584.

3. Scully RE, Schoenfeld AJ, Jiang W, et al. Defining optimal opioid pain medication prescription length following common surgical procedures. *JAMA Surg.* 2018;153(1):37-43.

4. Nguyen LL, Smith AD, Scully RE, et al. Provider-induced demand in the treatment of carotid artery stenosis: variation in treatment decisions between private sector fee-for-service vs salary-based military physicians. *JAMA Surg.* 2017;152(6):565-572. Medline:28249083.

5. Schoenfeld AJ, Jiang W, Harris MB, et al. Association between race and postoperative outcomes in a universally insured population vs patients in the state of California. *Ann Surg.* 2017;266(2):267-273. Medline:27501169.

6. Gimbel RW, Pangaro L, Barbour G. America's "undiscovered" laboratory for health services research. *Med Care.* 2010;48(8):751-756. Medline:20613659.

7. Henry AJ, Hevelone ND, Lipsitz S, Nguyen LL. Comparative methods for handling missing data in large databases. *J Vasc Surg.* 2013;58(5):1353-1359.e6. Medline:23830314.

Practical Guide to Surgical Data Sets: Veterans Affairs Surgical Quality Improvement Program (VASQIP)

Nader N. Massarweh, MD, MPH,
Amy H. Kaji, MD, PhD, and
Kamal M. F. Itani, MD

IN THIS CHAPTER

Advent of the Veterans Affairs Surgical Quality Improvement Program

Data Considerations

Patients

Procedure

Hospital

Outcomes

Utility and Unique Features of VASQIP

Statistical Considerations

Conclusions

This JAMA Guide to Statistics and Methods summarizes the advent, data considerations, utility and unique features, and statistical considerations of the Veterans Affairs National Surgical Quality Improvement Program (VASQIP) for use in surgical quality improvement research.

ADVENT OF THE VETERANS AFFAIRS SURGICAL QUALITY IMPROVEMENT PROGRAM

Since the early 1990s, US Veterans Affairs (VA) has been at the vanguard of national efforts to measure hospital-level performance and ensure quality care for veterans. In response to a congressional mandate that "the VA should report its surgical outcomes in comparison to the national average…with risk adjustment," the initial VA National Surgical Quality Improvement Program (NSQIP) was created to accurately collect clinical data using standardized methodology and incorporating robust risk adjustment.[1] Renamed the VA Surgical Quality Improvement Program (VASQIP) after merging the cardiac and noncardiac surgery components of NSQIP, this mandatory, VA-wide program has remained a model for national quality improvement (QI) efforts and was the template used to develop the private sector American College of Surgeons–NSQIP.

DATA CONSIDERATIONS

Cases abstracted by trained local VASQIP nurses are identified on an 8-day cycle to ensure data collection periods begin on different days of the week and provide a more representative sample of cases performed at each hospital. Data abstraction involves a thorough review of the electronic medical record and abstraction of preoperative, intraoperative, and postoperative variables based on standardized definitions. All patients are followed for a full 30 days after surgery, regardless of the duration of the postoperative in-hospital length of stay. Abstraction of certain higher-volume cases, such as inguinal hernia repair, is limited to no more than 5 per cycle. Data are collected for up to a maximum of 36 cases per cycle.

The Veterans Affairs Surgical Quality Improvement Program (Box 7) is a rich and accurate source of data for QI and surgical research.[2] A complete VASQIP assessment includes more than 200 variables with 78 manually abstracted for each case. In 2009, *The American Journal of Surgery* dedicated an issue to comprehensively summarize the first 15 years of NSQIP.[3] Below is a brief synopsis of the type of data available in VASQIP.

BOX 7

Best Practices for Using VASQIP

1. For patients with more than 1 operation in the data, only evaluate the first operation in each 30-day follow-up interval.
2. Review the definitions of each individual data point and outcome to avoid misinterpretation.
3. Given the large sample size, correlate clinical significance of findings with statistical significance.
4. Crosslinking of VASQIP to other available databases at the patient level is a unique resource for research within the VA.
5. Use judicious empirical selection of model covariates based on established evidence or biologic/clinical plausibility to avoid overfitting.
6. Consider hierarchical models and reliability adjustment to account for patient clustering and statistical noise from small sample size, respectively.

Abbreviations: VA, Veterans Affairs; VASQIP, Veterans Affairs Surgical Quality Improvement Program.

Patients

Depending on the research goals, patients in VASQIP can be identified using either their social security number (SSN), a scrambled SSN, or a unique patient identifier. Justification must be provided for data requests to obtain SSNs. In addition to basic demographic information, VASQIP provides numerous variables describing patients' preoperative condition (eg, the data provide information on the presence of diabetes and the severity of the disease) as well as a variety of laboratory values.

Procedure

Cases are identified for VASQIP data collection based on the principal *Current Procedural Terminology* (*CPT*) code. In addition to the principal *CPT* code, up to 10 other *CPT* codes for concurrently performed procedures are provided. A variety of different variables also characterize the nature of the principal procedure, such as time and date stamps for the start and end of the operation, type of anesthesia administered, presence of postgraduate trainees, wound classification, and associated relative value units. These variables allow for comparative analyses across procedures of varying complexity.

Hospital

Although the American College of Surgeons–NSQIP Participant User File does not uniquely identify individual hospitals, VASQIP does provide a unique hospital identifier allowing for hospital-level analyses. Additionally, in 2010, the VA National Surgery Office assigned each hospital an operative complexity level, allowing the facility to be identified as an ambulatory surgery center (basic or complex) or inpatient facility (standard, intermediate, or complex). This in turn allows for more measured comparisons across hospitals with similar resources and performing procedures of similar complexity.

Outcomes

The Veterans Affairs Surgical Quality Improvement Program primarily provides information on 30-day perioperative outcomes, including morbidity and mortality. With regard to morbidity, data are currently available on a standardized set of 22 different postoperative complications of varying severity. Additional outcomes include reoperation within 30 days of the index procedure, postoperative length of stay, and 30-day or 14-day readmission for inpatient or outpatient procedures, respectively. Furthermore, unlike American College of Surgeons–NSQIP, long-term mortality is available throughout the entire VA system allowing ascertainment of postoperative death beyond the standard 30-day window. Specific dates for each listed outcome are also available.

UTILITY AND UNIQUE FEATURES OF VASQIP

The Veterans Affairs Surgical Quality Improvement Program provides unique research opportunities not available outside the VA. Using either a patient's SSN or scrambled SSN, VASQIP can be easily linked to each patient's information in more than 60 other VA data sources or to Medicare claims for patients receiving part of their care outside the VA. Linked data sets can then help to overcome inherent limitations of each individual data set. For example, linkage to VA Central Cancer Registry can provide data on cancer staging information not provided by VASQIP and robust data on perioperative morbidity not available in cancer registries. Furthermore, although administrative data sources are commonly used for conducting surgical outcomes and health services research, the rigor of VASQIP data collection ensures the validity of abstracted outcomes. Compared with VASQIP, the sensitivity and positive predictive value when using claims data to identify commonly occurring complications are poor.[4]

STATISTICAL CONSIDERATIONS

Studies using VASQIP should be described as retrospective (observational) analyses. The Veterans Affairs Surgical Quality Improvement Program is a systematic sample of cases performed at each hospital; therefore, hospital volume can only be calculated for certain cases for which data collection is mandatory (eg, bariatric procedures, esophageal resections, pancreatic resections, cardiac cases). When preparing the data for analysis, investigators should be mindful that patients who undergo reoperation within 30 days of an index procedure will have data for both procedures abstracted. As such, duplicate records for the same episode of care will need to be purged so outcomes are not duplicative.

Because outcomes within hospitals are likely correlated, studies evaluating hospital-level variation should use multilevel (ie, hierarchical) modeling to account for clustering at the hospital-level by including the hospital identifier as the random effect in the model.[5] In addition, because certain outcomes are either uncommonly occurring or have decreased in frequency over time (eg, mortality), stratification of hospitals based on such outcomes could lead to misclassification (eg, categorizing hospitals based on mortality rates). As such, consideration should be given to reliability adjustment—a Bayesian approach in which observed outcome rates are shrunk toward the population mean with the degree of shrinkage proportional to each hospital's volume.[6] For example, the observed 30-day mortality rate at a very low-volume hospital would be expected to be subject to greater random variation and statistical noise (ie, less reliable) relative to a very high-volume hospital. Thus, reliability adjustment for the former would result in more shrinkage relative to the latter.

The approach to missing data is often an important consideration in observational studies. The Veterans Affairs Surgical Quality Improvement Program variables relating to demographic or preoperative comorbid conditions are generally complete for all patients because, as part of data quality control, missing data points are flagged and the field(s) completed. By comparison, variables like laboratory values are frequently missing because they may not have been drawn. The pattern of missingness and the degree to which missing data are informative should be considered and used to decide how best to address missing covariates by using techniques such as multiple imputation when appropriate.[7]

CONCLUSIONS

Given the emphasis currently placed on the quality of US health care, VASQIP will remain an important data source for investigations into surgical quality and the general care of veterans. The infrastructure of the VA health system and the data sources available therein provide unique opportunities to evaluate how system-level changes can potentially improve the value of surgical care.

Acknowledgment

The following disclosures were reported at the time this original article was first published.

Conflict of Interest Disclosures: None reported.

Funding/Support: This work was supported by the Department of Veterans Affairs, Veterans Health Administration, Office of Research and Development, and the Center for Innovations in Quality, Effectiveness and Safety (CIN 13-413).

Role of the Funder/Sponsor: The funders had no role in the design and conduct of the study; collection, management, analysis, and interpretation of the data; preparation, review, or approval of the manuscript; and decision to submit the manuscript for publication.

References

1. Veterans' Administration Health-Care Amendments of 1985, HR 505, 99th Cong (1985).
2. Davis CL, Pierce JR, Henderson W, et al. Assessment of the reliability of data collected for the Department of Veterans Affairs national surgical quality improvement program. *J Am Coll Surg*. 2007;204(4):550-560. Medline:17382213
3. A Festschrift Honoring Shukri F. Khuri, MD: Celebrating 15 Years of NSQIP. *Am J Surg*. http://www.americanjournalofsurgery.com/issue/S0002-9610(09)X0012-7. Published November 2009. Accessed February 20, 2018.
4. Best WR, Khuri SF, Phelan M, et al. Identifying patient preoperative risk factors and postoperative adverse events in administrative databases: results from the Department of Veterans Affairs National Surgical Quality Improvement Program. *J Am Coll Surg*. 2002;194(3):257-266. Medline:11893128
5. Massarweh NN, Kougias P, Wilson MA. Complications and failure to rescue after inpatient noncardiac surgery in the Veterans Affairs health system. *JAMA Surg*. 2016;151(12):1157-1165. Medline:27653498
6. Dimick JB, Ghaferi AA, Osborne NH, Ko CY, Hall BL. Reliability adjustment for reporting hospital outcomes with surgery. *Ann Surg*. 2012;255(4):703-707. Medline:22388108
7. Newgard CD, Lewis RJ. Missing data: how to best account for what is not known. *JAMA*. 2015;314(9):940-941. Medline:26325562

# Practical Guide to Surgical Data Sets: National Surgical Quality Improvement Program (NSQIP) and Pediatric NSQIP

Mehul V. Raval, MD, MS, and
Timothy M. Pawlik, MD, MPH, PhD

IN THIS CHAPTER

Introduction

Data Elements and Considerations

Access and Logistics

Variables and Outcomes

Statistical Methodology

Limitations

Conclusions

This JAMA Guide to Statistics and Methods summarizes the National Surgical Quality Improvement Program (NSQIP) and its pediatric offshoot for use in surgical research.

INTRODUCTION

For more than 100 years, the American College of Surgeons (ACS) has set the standard for the delivery of high-quality medical and surgical care. Based on programs originally created at the US Department of Veterans Affairs, the ACS developed and implemented the National Surgical Quality Improvement Program (NSQIP) in 2004.[1] Since its inception, the NSQIP has spread to nearly 700 hospitals and captures more than 1 million incident cases annually.

A major strength of the ACS NSQIP program is the means that it provides to report national, clinically abstracted, highly reliable, risk-adjusted, and case-mix–adjusted surgical data that facilitates validated peer-comparison. As such, the ACS NSQIP is widely recognized as the premier surgical quality and outcomes assessment program (Box 8). Via the ACS NSQIP, hospitals and clinicians have access to granular, actionable data that have led to improvements in morbidity and mortality, cost savings from prevention of complications, and a platform for disease-specific, procedure-specific, or regional or system-based collaboratives.

In parallel, the ACS NSQIP Pediatric (NSQIP-P) program was piloted in 2008 to address surgical quality improvement for children undergoing surgery.[2] The ACS NSQIP-P now includes more than 100 sites and captures more than 150 000 pediatric cases annually.

> ## BOX 8
> ### Best Practices for Using NSQIP Data
>
> 1. Identify a hypothesis-driven question and ensure that the NSQIP data set is the appropriate source to address questions on the target population and outcomes.
> 2. Secure data access and examine all variables and outcomes for definition continuity over time.
> 3. Define an analytic plan to appropriately exclude preexisting conditions, account for missing data, and risk adjust for comorbidities and procedural case mix.
> 4. Perform sensitivity analyses to address confounding.
> 5. Interpret results understanding the limitations related to missing clinician-level and hospital-level clustering of outcomes, length of follow-up periods, and generalizability beyond the hospitals participating in the program.
>
> Abbreviation: NSQIP, National Surgical Quality of Improvement Program.

DATA ELEMENTS AND CONSIDERATIONS

Access and Logistics

More than 1500 peer-reviewed articles associated with the use of ACS NSQIP data have been published. Researchers can access the data through a Health Insurance Portability and Accountability Act-compliant Participant Use File (PUF) (https://www.facs.org/quality-programs/acs-nsqip/participant-use). Pending approval and permission by local administration and quality leaders, PUF access incurs no cost to researchers at a participating ACS NSQIP hospital. While the PUF contains deidentified patient-level aggregate data, the ACS does not provide hospital or clinician identifiers. In addition, there is a data use agreement that prohibits the attempted identification of patients, clinicians, or hospitals. The PUFs are available by calendar year or as separate procedure-targeted PUFs. Procedure-targeted PUFs contain unique procedure-specific variables based on center participation.

Variables and Outcomes

The standard variable definition and rigorous clinical abstraction available through the ACS NSQIP provide reliable and valid surgical outcomes measures. Complication data available in the ACS NSQIP data sets are more accurate than data obtained from administrative claims data sources or other registry-based data sets.[3] In addition, a broad range of 30-day outcomes are documented in the ACS NSQIP, including mortality, readmissions, and length of stay. Composite morbidity outcomes are often used to create tiers of morbidity (eg, serious morbidity vs any morbidity) or group clinically related occurrences (eg, wound complications that combine various forms of surgical site infection with wound disruption).

The ACS NSQIP data provide the ability to account for preoperative comorbidities, as well as complications that occur in the perioperative period, such as surgical site infections, renal failure, urinary tract infections, ventilator dependence, and pneumonia. Excluding preexisting conditions that may be present on admission provides a more accurate assessment of postoperative outcomes. Research on specific outcomes, such as readmission, as well as factors associated with these outcomes, including timing of post-discharge complications, has highlighted policy shortcomings that often aim to tie quality metrics to financial penalties. Data on practice patterns and quality metrics using ACS NSQIP can drive more efficient care and judicious resource utilization.

Statistical Methodology

Most studies that use the ACS NSQIP PUF define the study population with *Current Procedural Terminology* codes and then validate this population using the *International Classification of Diseases, Ninth Revision (ICD-9)* or *ICD-10* diagnostic codes. Beyond standard statistical analyses that compare continuous and categorical variables with modifications based on data distribution, most studies use multivariable logistic regression models. To account for missing data, imputation or sensitivity analyses should be performed. Trends over time can be studied using multiple years of data. Furthermore, observed-to-expected event ratios can be created for various cohorts within the data source based on available demographic or clinical variables.

The large sample sizes and clinically granular data facilitate quality improvement and comparative effectiveness research. For example, in 1 study, Lancaster and Hutter[4] not only compared outcomes of open vs laparoscopic approaches to bariatric surgery, but also outcomes of bypass vs banding procedures. Specific clinical comorbidities can be studied across a wide spectrum of populations and procedures to identify targeted areas for quality improvement. To this end, Merrill and Millham[5] demonstrated that patients with inflammatory bowel disease were at an increased risk for developing postoperative complications, such as deep vein thrombosis or pulmonary embolism. Similarly, ACS NSQIP data have been used to demonstrate risk factors such as poor nutrition and smoking increase the risk of postoperative complications. Emerging research in predictive modeling has resulted in an expanding body of work around risk-assessment tools based on comorbidities to help counsel patients and clinicians prior to surgery.[6]

Operative factors collected in the ACS NSQIP provide an opportunity to assess risk for developing specific complications. Examples of intraoperative factors that influence outcomes that have been examined include duration of procedure and intraoperative presence of resident trainees.[7]

Limitations

There are several weaknesses of the ACS NSQIP data sets. First, current policies prohibit the sharing of hospital or clinician identifiers, even in a blinded fashion. In turn, researchers cannot study variations among specific clinicians or account for clustering of outcomes. Exclusion of specific dates and times precludes evaluation of time-of-day or day-of-week effects. Most outcomes in the ACS NSQIP data are limited to a 30-day follow-up period, even though many procedure-specific outcomes of interest may extend beyond 30 days. Cases included in the ACS NSQIP data are also typically selected using random sampling to provide a hospital-level quality assessment, and they may not adequately capture rare outcomes or accurately portray outcomes for rare cases. To this end, many hospitals now participate in a more modular program that oversamples specific cases and captures procedure-specific outcomes. Another weakness of the data source is that a select number of variables are missing or have undergone evolution over time, thereby making analysis difficult or impossible. Therefore, special attention should be paid to data definition dictionaries provided by the program for each PUF release and to methods that can account for missing data.

Despite absence of financial outcomes prohibiting cost-effectiveness studies using the PUF, several ACS NSQIP studies have used individual hospital data to estimate cost-effectiveness of the program or cost savings from avoided complications. Patient-reported outcomes such as patient satisfaction and quality of life assessments are also missing from the ACS NSQIP, although efforts are underway to incorporate these outcomes into the program. Finally, all PUF data are from ACS NSQIP hospitals and do not represent a statistically valid nationally representative sample.

CONCLUSIONS

The ACS NSQIP provides a data source of clinically granular data that allows researchers to study both adult and pediatric surgical populations. The availability of the PUF provides an opportunity for researchers at participating sites to use these data for quality improvement and academic endeavors. As the quality focus of the ACS NSQIP continues to expand toward procedure targeted preoperative, intraoperative, and postoperative factors, patient-reported outcomes, and value-based care, the role of ACS NSQIP data in outcomes research will continue to increase.

Acknowledgment

The following disclosures were reported at the time this original article was first published.

Conflict of Interest Disclosures: Dr Raval reports receiving personal fees as a research scholar at the American College of Surgeons as well as personal fees and research funding from the Emory University and Children's Healthcare of Atlanta Pediatric Research Alliance, the Department of Surgery at Emory University, the Agency for Healthcare Research and Quality, and the Robert Wood Johnson Foundation. No other disclosures were reported.

References

1. Fink AS, Campbell DAJr, Mentzer RMJr, et al. The National Surgical Quality Improvement Program in non-veterans administration hospitals: initial demonstration of feasibility. *Ann Surg*. 2002;236(3):344-353. Medline:12192321

2. Raval MV, Dillon PW, Bruny JL, et al. ACS NSQIP Pediatric Steering Committee. American College of Surgeons National Surgical Quality Improvement Program Pediatric: a phase 1 report. *J Am Coll Surg*. 2011;212(1):1-11. Medline:21036076

3. Lawson EH, Louie R, Zingmond DS, et al. A comparison of clinical registry versus administrative claims data for reporting of 30-day surgical complications. *Ann Surg*. 2012;256(6):973-981. Medline:23095667

4. Lancaster RT, Hutter MM. Bands and bypasses: 30-day morbidity and mortality of bariatric surgical procedures as assessed by prospective, multi-center, risk-adjusted ACS-NSQIP data. *Surg Endosc*. 2008;22(12):2554-2563. Medline:18806945

5. Merrill A, Millham F. Increased risk of postoperative deep vein thrombosis and pulmonary embolism in patients with inflammatory bowel disease: a study of National Surgical Quality Improvement Program patients. *Arch Surg*. 2012;147(2):120-124. Medline:22006853

6. Bilimoria KY, Liu Y, Paruch JL, et al. Development and evaluation of the universal ACS NSQIP surgical risk calculator: a decision aid and informed consent tool for patients and surgeons. *J Am Coll Surg*. 2013;217(5):833-42.e1, 3. Medline:24055383

7. Daley BJ, Cecil W, Clarke PC, Cofer JB, Guillamondegui OD. How slow is too slow? Correlation of operative time to complications: an analysis from the Tennessee Surgical Quality Collaborative. *J Am Coll Surg*. 2015;220(4):550-558. Medline:25728140

Practical Guide to Surgical Data Sets: Metabolic and Bariatric Surgery Accreditation and Quality Program (MBSAQIP)

Dana A. Telem, MD, MPH, and
Justin B. Dimick, MD, MPH

IN THIS CHAPTER

Introduction

Data Considerations for the MBSAQIP Participant Use File

Deidentification of Patients, Facilities, and Clinicians

MBSAQIP PUF Content

Outcomes

Statistical Considerations

MBSAQIP PUF Advantages and Limitations

Conclusions

This JAMA Guide to Statistics and Methods details the Metabolic and Bariatric Surgery Accreditation and Quality Improvement Program (MBSAQIP) participant use file data set for quality and outcomes reporting.

INTRODUCTION

This chapter details important considerations for quality and outcomes reporting in bariatric surgery with the Metabolic and Bariatric Surgery Accreditation and Quality Improvement Program (MBSAQIP) participant use file (PUF) data set. In 2012, the American College of Surgeons (ACS) and the American Society for Metabolic and Bariatric Surgery (ASMBS) merged their respective bariatric surgery accreditation programs into a single unified program, the MBSAQIP.[1] This program is responsible for accrediting inpatient and outpatient bariatric surgery centers in the United States and Canada. To date, 780 bariatric surgery programs are MBSAQIP-accredited; together, these account for 94% of bariatric programs in these countries.[1] As part of accreditation, centers are required to input prospectively collected patient data into the MBSAQIP national data registry platform.[2]

Every metabolic and bariatric operation and intervention performed at an MBSAQIP-accredited center, including primary operations, reoperations, reinterventions, and endoluminal therapeutic interventions, must be captured within the MBSAQIP data registry. Data entry is performed by rigorously trained metabolic and bariatric surgical clinical reviewers via patient medical record review. The data registry collects prospective, clinically rich data on more than 200 preoperative, intraoperative, and postoperative variables with standardized definitions.[2] Longitudinal patient data are collected at 30-day,

6-month, and 1-year points and yearly thereafter. More than 150 000 bariatric cases are captured annually within this data registry. To ensure high-quality data, MBSAQIP conducts data integrity audits of participating centers. Collected data are then adjusted for risk and reliability across centers.[2]

In January 2017, the inaugural participant use file (PUF) (Box 9) from the MBSAQIP data registry was made available to participating MBSAQIP centers. This PUF was released for the express purpose of providing researchers a data resource to investigate and advance the quality of care delivered to patients undergoing metabolic and bariatric surgeries.

BOX 9

Attributes of MBSAQIP Data

1. The MBSAQIP PUF captures high-quality, validated data from more than 90% of the bariatric procedures performed in the United States and Canada.
2. This data set is an important resource for capturing 30-day outcomes, particularly for low-frequency events.
3. When considering this data set for use in research, it is important to note that the PUF contains deidentified, patient-level, aggregated data and does not provide data on individual hospitals, clinicians, and patients.
4. This data set may not be linked to other existing data sets and patients cannot be longitudinally tracked across years.
5. Consideration should be given to ensure appropriate statistical methodology, particularly for handling missing data in variables with a high level of performance inconsistency.

Abbreviations: MBSAQIP, Metabolic and Bariatric Surgery and Quality Improvement Program; PUF, participant use file.

DATA CONSIDERATIONS FOR THE MBSAQIP PARTICIPANT USE FILE

All metabolic and bariatric cases with operation dates between January 1, 2015, and December 31, 2015, were included in the inaugural PUF release. Data from additional years are forthcoming. The 2016 PUF was recently released in Fall 2017. Prior to using this data set for research, a few important issues require discussion.

Deidentification of Patients, Facilities, and Clinicians

In contrast to the MBSAQIP data registry, the MBSAQIP PUF contains deidentified patient-level and aggregate data and does not identify individual hospitals, clinicians, or patients. To comply with Health Insurance Portability and Accessibility Act provisions, all absolute dates have been removed, as have facility identifiers, clinician information, patient-level data, and geographic information, to comply with the participation agreement between the ACS and participating centers. This limits studies addressing variation in the provision of care and the identification of outliers for targeted, national quality improvement initiatives. This also prevents linkage of this data set to other national data sets (eg, the National Inpatient Sample, American Hospital Association).

MBSAQIP PUF Content

The PUF includes 5 data sets (Table 5). The main PUF is a flat file in which each row represents a case, and it contains 135 associated variables (eg, demographics, preoperative patient characteristics, operative information, outcomes, and other case descriptors). The 4 additional data sets contain additional event-specific variables (approximately 10 variables per data set) for reoperations, readmissions, interventions, and postoperative

TABLE 5

Broad Characterization of Data Files Available in the Metabolic and Bariatric Surgery Accreditation and Quality Improvement Program Participant Use File

Data Set[a]	File Type	Included Information
Main	Flat file (1 row per case)	Preoperative, intraoperative, procedural, and postoperative characteristics
Reoperation	Long-form (multiple rows per case)	Detailed information on 30-d reoperation
Readmission	Long-form (multiple rows per case)	Detailed information on 30-d readmission
Intervention	Long-form (multiple rows per case)	Detailed information on 30-d intervention
BMI	Long-form (multiple rows per case)	Detailed information on BMI (0-150 days from index procedure)

Abbreviation: BMI, body mass index.
[a]All data are available as text files and files compatible with SAS and SPSS software programs.

body mass index (BMI) measurements. Each observation in the readmission, reoperation, intervention, and BMI data sets may be merged with a case in the main data set using a key-matching variable. Merging these data sets is important when cleaning and constructing data analyzable for a particular research question.

Outcomes

Released data in the PUF are limited to 30-day outcomes and exclude the longer-term data variables collected within the MBSAQIP data registry. This limits long-term analyses assessing efficacy, safety, and durability of surgery beyond the perioperative period. Additionally, data on costs of an episode of care, patient out-of-pocket costs, insurance plans, or other associated health care expenditures are unavailable within this data set. Thus, analyses of resource use are not possible.

STATISTICAL CONSIDERATIONS

For many studies, depending on the hypothesis, descriptive statistics, and univariate analysis may be sufficient for quantitative analysis. Various forms of regression models (eg, logistic regression, linear regression) may also be used to estimate the effects of multiple variables on the outcome of interest. For comparative effectiveness research, propensity scores are often used for matching or adjustment of differences in patient characteristics between treatment groups. Of course, multivariate adjustment and propensity scores can only adjust for variables that are present in the data set, leaving the possibility of confounding by unobserved patient factors.

Another important consideration is missing data. Overall, there is a small percentage of missing data for mandatory variables (eg, preoperative body mass index age, reason for readmission). Variables with a high level of performance inconsistency (eg, laboratory studies, radiographic imaging) between patients, however, result in higher percentages of missing values (10% to 30%, depending on the variable[3]). This can be problematic within traditional regression models and many other types of analysis. Missing data may be handled by either excluding the variable or observation of interest or through various imputation methods.[4]

MBSAQIP PUF ADVANTAGES AND LIMITATIONS

One of the strongest advantages of the MBSAQIP data set is that it captures high-quality data for the majority of bariatric cases performed in the United States and Canada. The large sample size accrued from 780 institutions allows for increased external validity, a focus on effectiveness rather than efficacy, and the ability to capture rare or low frequency events. The rigorous data collection, validation, and assurance processes developed by the MBSAQIP ensures that the data collected are accurate, complete, and of the highest quality.

Several limitations of the MBSAQIP PUF data are noted in addition to what has previously been discussed. The observed operations and interventions that patients underwent were not randomly assigned. Decisions made by individual clinicians based on unique characteristics of the patient, clinician, and/or patient preferences, and other clinical factors, are not captured within the data set. Thus, treatment bias confounds direct comparisons between groups, and studies should be designed to address and reduce this bias. Additional limitations include selection bias and the systematic differences in accredited vs nonaccredited hospitals in the MBSAQIP data sets, though this is likely less significant as most facilities performing bariatric surgery in the United States are accredited.

CONCLUSIONS

The MBSAQIP PUF is a promising new data set that will allow researchers to evaluate quality and outcomes for patients undergoing bariatric surgery. While there are many advantages to this data set, researchers must be mindful of the limitations when using these data to test research hypotheses.

Acknowledgment

The following disclosures were reported at the time this original article was first published.

Conflict of Interest Disclosures: Dr Dimick is a cofounder of ArborMetrix, a company that makes software for profiling hospital quality and efficiency. Dr Telem serves on the MBSAQIP data registry and reporting subcommittee. Dr Telem reports receiving personal fees from Medtronic outside the submitted work. No other disclosures were reported.

References

1. The Metabolic and Bariatric Surgery Accreditation and Quality Improvement Program. Website. https://www.facs.org/quality-programs/mbsaqip. Published 2016. Accessed September 9, 2017.
2. The Metabolic and Bariatric Surgery Accreditation and Quality Improvement. Program standards manual version 2.0. https://www.facs.org/~/media/files/qualityprograms/bariatric/mbsaqipstandardsmanual.ashx. Published 2016. Accessed February 27, 2018.
3. The Metabolic and Bariatric Surgery Accreditation and Quality Improvement Program. User guide for the 2015 participant use data file. https://www.facs.org/~/media/files/quality%20programs/bariatric/mbsaqip_2015_puf_user_guide.ashx. Published January 2017. Accessed February 27, 2018.
4. Pedersen AB, Mikkelsen EM, Cronin-Fenton D, et al. Missing data and multiple imputation in clinical epidemiological research. *Clin Epidemiol*. 2017;9:157-166. Medline:28352203

Practical Guide to Surgical Data Sets: National Cancer Database (NCDB)

Ryan P. Merkow, MD, MS,
Alfred W. Rademaker, PhD, and
Karl Y. Bilimoria, MD, MS

IN THIS CHAPTER

Introduction

Data Element Considerations

Hospital Variables

Tumor Characteristics

Treatment Variables

Outcomes

Analytic and Statistical Considerations

Conclusions

This JAMA Guide to Statistics and Methods summarizes the characteristics and uses of the National Cancer Database (NCDB) for use in surgical research.

INTRODUCTION

The National Cancer Database (NCDB) is a joint program of the American College of Surgeons Commission on Cancer (CoC) and the American Cancer Society (Box 10).[1] The NCDB is a hospital-based clinical cancer registry established in 1989 that collects data from more than 1500 hospitals in the United States, capturing more than 70% of all newly diagnosed cancers.

BOX 10

Best Practices for Using the National Cancer Database (NCDB)

1. Ensure the NCDB is the appropriate data set to address the question of interest.
2. Consult an experienced user of the NCDB early.
3. Examine all variables and data definitions before beginning the project and define an analytic plan a priori. Keep in mind that variables may change over time.
4. The strengths of the NCDB are in examining treatment patterns and trends over time across the United States. Focus projects on these research questions.
5. Perform extensive sensitivity analyses to evaluate and address confounding and selection biases.
6. Thoughtful handling of missing data is necessary when using the NCDB.

In 2013, the American College of Surgeons CoC began to make available the participant use file (PUF) to CoC member facilities. This led to an exponential growth in the number and breadth of publications using the NCDB. With the continued expansion and access to NCDB, it is expected that the number of publications will continue to increase.

Given the power of the NCDB, it is of primary importance to ensure that appropriate methods are used during data analysis and reporting. Like all secondary data sets, there are unique nuances and challenges that may introduce significant confounding and bias into study results. Our objectives are to present an overview of unique data elements in the NCDB and provide an analytic framework when using the data set for the purposes of research.

DATA ELEMENT CONSIDERATIONS

The NCDB PUF includes a range of data elements that include patient characteristics and comorbidities, staging data, treatment information, and survival outcomes. Specific variables and definitions can be found elsewhere.[2,3] Although describing each variable is beyond our scope and purpose, we will discuss a few important issues.

Hospital Variables

The PUF data set contains 2 hospital-specific variables. First, there is an anonymous randomly generated "facility ID." This variable can be used for hospital-specific calculations, including hospital and procedure volume metrics. It is important to understand how volume calculations may change over the study period. It is common to exclude hospitals if they did not submit at least 1 case to the data set every year of the study to ensure a consistent population of hospitals. A second variable, "facility type," details the type of cancer center (eg, community, comprehensive, academic). It can be combined with a hospital's volume status (eg, high-volume academic, low-volume academic) or considered separately. An additional variable, "class of case," should also be considered when calculating volume metrics. This variable indicates whether diagnosis, treatment, or both were performed at the index facility. If a patient received treatment at a nonindex hospital, the observation should likely be excluded from analysis.

Tumor Characteristics

There are numerous tumor characteristic variables that should be reported. A unique aspect of the NCDB is the inclusion of clinical and pathologic stages. Depending on the study, clinical (eg, study of neoadjuvant therapy use) or pathologic stage (eg, study of adjuvant therapy use) may be used to select patients. In addition, there is a summary stage variable that is a combination of the clinical and pathologic stages. This variable is generated to minimize missing staging information. It is essential to select the most appropriate staging variable and then standardize the way it is used throughout a multiyear study.

Treatment Variables

Many treatment variables are reported, including the receipt of chemotherapy, radiation therapy, and surgery. The NCDB only reports treatment that was used in the first 6 months after diagnosis. For example, if a patient was treated with neoadjuvant imatinib for a gastrointestinal stromal tumor for 8 months after diagnosis (prior to resection), the NCDB will only report the use of imatinib and not surgery.[4] In addition, surgical procedures entered will also only include the most definitive intervention. For example, if an endoscopic mucosal resection was performed before an esophagectomy, the esophagectomy will be reported.[5] One approach to determining if this limitation is present is to use the "time from diagnosis to treatment" variables.

Outcomes

The primary outcome variable collected is "vital status" (ie, alive or dead) and therefore both short- (30-, 60-, and 90-day mortality) and long-term 5-year overall survival is available for analysis. Conclusions based on overall survival analyses using the NCDB should be interpreted with consideration of the confounding and biases that may be present.

An additional outcome variable is readmission. This variable captures only patients who were readmitted to the same hospital within 30 days of discharge, and therefore reporting bias is a significant problem. Because readmission assessment may not be reliable with the NCDB, it should be interpreted with caution and discussed as a study limitation.

ANALYTIC AND STATISTICAL CONSIDERATIONS

Statistical analyses using the NCDB have both similarities and differences to other large cancer registry, administrative, and clinical data sets. First, it should be noted that the NCDB is not population based and results cannot be projected beyond the CoC hospitals included in the analysis. Nevertheless, because CoC hospitals report more than 70% of new patients with cancer, the results are representative of care across the United States.[6]

Managing confounding and bias is a primary concern when working with observational data sets. Most issues should be clarified during the exploration phase of the analysis, as discussed previously. Nevertheless, during the analytic phase, it is important to include and report (as necessary) sensitivity analyses. It is particularly important in the NCDB, when the study spans many years, to determine whether the period qualitatively changes the study results. If present, consider a stratified analysis, including time as a variable, and/or only studying the most recent period. When applicable, a propensity score analysis is another technique that should be considered. This analytic tool helps balance comparative groups based on known confounding variables in an attempt to minimize selection bias.

Handling missing data is an especially important issue when using the NCDB. Certain variables, such as many site-specific factors (eg, carcinoembryonic antigen, carbohydrate antigen 19-9), may not have any or less than 50% of data available for analysis. These variables should be discarded. Other variables may have substantial amounts of missing information (greater than 10% but less than 50%) but may still be informative. Options for managing missing data include coding dummy variables, excluding observations with missing data, simply not using the variable in the analysis, or using a preferred method of imputation.[7]

Estimating hospital-level practice patterns and outcomes is another important consideration. Deciphering statistical noise from meaningful differences between hospitals is not straightforward, particularly for lower-volume hospitals. For example, if 1 hospital performs 5 pancreatectomy cases per year and 1 patient dies, the mortality rate is 20%. However, a larger volume hospital may perform 100 cases per year and experience 5 deaths with a mortality rate of 5%. Such imbalances in the signal-to-noise ratio, even after risk adjustment, make interpreting results challenging. However, a statistical technique using multilevel modeling using "facility ID" as the random effect allows for more fair and reliable estimates. This type of adjustment should be considered in NCDB studies when examining hospital-level differences.

CONCLUSIONS

The NCDB is a well-established data set that has had a meaningful effect on cancer care in the United States.[1,6] With the release of the PUF and increasing acceptance of its relevance, the number of researchers using the NCDB will continue to expand. The data set does have several limitations that should be considered during cleaning, analyzing, and reporting data. By understanding the strengths and weaknesses of the NCDB, future work will continue to improve the care of patients with cancer in the United States and around the world.

Acknowledgment

The following disclosures were reported at the time this original article was first published.

Conflict of Interest Disclosures: None reported.

References

1. American College of Surgeons. National cancer database. http://www.facs.org/quality-programs/cancer/ncdb. Accessed August 1, 2017.
2. American College of Surgeons. National cancer database—data dictionary PUF. http://ncdbpuf.facs.org/node/259?q=print-pdf-all. Accessed August 1, 2017.
3. Boffa DJ, Rosen JE, Mallin K, et al. Using the National Cancer Database for Outcomes Research: a review. *JAMA Oncol*. 2017;3(12):1722-1728. Medline:28241198
4. Bilimoria KY, Wayne JD, Merkow RP, et al. Incorporation of adjuvant therapy into the multimodality management of gastrointestinal stromal tumors of the stomach in the United States. *Ann Surg Oncol*. 2012;19(1):184-191. Medline:21725688
5. Merkow RP, Bilimoria KY, Keswani RN, et al. Treatment trends, risk of lymph node metastasis, and outcomes for localized esophageal cancer. *J Natl Cancer Inst*. 2014;106(7):dju133. Medline:25031273
6. Bilimoria KY, Stewart AK, Winchester DP, Ko CY. The National Cancer Data Base: a powerful initiative to improve cancer care in the United States. *Ann Surg Oncol*. 2008;15(3):683-690. Medline:18183467
7. Hamilton BH, Ko CY, Richards K, Hall BL. Missing data in the American College of Surgeons National Surgical Quality Improvement Program are not missing at random: implications and potential impact on quality assessments. *J Am Coll Surg*. 2010;210(2):125-139.e2. Medline:20113932

Practical Guide to Surgical Data Sets: National Trauma Data Bank (NTDB)

Zain G. Hashmi, MBBS, Amy H. Kaji, MD, PhD, and Avery B. Nathens, MD, MPH, PhD

IN THIS CHAPTER

Introduction

Data Compilation and Structure

Methods

Limitations

Recommended Reading

Conclusions

This JAMA Guide to Statistics and Methods summarizes the data compilation, structure, and methods of the National Trauma Data Bank (NTDB) for use in surgical research.

INTRODUCTION

Trauma remains a leading cause of death and disability and accounts for a substantial portion of health care expenditures.[1] Therefore, research to improve trauma care is a leading public health priority.

Spearheading this effort, the American College of Surgeons Committee on Trauma coordinated a landmark multi-institutional endeavor, the Major Trauma Outcomes Study.[2] On its completion in 1989, the American College of Surgeons Committee on Trauma recognized the importance of national trauma data aggregation to inform quality improvement. In 1997, it formed a subcommittee to develop the National Trauma Data Bank (NTDB), a standardized collection of national trauma data (Box 11). Today, to our knowledge, the NTDB is the world's largest trauma data repository, with more than 7.5 million electronic records from more than 900 trauma centers.

DATA COMPILATION AND STRUCTURE

Annually, between February and May, the NTDB collects voluntarily submitted data from individual hospitals, concordant with the National Trauma Data Standard, a set of standardized data definitions.[3] Inclusion/exclusion criteria are based on *International Statistical Classification of Diseases, Tenth Revision, Clinical Modification* diagnoses codes and certain admission characteristics.[4] The NTDB is an incident-based record; each incident is recorded independently of repeated

> **BOX 11**
>
> ## Attributes of the National Trauma Data Bank
>
> 1. The National Trauma Data Bank (NTDB) is the world's largest trauma data repository with more than 7.5 million electronic records.
> 2. The NTDB is considered a convenience sample because of voluntary trauma data submission.
> 3. The large sample size of NTDB facilitates hypothesis-generating research and the study of rare injuries, procedures, and outcomes.
> 4. The NTDB contains prehospital and in-hospital injury data, including anatomic and physiologic severity.
> 5. The NTDB does not include data on costs, laboratory values, readmissions, or long-term outcomes.
> 6. Careful study design, sample selection, and analytics can help mitigate NTDB limitations resulting from missing data and selection/information bias.

injuries. Validation rules mitigate the submission of missing or nonsensical data. A fully deidentified data set is reported annually in compliance with the Health Insurance Portability and Accountability Act, such that no patient can be identified.

Data quality in the NTDB has improved significantly since the adoption of the National Trauma Data Standard in 2007 and the implementation of American College of Surgeons Trauma Quality Improvement Program (ACS TQIP) in 2010, which is based on NTDB data. Over time, ACS TQIP has added several fields that are only required for participating centers. Further, ACS TQIP has focused significantly on registrar education to achieve greater data standardization. The quality of data in the NTDB has improved significantly as the number of centers participating in ACS TQIP has increased. Data from ACS TQIP centers represent a large subset of NTDB data, which differ from the non-TQIP centers by virtue of (1) higher-quality data and (2) expanded fields. Researchers may access the data in the form of the research data set after completing a brief project proposal and payment of the data set fee. This includes data from all centers (TQIP and non-TQIP) but excludes the expanded fields. Investigators from TQIP centers may request the public use file, which includes only TQIP centers along with the expanded fields.

The research data set exists as a set of relational tables that can be imported using most statistical software. The user manual describes each file and its contents.[4] Because of aforementioned changes, we caution against combining 2002 to 2006 data with later years and recommend using data from 2007 to the present.

METHODS

Retrospective, cross-sectional and matched case-control study designs have commonly been used to analyze outcomes such as mortality, length of stay, and complications. The NTDB's large size facilitates the study of rare injuries, procedures, and outcomes.

A brief description of NTDB should be included to inform the reader about the characteristics of this data set. The rationale for using NTDB vs other available data should also be provided.

Sample inclusion/exclusion criteria should be explicitly stated. We recommend including a flow diagram of sample selection along with reasons for exclusions, documenting a stepwise derivation of the final sample.[5]

All predictor and outcome variables should be defined a priori. A justification should be provided regarding categorizing continuous variables. When studying mortality, at a minimum age, hypotension, pulse, total Glasgow Coma Scale score, the mechanism of injury, and injury severity score should be considered.[6]

Mortality is an important end point for trauma and therefore requires diligence to ensure that ascertainment is adequate. Currently, data capture ceases at the time of discharge and deaths occurring after administrative discharge are not identified. For example, if a patient with severe traumatic brain injury was transferred to hospice (even in the same institution), he or she would first be discharged and then readmitted to hospice. For this reason, investigators have recommended that transfers-to-hospice be treated as deaths in this data set.[7] Additionally, patients arriving with no signs of life (dead on arrival) may need to be excluded depending on the nature of the analysis.[4]

Standard statistics should be used to report descriptive, univariate, and multivariate analyses. For risk-adjusted analyses, we recommend specifying the model type (eg, logistic or Poisson regression) with a description of its theoretical underpinnings/assumptions. Variable selection should be based on prior evidence and biological/clinical plausibility.[6] If selection is based on statistical significance criteria, the model should be presented as being hypothesis-generating rather than conclusive. Additionally, model performance statistics and whether multicollinearity and effect modification were assessed should be specified. If data include a facility identifier, hierarchical analyses should be used to account for correlated patient outcomes, as patients are nested within facilities.

LIMITATIONS

The NTDB is a convenience sample of voluntarily submitted data and therefore is not nationally representative. However, virtually all level I/II trauma centers now submit data to the NTDB and the data can be considered nationally representative of those facilities. The NTDB does not include data on costs, laboratory values, and long-term outcomes including readmissions and functional outcomes.

Selection bias refers to the differences between groups due to differences in inclusion. Two important sources of selection bias in the NTDB arise because of differences in hospital-level inclusion of isolated hip fractures and transferred patients.[8] Researchers should be cognizant of these and other distinct patient subpopulations that can alter their results. Strategies to mitigate this bias may involve including an indicator variable in the model or using sensitivity analyses.

Information bias refers to differences between groups due to differential data availability. This may be caused by missing data or variations in data abstraction. For example, an injury severity score is manually abstracted and depends on diagnostic aggressiveness. Hospitals with more liberal imaging protocols may detect more incidental, clinically insignificant injuries and subsequently report higher injury severity scores than other centers. Further, patients who die shortly after arrival to the emergency department, before operative or radiologic evaluation, will have inadequate injury ascertainment, and severity scores might be challenging to interpret. Additionally, injury severity scores may be recorded differently depending on which registry software was used. To mitigate this, NTDB now requires the use of the Abbreviated Injury Scale 2005 to standardize injury severity data.[4]

Most of the demographic and injury data included in the NTDB are considered robust. However, certain data, like emergency medical services parameters, comorbidities, and complications, may not be adequately captured, especially at some trauma centers. As previously mentioned, missing data in the NTDB can pose a significant challenge. We advise researchers to undertake thorough exploratory analyses to understand and describe patterns of "missingness" (missing completely at random, missing not at random). Strategies to mitigate these include restricting the analyses to hospitals with known superior data-quality (level I/II trauma centers, centers reporting >100 cases per year and/or at least >1 outcome of interest) and using multiple imputation techniques.[9]

RECOMMENDED READING

The NTDB Data Manual is a comprehensive resource providing detailed insight into several methodological issues highlighted here.[4] Additionally, several high-impact publications, such as those by Galvagno et al[5] and Haider et al,[6] serve as excellent examples of appropriate data use and presentation.[10]

CONCLUSIONS

The NTDB is a powerful repository providing increasingly granular insight into trauma care and is considered a robust hypothesis-generating resource to guide future research. An in-depth understanding of its characteristics is essential to harness its true potential.

Acknowledgment

The following disclosures were reported at the time this original article was first published.

Conflict of Interest Disclosures: Dr Nathens works for the American College of Surgeons as the director of the Trauma Quality Improvement Program. No other disclosures were reported.

References

1. Rhee P, Joseph B, Pandit V, et al. Increasing trauma deaths in the United States. *Ann Surg*. 2014;260(1):13-21. Medline:24651132
2. Champion HR, Copes WS, Sacco WJ, et al. The Major Trauma Outcome Study: establishing national norms for trauma care. *J Trauma*. 1990;30(11):1356-1365. Medline:2231804
3. American College of Surgeons. National trauma data standard. https://www.facs.org/~/media/files/quality%20programs/trauma/ntdb/ntds/data%20dictionaries/ntds%20data%20dictionary%202018.ashx. Accessed July 24, 2017.

4. American College of Surgeons. National Trauma Data Bank research data set user manual and variable description list. https://www.facs.org/~/media/files/quality%20programs/trauma/ntdb/ntdb%20rds%20user%20manual%20all%20years.ashx. Accessed July 24, 2017.

5. Galvagno SMJr, Haut ER, Zafar SN, et al. Association between helicopter vs ground emergency medical services and survival for adults with major trauma. *JAMA*. 2012;307(15):1602-1610. Medline:22511688

6. Haider AH, Hashmi ZG, Zafar SN, et al. Developing best practices to study trauma outcomes in large databases: an evidence-based approach to determine the best mortality risk adjustment model. *J Trauma Acute Care Surg*. 2014;76(4):1061-1069. Medline:24662872

7. Kozar RA, Holcomb JB, Xiong W, Nathens AB. Are all deaths recorded equally? The impact of hospice care on risk-adjusted mortality. *J Trauma Acute Care Surg*. 2014;76(3):634-639. Medline:24553529

8. Gomez D, Haas B, Hemmila M, et al. Hips can lie: impact of excluding isolated hip fractures on external benchmarking of trauma center performance. *J Trauma*. 2010;69(5):1037-1041. Medline:21068608

9. Oyetunji TA, Crompton JG, Ehanire ID, et al. Multiple imputation in trauma disparity research. *J Surg Res*. 2011;165(1):e37-e41. Medline:21067775

10. Haider AH, Hashmi ZG, Zafar SN, et al. Minority trauma patients tend to cluster at trauma centers with worse-than-expected mortality: can this phenomenon help explain racial disparities in trauma outcomes? *Ann Surg*. 2013;258(4):572-579. Medline:23979271 doi:10.1097/SLA.0b013e3182a50148

Practical Guide to Surgical Data Sets: Society for Vascular Surgery Vascular Quality Initiative (SVS VQI)

Sapan S. Desai, MD, PhD, MBA,
Amy H. Kaji, MD, PhD, and
Gilbert Upchurch, Jr, MD

IN THIS CHAPTER

Features of the Data Set

Statistical Considerations

Conclusions

This JAMA Guide to Statistics and Methods details use of the Society for Vascular Surgery's Vascular Quality Improvement Program, a robust database that provides detailed data of common vascular procedures.

The Vascular Quality Initiative (VQI) was developed by the Society for Vascular Surgery in 2011 to improve the safety and effectiveness of 12 common vascular procedures (Box 12). The VQI operates within the structure of a patient safety organization, which protects the quality improvement activities as patient safety work product and thus provides a degree of privilege and confidentiality for the data. Because the VQI is a member of the Society for Vascular Surgery patient safety organization, comparisons with regional and national institutions can be performed.

The VQI registries include carotid artery stenting, carotid endarterectomy, endovascular abdominal aortic aneurysm repair hemodialysis access, infrainguinal bypass, inferior vena cava filter, lower extremity amputations, open abdominal aortic aneurysm repair, peripheral vascular interventions, suprainguinal

---

BOX 12

Best Practices for Using the Vascular Quality Improvement Program

1. Use a flow diagram to demonstrate how the target population was selected.
2. Clearly delineate sample sizes, statistical techniques to mitigate selection bias, and the efficacy of the predictive model.
3. Emphasize practical clinical findings instead of incidental statistically significant results.
4. Include a power calculation.
5. Ensure clear methods to permit reproduction of results.

bypass, thoracic and complex endovascular abdominal aortic aneurysm repair, and varicose vein treatment. As of July 2017, 390 270 procedures were captured.[1] A total of 431 participating institutions represent more than 3200 physicians throughout the United States and Canada. There are 18 regional quality improvement groups that promote ownership of the quality improvement process and practical implementation of new clinical processes. Approximately 40% of the participating institutions are community hospitals, 29% are teaching hospitals, and 31% are academic hospitals.[2] Multiple physician specialties are represented within the database.

FEATURES OF THE DATA SET

Each VQI registry tracks demographic, physician, hospital, and patient-specific factors that are pertinent to the procedure being performed. Clinical care details are collected for the index procedure hospitalization and at 1 year, thus providing data on outcomes including mortality, reintervention, and postoperative complications. The VQI uses patient identifiers to match with other data sets such as the Social Security Death Index or Medicare claims. These data sources are used in conjunction with periodic billing data to ensure that 100% of the sample is being captured by each member institution.

The web-based system used for data entry is provided by M2S (M2S Inc), a subsidiary of Medstreaming, and is used to generate deidentified benchmark reports that allow participating centers and physicians to compare their outcomes with the regional and national benchmarks. Multiple users are able to navigate the data forms, and data capture can be integrated with some electronic health record systems.

The limitations of the data set include a selection bias manifest with the participation of a convenience sample of institutions and clinicians who provide self-reported information. Not all institutions or clinicians participate in all aspects of the registry, which may represent a further selection bias and emphasize this limitation. There may also be some debate about whether participation in a quality registry leads to meaningful improvement in institutional health care quality.[3]

Second, while the data collected within the VQI are prospective, the analysis is retrospectively done and thus cannot draw conclusions on causation. Third, not all potential independent predictors of outcomes can ever be captured by a single database, and this means that discriminatory ability of predictive models may be limited. Finally, the choice of registry is important because the procedural registries do not give information about patients not selected for the procedure, while the new vascular medicine registry does.[4] This may introduce a further element of selection bias.[5]

There are challenges associated with participation given the complexity of the data entry required. Use of dedicated data analysts may be required, thus representing an additional cost. Some potential solutions to this include a higher level of integration, with some third-party electronic health record systems, and the use of a third-party data conversion engine. Specific templates to assist with this integration have been developed by the Vascular Study Group of Greater New York.[6]

STATISTICAL CONSIDERATIONS

The statistical analysis for large databases can be complex, particularly for articles that analyze years of data and hundreds of different variables.[7] The connection between the hypothesis, main results, primary findings, and the clinical implications needs to be clear. The emphasis of the article should be on practical clinical findings, not incidental statistically significant results. This is particularly important for retrospective studies that use registries and databases. At a significance level of P less than .05, it is possible for an article that completes more than 20 statistical comparisons to have at least 1 significant finding that could have occurred by chance. For example, a statistically significant finding that may improve length of stay by 0.1 days may be practically meaningless, especially if implementation of the recommendations leads to a disproportionate increase in cost of care.

A flow diagram should be included that shows the number of patients included and excluded, along with reasons for exclusion. This helps improve the reproducibility of the study and also clearly delineates which population of patients the findings may affect. If a subgroup analysis was completed, it should be specified whether this was planned as part of the study or done post hoc. There must also be confirmation that all appropriate variables are normally distributed prior to analysis to ensure a large enough sample size. This analysis is especially important when working with large databases because there may be underlying bias in how the data are collected, which in turn will affect the relevance of the results.[8]

The sample size for each group should be included in the tables. A power calculation should be included when dealing with small subgroups; the findings for a subgroup may be susceptible to bias if the sample size is small. The data presented should have an appropriate level of precision such that it is consistent throughout the article and amenable to interpretation.

Each statistical method used should have sufficient background to permit a reader to reproduce the findings. Adjustments to predictive models based on clustering or repeated measures should be detailed. For logistic multivariate regression analysis, coefficients should be interpreted using odds ratios, while linear and Poisson models should incorporate effect size. For example, when discussing results related to stroke after carotid endarterectomy vs carotid stenting, presenting the results as odds ratios may be more applicable and intuitive to the reader.[9] Only clinically meaningful variables should be included in the model, not necessarily any variable that is statistically significant.

Multiple imputation for missing values should be used in the appropriate circumstances, and the assumptions should be detailed. Analyze whether the missing values are owing to an underlying bias in the data such that multiple imputation could skew the results. If cases with missing values are ignored, this should be clearly stated in the article, and analysis of the findings should be done with and without this data to confirm validity. Missing values in the data set may reflect an underlying bias, and simply eliminating these incomplete results may adversely affect the quality of the results. For example, smoking status in symptomatic carotid patients may be missing, and lack of inclusion may underestimate the effect of smoking on symptomatic disease.

CONCLUSIONS

The VQI is a robust database that provides detailed data of common vascular procedures. The large sample size of the procedures within the registry, inclusion of pertinent independent variables, and participation from a significant number of institutions allow a variety of outcomes analyses to be completed. As with the use of any large database, care must be taken in the statistical methods, and the results must be clearly presented such that the reader is able to reproduce the findings of any article.

Acknowledgment

The following disclosures were reported at the time this original article was first published.

Conflict of Interest Disclosures: None reported.

References

1. Regional Quality Groups. Vascular quality initiative. http://www.vascularqualityinitiative.org/wp-content/uploads/VQI-Summary-Slides-June-2017.pdf. Accessed July 23, 2017.
2. VQI 2017 Annual Report. http://www.vascularqualityinitiative.org/wp-content/uploads/VQI_2017-Annual-Report_DIGITAL_final.pdf. Accessed July 23, 2017.

3. Etzioni DA, Wasif N, Dueck AC, et al. Association of hospital participation in a surgical outcomes monitoring program with inpatient complications and mortality. *JAMA*. 2015;313(5):505-511. Medline:25647206

4. DeMartino RR, Brooke BS, Neal D, et al. Vascular Quality Initiative. Development of a validated model to predict 30-day stroke and 1-year survival after carotid endarterectomy for asymptomatic stenosis using the Vascular Quality Initiative. *J Vasc Surg*. 2017;66(2):433-444.e2. Medline:28583737

5. Hicks CW, Wick EC, Canner JK, et al. Hospital-level factors associated with mortality after endovascular and open abdominal aortic aneurysm repair. *JAMA Surg*. 2015;150(7):632-636. Medline:25970850

6. VSGGNY Data Management. https://www.vqi.org/components-of-the-vqi/regional-quality-groups/current-regional-quality-groups/vascular-study-group-greater-new-york/vsggny-data-management/. Accessed December 3, 2017.

7. Dua A, Kuy S, Lee CJ, Upchurch GR Jr, Desai SS. Epidemiology of aortic aneurysm repair in the United States from 2000 to 2010. *J Vasc Surg*. 2014;59(6):1512-1517. Medline:24560865

8. Dua A, Ali F, Traudt E, Desai SS. Utilization of the National Inpatient Sample for abdominal aortic aneurysm research. *Surgery*. 2017;162(4):699-706. Medline:28237647

9. Dua A, Romanelli M, Upchurch GR Jr, et al. Predictors of poor outcome after carotid intervention. *J Vasc Surg*. 2016;64(3):663-670. Medline:27209401

Practical Guide to Surgical Data Sets: Society of Thoracic Surgeons (STS) National Database

Farhood Farjah, MD, MPH, Amy H. Kaji, MD, PhD, and Danny Chu, MD

IN THIS CHAPTER

Introduction

Data Element Considerations

Adult Cardiac Surgery Database (ACSD)

Congenital Heart Surgery Database

General Thoracic Surgery Database

Data Source

Outcomes and Other Key Measures

Accessing Data

Statistical Considerations

Limitations

Conclusions

This JAMA Guide to Statistics and Methods describes the attributes, potential uses, and limitations of the Society of Thoracic Surgery National Database.

INTRODUCTION

The Society of Thoracic Surgeons (STS) National Database is a voluntary clinical registry created to facilitate a national quality improvement and safety initiative for cardiac surgery. This progressive initiative led to one of the earliest attempts to provide surgeons with nationally benchmarked, risk-adjusted outcomes. The database (Box 13) is now also used to facilitate the public reporting of outcomes and clinical research. It consists of 3 components, each focusing on a separate type of cardiothoracic surgery: adult cardiac surgery (established 1989), congenital heart surgery (1994), and general thoracic surgery (2002). Since 1999, the STS has contracted the Duke Clinical Research Institute to warehouse the data, conduct statistical analyses, and provide participants with performance reports.

DATA ELEMENT CONSIDERATIONS

Adult Cardiac Surgery Database (ACSD)

As of September 2016, the Adult Cardiac Surgery Database (ACSD) had more than 6.1 million patient records from 1119 participant health care centers (typically defined as an institutional surgical program, rather than a single hospital) encompassing 3100 surgeons from all 50 US states and 29 participants from 8 other countries.[1] Linkage analysis between ACSD and Centers for Medicare and Medicaid Services (CMS) data reveals high voluntary participation levels, with data on 94% of Medicare beneficiaries undergoing coronary artery bypass

> ## BOX 13
> ### Details of the STS National Database
>
> 1. The STS National Database measures demographic variables, specialty-specific covariates, and short-term outcomes such as morbidity, mortality, and length of stay.
> 2. Studies using the STS National Database are retrospective cohort designs. Consecutive cases are abstracted with longitudinal follow-up for short-term outcomes.
> 3. Like other observational study designs, confounding threatens validity; however, covariate breadth and specificity provide ample opportunity for adjustment through standard methods.
> 4. Limitations include the procedure-based (rather than disease-based) nature of the database; absence of clinician-level characteristics, long-term outcomes, and patient-reported outcomes; and possibly limited generalizability.
> 5. The STS National Database provides the most granular and specialty-specific data for performance feedback, voluntary public reporting outcomes, and clinical research on patients undergoing cardiothoracic surgery in the United States.
>
> Abbreviation: STS, Society of Thoracic Surgery.

grafting surgery and from 90% of the sites providing care to Medicare beneficiaries.

All STS data are subject to internal validation checks. Each year, a random sample of 10% of sites undergo an external audit, revealing 100% case ascertainment and 95% concordance between abstracted and audited data. Participants receive performance reports with risk-adjusted mortality rates for 7 major procedures; coronary artery bypass grafting surgery accounts for 69% of all cases. Using a 3-star system (in which 3 stars indicate the best performance), the STS calculates a composite score across 11 National Quality Forum indicators to publicly report participant-level performance.[1]

Congenital Heart Surgery Database

As of September 2016, the Congenital Heart Surgery Database (CHSD) contained data on 394 980 operations submitted by 120 participants, encompassing 392 surgeons from 39 US states and 3 other countries.[2] Hospitals participating in the CHSD include 95% of centers known to be performing congenital heart surgery in the United States. Participants receive risk-adjusted mortality and prolonged length of stay performance reports for 10 benchmark operations, of which ventricular septal defect is the most common. Public reporting of outcomes uses a 3-star system based on risk-adjusted mortality.[2]

General Thoracic Surgery Database

As of February 2016, the General Thoracic Surgery Database (GTSD) contained data on 482 432 operations submitted by 279 participants with 919 physicians (892 thoracic surgeons, 26 general surgeons, and 1 pulmonologist) and data from 2 other countries.[3] An independent external audit has determined that data in the GTSD is 95% accurate.[4] Participants receive performance reports on risk-adjusted mortality, morbidity, and a weighted composite score (combining morbidity and mortality) for lobectomy and esophagectomy. The GTSD also uses a 3-star system (based on the composite score) to publicly report outcomes.[3]

Data Source

Data managers at each site abstract information from the medical record into a standardized data collection form. The STS website has instructional web-based videos for data managers to facilitate uniform data collection. Training and standardized data collection is crucial to ensuring the reliability and validity of the data.

Outcomes and Other Key Measures

Additional outcome measures include specialty-specific complications, postoperative length of stay, and 30-day readmission in the ACSD; and length of stay in the GTSD. All databases collect demographic information, and each database collects granular specialty-specific covariates not found in other databases. For instance, the GTSD has information on functional status, pulmonary function test results, and variables describing the method by which clinical stage was determined. Because of inherent complexity, the Charlson, Elixhauser, and other comorbidity indices have not been validated for adult and congenital cardiac surgery. The STS database is a robust database that encompasses specific detailed clinically relevant preoperative and intraoperative patient-level characteristics unavailable in other administrative databases. A complete set of specialty-specific variables is described on the STS Data Managers website.[5]

Accessing Data

The principal investigator of a proposed research project does not necessarily have to be an STS database participant to access its database. However, the principal investigator or his or her institutional affiliate must either be a participant or the collaborator of a coinvestigator who is one.

Researchers can access STS data through the Access and Publications Committee or the participant use file (PUF). Twice a year, the Access and Publications committee selects several projects per specialty to undergo statistical analysis by the Duke Clinical Research Institute free of charge with a prespecified number of analyst hours. Selected investigators then receive aggregate data. The PUF program accepts proposals continuously from STS participants or their coinvestigators and reviews projects to avoid duplicative investigations and assess the feasibility of using STS data to test stated hypotheses. Project approval results in investigators receiving patient-level data after paying administrative and data volume-based fees. Approved PUF proposals require demonstration of local graduate-level statistical collaborators. Access and Publications and PUF committees both require a review of draft abstracts and/or manuscripts prior to submission for presentation or publication to ensure compliance with data use agreements.

Statistical Considerations

Since the STS database is based on medical record review performed by data collectors who perform complete consecutive case ascertainment with longitudinal outcome follow-up, investigations using the STS National Database are cohort studies. Like other observational study designs, confounding threatens the validity of STS database investigations. Yet the breadth and specificity of covariates provide ample opportunity for adjustment through standard methods (multivariable regression, propensity score, or propensity-matched methods[6] or instrumental variable analysis). Because of the large number of patients in the database, it is easy to discover statistically significant associations that are clinically unimportant. Therefore investigators should prespecify predictors, outcomes of interest, and the definition of a clinically important difference across variables. Conversely, despite large numbers of patients, Type 2 errors remain a possibility for rare events (eg, operative mortality), particularly when adjusting for many covariates.

Limitations

One limitation of the STS database is that it is a procedure-based (rather than disease-based) data set, making it difficult to perform comparative effectiveness research on surgical vs nonsurgical interventions. Some investigators have overcome this limitation through linkages to other databases (eg, CMS[1] and the American College of Cardiology Foundation National Cardiovascular Data Registry[7]). A second limitation of the STS database is a paucity of information on surgeon and hospital characteristics. The STS collects several clinician-level variables, but does not release them to investigators; it also prohibits analyses that could reveal the identity of a clinician. Thus, investigators generally cannot study the relationship between clinician characteristics and outcomes or adjust for potential confounding from these variables. A fourth limitation is the lack of data on long-term outcomes (eg, survival) and patient-reported outcomes. Finally, the STS database may be subject to self-reporting bias, although this is far less likely to be the case for the ACSD and CHSD, because there are no other specialties that perform cardiac surgery. For this reason, the GTSD is unlikely generalizable to the rest of the nation. An overwhelming majority of surgeons participating in the GTSD are board-certified thoracic surgeons with a dedicated thoracic practice, although cardiac and general surgeons also perform pulmonary and esophageal surgery.[3]

CONCLUSIONS

The STS National Database is the most comprehensive clinical registry for cardiothoracic surgery data, facilitating quality improvement, public reporting of outcomes, and research. Investigators can learn more through the STS website and annual reports.[1-3]

Acknowledgment

The following disclosures were reported at the time this original article was first published.
Conflict of Interest Disclosures: None reported.

References

1. D'Agostino RS, Jacobs JP, Badhwar V, et al. The Society of Thoracic Surgeons Adult Cardiac Surgery Database: 2017 update on outcomes and quality. *Ann Thorac Surg*. 2017;103(1):18-24. Medline:27884412

2. Jacobs ML, Jacobs JP, Hill KD, et al. The Society of Thoracic Surgeons congenital heart surgery database: 2017 update on research. *Ann Thorac Surg*. 2017;104(3):731-741. Medline:28760477

3. Seder CW, Raymond DP, Wright CD, et al. The Society of Thoracic Surgeons general thoracic surgery database 2017 update on outcomes and quality. *Ann Thorac Surg*. 2017;103(5):1378-1383. Medline:28431693

4. Magee MJ, Wright CD, McDonald D, Fernandez FG, Kozower BD. External validation of the Society of Thoracic Surgeons general thoracic surgery database. *Ann Thorac Surg*. 2013;96(5):1734-1739. Medline:23998406

5. Society of Thoracic Surgeons. Data managers website. https://www.sts.org/registries-research-center/sts-national-database. Published January 1, 2018. Accessed February 28, 2018.

6. McMurry TL, Hu Y, Blackstone EH, Kozower BD. Propensity scores: methods, considerations, and applications in the Journal of Thoracic and Cardiovascular Surgery. *J Thorac Cardiovasc Surg*. 2015;150(1):14-19. Medline:25963441

7. Weintraub WS, Grau-Sepulveda MV, Weiss JM, et al. Comparative effectiveness of revascularization strategies. *N Engl J Med*. 2012;366(16):1467-1476. Medline:22452338

GLOSSARY

Term	Definition
Absolute difference	The absolute difference in rates of good or harmful outcomes between experimental groups (experimental group risk [EGR]) and control groups (control group risk [CGR]), calculated as the risk in the control group minus the risk in the experimental group (CGR − EGR). For instance, if the rate of adverse events is 20% in the control group and 10% in the treatment group, the absolute difference is 20% − 10% = 10%.
ACS NSQIP-P	See National Surgical Quality Improvement Program Pediatric (NSQIP-P).
American College of Surgeon Trauma Quality Improvement Program (ACS TQIP)	Implemented in 2010 to improve the quality of care for trauma patients. See also National Trauma Data Bank (NTDB).
Analysis of covariance (ANCOVA)	The linear model used for covariate adjusting. It assumes, for all possible values of covariates, that covariate effect size (ES) is equal to typical ES; that is, that there is no interaction between the covariates and the treatment effect.
Analysis of variance (ANOVA)	Statistical method used to compare a continuous dependent variable and more than 1 nominal independent variable. Often used for analyzing longitudinal data. ANOVA does not have the flexibility of mixed models of analysis and can yield misleading results if its more rigid assumptions (eg, all effects are considered fixed) are not met.

Term	Definition
Area under the ROC curve (AUROC)	Technique used to measure the performance of a test plotted on a receiver operating characteristic (ROC) curve or to measure drug clearance in pharmacokinetic studies. When measuring test performance, the larger the AUC, the better the test performance. A model with perfect sensitivity and specificity would have an AUROC of 1. See also Receiver operating characteristic (ROC) curve.
Bayesian analysis	A statistical method that uses prior knowledge (eg, prior probability, conditional probability or likelihood) combined with data to obtain a new probability.
Bayesian hierarchical model (BHM)	A statistical procedure that integrates information across many levels, so multiple quantities are estimated simultaneously, and explicitly separates the observed variability into parts attributable to random differences and true differences.
Bias	Systematic deviation from the underlying truth because of a feature of the design or conduct of a research study (eg, overestimation of a treatment effect because of failure to randomize).
Bonferroni correction	A statistical adjustment to the threshold P value to adjust for multiple comparisons. The usual threshold for statistical significance (α) is 0.05. To perform a Bonferroni correction, one divides the critical P value by the number of comparisons being made. For example, if 10 hypotheses are being tested, the new critical P value would be $\alpha/10$, usually 0.05/10 or 0.005. The Bonferroni correction represents a simple adjustment but is very conservative (ie, less likely than other methods to give a significant result).

Term	Definition
C statistic	The C statistic is the probability that, given 2 individuals (one who experiences the outcome of interest and the other who does not or who experiences it later), the model will yield a higher risk for the first patient than for the second. The C is short for "concordance" between model estimates of risk and the observed events. See also Area under the ROC curve (AUROC) and Receiver operating characteristic (ROC) curve.
Calibration	The ability of the logistic regression model to assign the correct average absolute level of risk (ie, accurately estimate the probability of the outcome for a patient or group of patients). For risk prediction models, calibration measures how accurately the model's predictions match overall observed event rates. See also Discrimination.
Case-control study	A study designed to determine the association between an exposure and outcome in which patients are sampled by outcome. Those with the outcome (cases) are compared with those without the outcome (controls) with respect to exposure to the suspected harmful agent.
Center effects	Clinical trials sometimes need to use multiple clinical sites, and this can introduce complexity because outcomes at different sites may be systematically different, eg, due to differences in patient populations, ancillary treatment practices, or other factors. Such differences are referred to as *center effects*.
Clinical trial	See randomized clinical trial.

Term	Definition
Cluster randomized trial	A trial in which groups (eg, schools, clinics) rather than individuals are assigned to intervention and control groups. This approach is often used when assignment by individuals is likely to result in contamination (eg, if adolescents within a school are assigned to receive or not receive a new sex education program, it is likely that they will share the information they learn with one another; instead, if the unit of assignment is schools, entire schools are assigned to receive or not receive the new sex education program). Cluster assignment is typically randomized, but it is possible (though not advisable) to assign clusters to treatment or control by other methods.
Cohort study	A study of a group of individuals, some of whom are exposed to a variable of interest (eg, a drug treatment or environmental exposure), in which participants are followed up over time to determine who develops the outcome of interest and whether the outcome is associated with the exposure.
Collinearity	When multiple variables in a statistical model convey closely related information.
Common shocks assumptions	The 2 main assumptions of difference-in-differences analysis are parallel trends and common shocks. The common shocks assumptions state that any events occurring during or after the time the policy changed will equally affect the treatment and comparison groups. See also Parallel trends assumption.
Comparative effectiveness research	The direct comparison of health care interventions to determine which works best, for whom, and in what circumstances.

Term	Definition
Composite end points, composite outcomes	When investigators measure the effect of treatment on an aggregate of end points of various levels of importance, this is a composite end point. Inferences from composite end points are strongest in the rare situations in which (1) the component end points are of similar patient importance, (2) the end points that are more important occur with at least similar frequency to those that are less important, and (3) strong biologic rationale supports results that, across component end points, reveal similar relative risks with sufficiently narrow confidence intervals.
Confidence interval (CI)	The range of values within which it is probable that the true value of a parameter (eg, a mean, a relative risk) lies.
Confounder	A factor that is associated with the outcome of interest and is differentially distributed in patients exposed and unexposed to the outcome of interest. Unless it is possible to adjust for confounding variables, their effects cannot be distinguished from those of the factors being studied.
Confounding by indication	A particularly important type of confounding in clinical research is "confounding by indication," which occurs when the clinical indication for selecting a particular treatment (eg, severity of the illness) also affects the outcome.
Confounding by severity	When, for example, patients with more severe illness are likely to receive more intensive treatments and, when comparing the interventions, the more intensive intervention will appear to result in poorer outcomes, it is called *confounding by severity* to emphasize that the degree of illness is the confounder. See also Confounding by indication.

Term	Definition
Control	In a case-control study, the term *control* refers to an individual who did not have the outcome; in contrast, the same term in a clinical trial refers to a study participant who receives the standard (or placebo) treatment.
Convolution	Each filter in a convolution neural network is shifted sequentially to each location in the image and measures the degree to which the local properties of the image match the filter at each location, a process called *convolution*.
Convolutional neural networks (CNNs)	A type of machine learning being used to automate the reading of medical images. Successful neural networks for such a task are typically composed of multiple analysis layers; the term *deep learning* is also (synonymously) used to describe this class of neural networks.
Cost-effectiveness analysis	An economic analysis in which the consequences are expressed in natural units (eg, cost per life saved or cost per bleeding event averted). Sometimes, cost-utility analysis is classified as a subcategory of cost-effectiveness analysis.
Covariate adjusting	The linear model used for covariate adjusting assumes, for all possible values of covariates, that covariate effect size (ES) is equal to typical ES; that is, that there is no interaction between the covariates and the treatment effect. See also Effect size.
Covariate adjustment	There are 4 general ways propensity scores are used. One approach is covariate adjustment using the propensity score. For this approach, a separate multivariable model is developed, after the propensity score model, in which the study outcome serves as the dependent variable and the treatment group and propensity score serve as predictor variables. See also Propensity score matching, Stratification, and Inverse probability of treatment weighting.

Term	Definition
Cox proportional hazards model	A model used to assess rate data (number of items per unit time) as opposed to proportions, which are analyzed by logistic regression. In addition to an outcome such as alive or dead, the time it takes to experience that outcome (time to event) is incorporated in Cox proportional hazards regression, adding power to the analysis above that available from logistic regression.
Cross-sectional study	A study that identifies participants with and without the condition or disease under study and the characteristic or exposure of interest at the same point in time.
Crossover trial	A trial in which participants receive more than 1 of the treatments under investigation, usually in a randomly determined sequence, and with a prespecified amount of time (washout period) between sequential treatments.
Current Procedural Terminology (CPT) code	Uniform system of codes for medical, surgical, and diagnostic services and procedures.
Decision curve analysis (DCA)	A method for evaluating the benefits of a diagnostic test across a range of patient preferences for accepting risk of undertreatment and overtreatment to facilitate decisions about test selection and use.
Deep learning	See Convolutional neural networks (CNNs).
Delphi approach	An approach to decision making that uses expert consensus acquired through questionnaires.
Difference-in-differences	A statistical technique for comparison of differences in outcomes between groups (eg, a treatment and control group), before and after an intervention, by attempting to control for bias from potential confounders that remain fixed over time.

Term	Definition
Directed acyclic graphic	Graph that visually represents relationships between variables. For registry data, this graph can help a reader to understand the role of potential confounders and intermediates.
Discrimination	The ability of the logistic regression model to correctly assign a higher risk of an outcome to the patients who are truly at higher risk (ie, "ordering them" correctly). In time-to-event settings, discrimination is the ability of the model to predict who will develop an event earlier and who will develop an event later or not at all. See also Calibration.
Dose-finding trials	Dose-finding trials are studies conducted to identify the most promising doses or doses to use in later studies.
Dunnett method	A method for comparing multiple experimental drug doses against a single control in which the number of comparisons is reduced by never comparing experimental drug doses against each other.
Effect size	The difference in outcomes between the intervention and control groups divided by some measure of variability. It is the observed or expected change in outcome as a result of the intervention. Whereas statistical significance provides only an indication that a difference between groups exists, it does not provide an indication of how important that effect is. Effect size provides a measure of the magnitude of the differences between groups and should always be considered in addition to the statistical significance.

Term	Definition
Equipoise	The principle of equipoise states that, when there is uncertainty or conflicting expert opinion about the relative merits of diagnostic, prevention, or treatment options, allocating interventions to individuals in a manner that allows the generation of new knowledge (eg, randomization) is ethically permissible.
Expected harm	In decision curve analysis, the expected harm is represented by number of patients without the disease who would be treated in error (false positives) multiplied by a weighting factor based on the patient's threshold probability. The weighting factor captures the patient's values regarding the risks of undertreatment and overtreatment. Specifically, the false-positive rate is multiplied by the ratio of the threshold probability divided by 1 − the threshold probability. See also Net benefit.
Explanatory trials	Explanatory trials seek to maximize the probability that the intervention—and not some other factor—causes the study outcome. They seek to give the intervention the best possible chance to succeed by using experts to deliver it, delivering the intervention to patients who are most likely to respond, and administering the intervention in settings that provide expert after-care.
External validity	External validity refers to study results that apply outside the context of the study (eg, patients usually seen in clinical practice).

Term	Definition
E-value	The E-value is an alternative approach to sensitivity analyses for unmeasured confounding in observational studies that avoids making assumptions that, in turn, require subjective assignment of inputs for some formulas. Specifically, an E-value analysis asks the question: how strong would the unmeasured confounding have to be to negate the observed results? The E-value itself answers this question by quantifying the minimum strength of association on the risk ratio scale that an unmeasured confounder must have with both the treatment and outcome, while simultaneously considering the measured covariates, to negate the observed treatment–outcome association. If the strength of unmeasured confounding is weaker than indicated by the E-value, then the main study result could not be overturned to one of "no association" (ie, moving the estimated risk ratio to 1.0) by the unmeasured confounder. E-values can therefore help assess the robustness of the main study result by considering whether unmeasured confounding of this magnitude is plausible. The E-value provides a measure related to that *evidence*.
False discovery rate (FDR)	The expected proportion of false positives among all discoveries.
False positive	Those who do not have the target disorder, but the test incorrectly identifies them as having it.
False-positive inference	When a single statistical test is performed at the 5% significance level, there is a 5% chance of falsely concluding that a supposed effect exists when in fact there is none, known as a false discovery or false-positive inference.

Term	Definition
False-positive rate (FPR)	The mean number of false-positive results.
Family-wise error rate (FWER)	A probability that quantifies the risk of making any false-positive inference by a group, or family, of tests.
FINER (Feasible, Interesting, Novel, Ethical, Relevant) criteria	A format that can help in development of a meaningful research question.
Free-response operating characteristic (FROC) analysis	Free-response operating characteristic analysis assesses the ability of a medical test to identify abnormalities on an image. Examples include identifying tumors in radiographs or foci of malignancy on histological slides. See also Free-response receiver operating characteristic (FROC) curve.
Free-response receiver operating characteristic (FROC) curve	There are similarities between FROC curve analysis and the more commonly used receiver operating characteristic (ROC) curve analysis. Conventional ROC curves, however, evaluate the accuracy of a test for detecting the presence or absence of disease but do not evaluate whether a test correctly identifies the location. See also Receiver operating characteristic (ROC) curve.
Gatekeeping	A serial gatekeeping procedure controls the false-positive risk by requiring the multiple end points to be compared in a predefined sequence and stopping all further testing once a nonsignificant result is obtained. A given comparison might be considered positive if it were placed early in the sequence, but the same analysis would be considered negative if it were positioned in the sequence after a negative result. By restricting the pathways for obtaining a positive result, gatekeeping controls the risk of false-positive results but preserves greater power for the earlier, higher-priority end points.

Term	Definition
Healthcare Cost and Utilization Project (HCUP)	HCUP, pronounced *H-Cup,* is a collection of data sets that represent the largest collection of administrative, longitudinal health care data in the United States.
Hochberg sequential procedure	When all of the tests (the multiple comparisons) are performed and the resultant P values are ordered from largest to smallest on a list. If the FWER is fixed at 5% and the largest observed P value is less than .05, then all the tests are considered significant. Otherwise, if the next largest P value is less than 0.05/2 (.025), then all the tests except the one with the largest P value are considered significant. If not, and the third P value in the list is less than 0.05/3 (.017), then all the tests except those with the largest 2 P values are considered significant. This is continued until all the comparisons are made.
Hosmer-Lemeshow statistic	Test for evaluating the goodness of fit in a logistic regression model; often used in risk prediction models. The Hosmer-Lemeshow statistic depends on the number of risk groups into which the study population is divided in order to assess whether a logistic regression model is appropriately calibrated. There is no theoretical basis for the "correct" number of risk groups into which a population should be divided.
I^2 statistic	The I^2 statistic is a test of heterogeneity, commonly used in meta-analyses. I^2 can be calculated from Cochrane Q according to the formula: $I^2 = 100\% \times$ (Cochrane Q − degrees of freedom). Any negative values of I^2 are considered equal to 0, so that the range of I^2 values is 0% to 100%, indicating no heterogeneity to high heterogeneity, respectively.

Term	Definition
Incremental effect	When the risk factor in a logistic regression is discrete (eg, presence or absence of diabetes), the change may be called an incremental effect. See also Marginal effects.
Incremental cost-effectiveness ratio (ICER)	The price at which additional units of benefit can be obtained.
Individual error rate (IER)	The individual error rate represents the risk of making a false discovery in an individual test.
Intention-to-treat (ITT) analysis	Analysis of outcomes for individuals based on the treatment group to which they were randomized, rather than on which treatment they actually received and whether they completed the study.
Interaction	When the value of one predictor in a logistic regression analysis alters the effect of another, there is said to be an "interaction" between the 2 predictors.
Internal validity	Whether a study provides valid results depends on whether it was designed and conducted well enough that the study findings accurately represent the direction and magnitude of the underlying true effect (ie, studies that have higher internal validity have a lower likelihood of bias/systematic error).
International Statistical Classification of Diseases and Related Health Problems	International coding system for diseases, disorders, injuries, and other related health conditions.
Intracluster correlation coefficient (ICC)	The ICC quantifies the likeness within clusters in a cluster randomized trial and ranges from 0 to 1, although it is frequently in the 0.02 to 0.1 range.

Term	Definition
Inverse probability of treatment weighting	Statistical technique to account for biases due to observed confounders. For example, propensity scores are used to calculate statistical weights for each individual to create a sample in which the distribution of potential confounding factors is independent of exposure, allowing an unbiased estimate of the relationship between treatment and outcome. See also Propensity score matching, Stratification, and Covariate adjustment.
Kaplan-Meier plot	A method for analyzing time-to-event data that accounts for censored observations. A Kaplan-Meier curve plots the fraction of "surviving" patients (those who have not experienced an event) against time for each treatment group.
Last observation carried forward (LOCF)	A method for handling missing data. Typically, LOCF involves using the last recorded data point as the final outcome.
Logistic regression	A regression analysis used to analyze the relationship between a binary dependent variable and 1 or more dependent variables.
Longitudinal cohort study	This is an investigation in which a cohort of individuals who do not have evidence of an outcome of interest but who are exposed to the putative cause is compared with a concurrent cohort of individuals who are also free of the outcome but not exposed to the putative cause. Both cohorts are then followed forward in time to compare the incidence of the outcome of interest. When used to study the effectiveness of an intervention, it is an investigation in which a cohort of individuals who receive the intervention is compared with a concurrent cohort who does not receive the intervention, wherein both cohorts are followed forward to compare the incidence of the outcome of interest. Cohort studies can be conducted retrospectively in the sense that someone other than the investigator has followed patients, and the investigator obtains the database and then examines the association between exposure and outcome.

Term	Definition
Machine learning	Form of artificial intelligence in which "machines" (computers, software, systems) "learn" from data by following algorithms and models to identify patterns and make predictions or decisions without, or with minimal, human involvement.
Marginal effects	Marginal effects can be used to express how the predicted probability of a binary outcome changes with a change in a risk factor. Marginal effects often are reported with logistic regression analyses to communicate and quantify the incremental risk associated with each factor.
Mediation analysis	Mediation analysis assesses variables in a pathway in which 1 variable is related to a second variable that, in turn, is related to a third variable. The second intervening variable may mediate a relationship between the first and third variables.
Medicare claim data	The Centers for Medicare and Medicaid Services administers Medicare, the primary US health insurance program for people aged 65 years and older and people who qualify for Social Security Administration disability benefits. Data from Medicare may be useful in comparative effectiveness research and health policy analysis.
Mendelian randomization	Mendelian randomization uses genetic variants to determine whether an observational association between a risk factor and an outcome is consistent with a potential causal effect.
Meta-analysis	A statistical technique for quantitatively combining the results of multiple studies that measure the same outcome into a single pooled or summary estimate.

Term	Definition
Metabolic and Bariatric Surgery Accreditation and Quality Improvement Program (MBSAQIP)	This program is responsible for accrediting inpatient and outpatient bariatric surgery centers in the United States and Canada.
Military Health System Data Repository (MDR)	Tricare claims data are maintained by the US Military Health System Data Repository. See also Tricare.
Minimal clinically important difference (MCID)	The smallest difference in a patient-important outcome that patients perceive as beneficial and that would mandate, in the absence of troublesome adverse effects and excessive cost, a change in the patient's health care management.
Minimum detectable difference (MDD)	The smallest possible rate difference in a trial that is feasible to detect.
Mixed models	Mixed models explicitly account for the correlations between repeated measurements of an outcome within each study participant. Mixed models are ideally suited to settings in which the individual trajectory of a particular outcome for a study participant over time is influenced both by factors that can be assumed to be the same for many patients (eg, the effect of an intervention) and by characteristics that are likely to vary substantially from patient to patient (eg, the severity of the ankle fracture, baseline level of function, and quality of life).
Modified intention-to-treat (MITT) analysis	While the definition of an MITT analysis varies from study to study, the MITT approach deviates from the intention-to-treat approach by eliminating patients or reassigning patients to a study group other than the group to which they were randomized. See also Intention-to-treat (ITT) analysis.

Term	Definition
Multicenter clinical trials	Clinical trials that involve many sites or centers, often because one center rarely can enroll sufficient numbers of patients to complete the trial.
Multiple comparisons	Problems can arise when researchers try to assess the statistical significance of more than 1 test in a study. In a single test, statistical significance is often determined based on an observed effect or finding that is unlikely (< 5%) to occur due to chance alone. When more than 1 comparison is made, the chance of falsely detecting a nonexistent effect increases. This is known as the problem of multiple comparisons.
Multiple imputation	Imputation is the process of replacing missing data with 1 or more specific values to allow statistical analysis that includes all participants and not just those who do not have any missing data. Multiple imputation, as compared with single-value imputation, better handles missing data by estimating and replacing missing values many times.
National Cancer Database (NCDB)	A joint program of the American College of Surgeons Commission on Cancer and the American Cancer Society that collects data from hospitals in the United States to capture newly diagnosed cancers.
National Inpatient Sample (NIS)	Formerly Nationwide Inpatient Sample. The NIS is designed to be representative of health care use in the United States overall, making it ideal for performing basic descriptive studies, deriving national estimates, studying costs, studying rare disease, and understanding trends over time.
National Surgical Quality Improvement Program (NSQIP)	US national program designed to measure and improve the quality of surgical care. See also VA Surgical Quality Improvement Program (VASQIP).

Term	Definition
National Surgical Quality Improvement Program Pediatric (NSQIP-P)	US national program to address surgical quality improvement for children undergoing surgery.
National Trauma Data Bank (NTDB)	A standardized collection of US national trauma data developed by the American College of Surgeons Committee on Trauma.
Negative predictive value (NPV)	The proportion of patients whom the model predicts will not have an event who actually do not experience the event.
Net benefit	A concept in decision curve analysis. The net benefit, or "benefit score," is determined by calculating the difference between the expected benefit and the expected harm associated with each proposed testing and treatment strategy. The expected benefit is represented by the number of patients who have the disease and who will receive treatment (true positives) using the proposed strategy. See also Expected harm.
Neural network	The application of nonlinear statistics to pattern-recognition problems. Neural networks can be used to develop clinical prediction rules. The technique identifies those predictors most strongly associated with the outcome of interest that belong in a clinical prediction rule and those that can be omitted from the rule without loss of predictive power.

Term	Definition
N-of-1 trial	An experiment designed to determine the effect of an intervention or exposure on a single study participant. In one n-of-1 design, the patient undergoes pairs of treatment periods organized so that 1 period involves the use of the experimental treatment and 1 period involves the use of an alternate treatment or placebo. The patient and clinician are blinded if possible, and outcomes are monitored. Treatment periods are replicated until the clinician and patient are convinced that the treatments are definitely different or definitely not different.
Noninferiority trial	Noninferiority trials address whether the effect of an experimental intervention is not worse than a standard intervention by more than a specified margin. This contrasts with equivalence trials, which aim to determine whether an intervention is similar to another intervention. Noninferiority of the experimental intervention with respect to the standard treatment may be of interest if the new intervention has some other advantage, such as greater availability, reduced cost, less invasiveness, fewer harms, or decreased burden—or a potential for increased income for the sponsor.
Null hypothesis	A statement used in statistics asserting that no true difference exists between comparison groups. In the hypothesis-testing framework, this is the starting hypothesis that the statistical test is designed to consider and possibly reject, which contends that there is no association among the variables under study.

Term	Definition
Number needed to treat (NNT)	The number of patients who need to be treated during a specific period to achieve 1 additional good outcome. When NNT is discussed, it is important to specify the intervention, its duration, and the desirable outcome. If an NNT calculation results in a decimal, round up as per Cochrane guidance (http://www.cochrane-net.org/openlearning/html/mod11-6.htm). It is the inverse of the absolute risk reduction (ARR), expressed as a percentage (100/ARR).
O'Brien-Fleming method	A method for determining early stopping criteria that requires very small P values to declare success early in the trial and then maintains a final P value very close to the traditional .05 level at the final analysis. Using this method, very few trials could be successful at the interim analyses that would not have been successful at the final analysis. Thus, there is a minimal "penalty" for the interim analyses. The more conservative the early stopping criteria, the more assurance there is that an early stop for success is not a false-positive result.
Odds	The ratio of events to nonevents; the ratio of the number of study participants experiencing the outcome of interest to the number of study participants not experiencing the outcome of interest.
Odds ratio	A ratio of the odds of an event in an exposed group to the odds of the same event in a group that is not exposed.

Term	Definition
P value	Probability of obtaining the observed data (or data that are more extreme) if the null hypothesis were exactly true. Also expressed as the probability that the observed result was obtained by chance alone. Although hypothesis testing often results in the *P* value, *P* values themselves can only provide information about whether the null hypothesis is rejected. Confidence intervals (CIs) are much more informative because they provide a plausible range of values for an unknown parameter, as well as some indication of the power of the study as indicated by the width of the CI. See also Confidence interval (CI).
Parallel trends assumption	The 2 main assumptions of difference-in-differences analysis are parallel trends and common shocks. The parallel trends assumption states that the trends in outcomes between the treated and comparison groups are the same prior to the intervention. If true, it is reasonable to assume that these parallel trends would continue for both groups even if the program was not implemented. See also Common shocks assumptions.
Participant use file (PUF)	Deidentified data file containing cases submitted to the American College of Surgeons National Surgical Quality Improvement Program (ACS NSQIP). The PUF contains patient-level, aggregate data and does not identify patients, health care professionals, or health care institutions.
Permuted block randomization	A restricted randomization method used to help ensure the balance of the number of patients assigned to each treatment group.

Term	Definition
Per-protocol analysis	Includes the subset of patients who complete the entire clinical trial according to the protocol. This approach compromises the prognostic balance that randomization achieves and is therefore likely to provide a biased estimate of treatment effect.
PICO	Acronym for Patient, Population, or Problem; Intervention, Prognostic Factor, or Exposure; Comparison or Intervention; and Outcome. A method for answering clinical questions.
Pleiotropy	*Pleiotropy* refers to a genetic variant influencing the outcome through pathways independent of the risk factor.
Positive predictive value (PPV)	The proportion of patients in whom the model predicts an event will occur who actually have an event. See also Negative predictive value (NPV).
Pragmatic trials	Trials intended to help typical clinicians and typical patients make difficult decisions in typical clinical care settings by maximizing the chance that the trial results will apply to patients who are usually seen in practice.
Preferred Reporting Items for Systematic Reviews and Meta-analyses (PRISMA)	A reporting guideline for systematic reviews and meta-analyses.
Preferred Reporting Items for Systematic Reviews and Meta-analyses Protocols (PRISMA-P)	A reporting standard for meta-analysis protocols.
Probability threshold	A level of diagnostic certainty above which the patient would choose to be treated.

Term	Definition
Propensity score	The propensity score is the probability that a patient receives a specific treatment based on his or her characteristics and the clinical indications determined by the treating physician.
Propensity score matching	There are 4 general ways propensity scores are used. The most common is propensity score matching, which involves assembling 2 groups of study participants, one group that received the treatment of interest and the other that did not, while matching individuals with similar or identical propensity scores. See also Stratification, Covariate adjustment, and Inverse probability of treatment weighting.
Propensity score methods	Propensity score methods are used to reduce the bias in estimating treatment effects and allow investigators to reduce the likelihood of confounding when analyzing nonrandomized, observational data.
PROSPERO	A registry for systematic reviews and meta-analyses.
Pseudo-R^2	The pseudo-R^2 is meant to mimic the R^2 calculated for linear regression models, a measure of the fraction of the variability in the outcome that is explained by the model.
Publication bias	Occurs when the publication of research depends on the direction of the study results and whether they are statistically significant.
Quality-adjusted life-year (QALY)	A unit of measure for survival that accounts for the effects of suboptimal health status and the resulting limitations in quality of life. For example, if a patient lives for 10 years and his or her quality of life is decreased by 50% because of chronic lung disease, survival would be equivalent to 5 quality-adjusted life-years (QALYs).

Term	Definition
Quality improvement (QI)	An approach to defining, measuring, improving, and controlling practices to maintain or improve the appropriateness of health care services.
R^2	Correlational coefficient that measures heterogeneity of variables. When a test has results that are heterogeneous, the R^2 statistic can quantify how much of the variability between studies can be attributed to a covariate.
Random-effects meta-analysis	In a random-effects meta-analysis, the statistical model estimates multiple parameters. First, the model estimates a separate treatment effect for each trial, representing the estimate of the true effect for the trial. The assumption that the true effects can vary from trial to trial is the foundation for a random-effects meta-analysis. Second, the model estimates an overall treatment effect, representing an average of the true effects over the group of studies included. Third, the model estimates the variability or degree of heterogeneity in the true treatment effects across trials.
Randomized clinical trial (RCT)	An experiment in which individuals are randomly allocated to receive or not receive an experimental diagnostic, preventive, therapeutic, or palliative procedure and then followed up to determine the effect of the intervention.
Receiver operating characteristic (ROC) curve	A figure depicting the power of a diagnostic test. The receiver operating characteristic (ROC) curve presents the test's true-positive rate (ie, sensitivity) on the horizontal axis and the false-positive rate (ie, 1 – specificity) on the vertical axis for different cut points dividing a positive from a negative test result. An ROC curve for a perfect test has an area under the curve of 1.0, whereas a test that performs no better than chance has an area under the curve of only 0.5. See also Area under the ROC curve (AUROC).

Term	Definition
Regression model diagnostics	Regression model diagnostics measure how well models describe the underlying relationships between predictors and patient outcomes existing within the data, either the data on which the model was built or data from a different population.
Relative risk (RR) (or risk ratio)	The ratio of the risk of an event among an exposed population to the risk among the unexposed.
Risk prediction model	Risk prediction models help clinicians develop personalized treatments for patients. The models generally use variables measured at one time point to estimate the probability of an outcome occurring within a given time in the future.
Risk ratio	See Relative risk.
Sensitivity analysis	Any test of the stability of the conclusions of a health care evaluation over a range of probability estimates, value judgments, and assumptions about the structure of the decisions to be made. This may involve the repeated evaluation of a decision model in which one or more of the parameters of interest are varied.
Sharing strength	In statistics, the ability to share data.
Single-value imputation	Single-value imputation methods are those that estimate what each missing value might have been and replace it with a single value in the data set. Single-value imputation methods include mean imputation, last observation carried forward, and random imputation. These approaches can yield biased results and are suboptimal. Multiple imputation better handles missing data by estimating and replacing missing values many times.

Term	Definition
Society of Thoracic Surgeons (STS) National Database	A voluntary clinical registry created to facilitate a national quality improvement and patient safety among cardiothoracic surgeons.
Statistical power	Power can be thought of as the probability of the complement of a type II error. If we accept a 20% type II error for a difference in rates of size d, we are saying that there is a 20% chance that we do not detect the difference between groups when the difference in their rates is d. The complement of this, $0.8 = 1 - 0.2$ is the statistical power. It means that when a difference of d exists, there is an 80% chance that our statistical test will detect it.
Stratification	There are 4 general ways propensity scores are used. One approach is stratification on the propensity score. This technique involves separating study participants into distinct groups or strata based on their propensity scores. Five strata are commonly used, although increasing the number can reduce the likelihood of bias. See also Propensity score matching, Covariate adjustment, and Inverse probability of treatment weighting.
Stratified randomization	A restricted randomization method used to balance one or a few prespecified prognostic characteristics between treatment groups.
Stepped-wedge design	The sequential rollout of a quality improvement (QI) intervention to study units (clinicians, organizations) during a number of periods so that by the end of the study all participants have received the intervention. The order in which participants receive the intervention may be randomized (similar rigor to cluster randomized designs). Data are collected and outcomes measured at each point at which a new group of participants ("step") receives the QI intervention. Observed differences in outcomes between the control section of the wedge with those in the intervention section are attributed to the intervention.

Term	Definition
Strengthening the Reporting of Observational Studies in Epidemiology (STROBE) reporting guidelines	Guidelines for reporting the results of observational studies, such as cohort and cross-sectional studies.
Surveillance, Epidemiology, and End Results (SEER) database	A publicly available, US federally funded cancer reporting system that provides information on cancer statistics in an effort to reduce the cancer burden among the US population; it represents a collaboration between the US Centers for Disease Control and Prevention, the National Cancer Institute, and regional and state cancer registries.
Survival analysis	A statistical procedure used to compare the proportion of patients in each group who experience an outcome or end point at various intervals throughout the study (eg, death). Also known as a time-to-event analysis.
Time horizons	For cost-effectiveness analysis, the time horizon is the time over which the costs and effects are measured.
Time-to-event analysis	A statistical procedure used to compare the proportion of patients in each group who experience an outcome or end point at various intervals throughout the study (eg, death). Also known as a survival analysis.
Tricare	Often styled TRICARE. The insurance product owned and operated by the US Department of Defense.
Tricare claims data	Tricare claims are maintained by the US Military Health System Data Repository. Tricare is the insurance product owned and operated by the US Department of Defense.

Term	Definition
Type I error	An error created by rejecting the null hypothesis when it is true (ie, investigators conclude that an association exists among variables when it does not).
Type II error	An error created by accepting the null hypothesis when it is false (ie, investigators conclude that no association exists among variables when, in fact, an association does exist).
VA National Surgical Quality Improvement Program (NSQIP)	The initial VA National Surgical Quality Improvement Program was created to accurately collect clinical data using standardized methodology and incorporating robust risk adjustment. Renamed the VA Surgical Quality Improvement Program (VASQIP) after merging the cardiac and noncardiac surgery components of NSQIP, this mandatory, VA-wide program has remained a model for national quality improvement efforts and was the template used to develop the private sector American College of Surgeons–NSQIP.
Vascular Quality Initiative (VQI)	Developed by the Society for Vascular Surgery in 2011 to improve the safety and effectiveness of 12 common vascular procedures.
VA Surgical Quality Improvement Program (VASQIP)	The initial VA National Surgical Quality Improvement Program was created to accurately collect clinical data using standardized methodology and incorporating robust risk adjustment. Renamed the VA Surgical Quality Improvement Program (VASQIP) after merging the cardiac and noncardiac surgery components of NSQIP, this mandatory, VA-wide program has remained a model for national quality improvement efforts and was the template used to develop the private sector American College of Surgeons–NSQIP.

INDEX

A

ACS NSQIP. *See* **National Surgical Quality Improvement Program (NSQIP)**
ACS NSQIP Pediatric (NSQIP-P), 392
ACS TQIP, 417-418
ACSD. *See* **Adult Cardiac Surgery Database (ACSD)**
Adjusting for covariates, 255-260
   analysis of covariance (ANCOVA), 257
   collinearity, 258
   post hoc hypothesis testing, 258, 259
   propensity score methods, 272
   typical effect size (ES)/covariate effect size (ES), 257, 258
Administrative data sets, 350, 354
Adult Cardiac Surgery Database (ACSD), 432-434, 437
Agency for Healthcare Research and Quality Healthcare Cost and Utilization Project (HCUP), 350. *See also* **HCUP data sets**
Analysis of covariance (ANCOVA), 257
Anchor-based methods, 51, 52
ANCOVA. *See* **Analysis of covariance (ANCOVA)**
Arbitrary scaling factor, 242, 244
Area under the ROC curve (AUROC), 123, 303. *See also* **Receiver operating characteristic (ROC) curve analysis**
AUROC. *See* **Area under the ROC curve (AUROC)**
Autoregressive correlation structure, 108

B

Baseline observation carried forward, 90-91
Bayesian analysis, 169-174, 294. *See also* **Prior information**
Bayesian hierarchical model (BHM), 293-300
   analyses to be conducted on subgroups separately, 299
   assumptions, 298
   defined, 294
   heterogeneity, 297
   how was BHM used in this case?, 298-299
   interpretation of study's findings, 299
   key characteristics, 295
   limitations, 298
   prior information, 295
   rare diseases, 298
   shrinkage estimation, 297
   why is BHM used?, 296-298
BHM. *See* **Bayesian hierarchical model (BHM)**
Bias. *See also* **Confounding**
   adjusting for covariates, 258
   blinding, 67
   case-control study, 195
   cluster randomized trials, 31
   complete case analysis, 93
   early stopping, 165
   HCUP data sets, 355
   intention-to-treat (ITT), 101
   mediation analysis, 235
   mendelian randomization, 210
   meta-analysis, 200

Bias. *See also* **Confounding**
(*continued*)
missing data, 93
multiple comparison procedures, 144
National Cancer Database (NCDB), 411-412
National Trauma Data Bank (NTDB), 420
permuted blocks and stratified randomization, 60-61
randomization, 67
stepped-wedge clinical trial, 35
STS National Database, 437
time-to-event analysis, 75
Vascular Quality Initiative (VQI), 425-426
Big data. *See* **Surgical database research**
Blinding
bias, 67
pragmatic trials, 21
Bonferroni procedure
gatekeeping strategies, 147
multiple comparison procedures, 139, 140, 141 (table)
Brief negotiated interview, 138, 142. *See also* **Multiple comparison procedures**
Brier score, 306

C

C statistic, 123, 301-307
alternatives to, 306
area under ROC curve, 303
calibration, 302
caveats, 306
defined, 302
discrimination, 302
familiar first-glance summary, 306
interpretation of study's findings, 304-305
limitations, 304
positive predictive value (PPV)/negative predictive value (NPV), 303
time-to-event data/competing risk settings, 306
why is C statistic used?, 302-303
why was C statistic used in this study?, 304-305
CAC testing. *See* **Coronary artery calcification (CAC) testing**
Calibration, 123, 124-125, 302
Calibration plot, 125
CAMELYON16 competition, 279 (figure), 282
Cancer database. *See* **National Cancer Database (NCDB)**
Cancer reporting system. *See* **Surveillance, epidemiology, and end results (SEER) database**
Cancer-specific survival, 365
Cardiac surgery. *See* **Society of Thoracic Surgeons (STS) National Database**
Case-control study, 191-198
advantages, 196
bias, 195
causality, 197
defined, 191
goal/objective, 191, 196
how was the method applied in this case?, 197
hypothetical example, 192 (figure)
interpretation of study's findings, 197
marginal effects, 251
nested study, 194, 195
odds ratio (OR), 194-196
randomized clinical trial (RCT), compared, 196
relative risk (RR), 196
retrospective nature of, 195
what is case-control study used?, 195

working backward from outcome to exposure, 191
Censoring
missing data, 92
time-to-event analysis, 75, 77, 78
Center effects, 263-264. *See also* **Treatment effects in multicenter trials**
Charlson comorbidity indices, 378
CHSD. *See* **Congenital Heart Surgery Database (CHSD)**
CLEAN-TAVI study, 146, 147, 150, 151
Clinical classifications software tools, 357
Clinical registries, 354
Clinical trials. *See also* **Cluster randomized trials, Noninferiority trial, Randomized clinical trial (RCT, Stepped-wedge clinical trial)**
cluster randomization, 25-32
permuted blocks and stratified randomization, 57-64
phases, 10
pragmatic trials, 17-24
primary goal, 225
stepped-wedge design, 33-39
stopping early, 161-167
Cluster randomized trials, 25-32
bias, 31
caveats, 30-31
defined, 26
interpretation of study's findings, 30
intracluster correlation coefficient (ICC), 29, 31
limitations, 28-29
randomized clinical trial (RCT), contrasted, 26
RESTORE trial, 27-30
why is cluster randomization used?, 27-28
why was cluster randomized used in this instance?, 29-30

CNN. *See* **Convolutional neural network (CNN)**
Cochran Q test, 211 (figure)
Cohort study, 228, 302
Collinearity
adjusting for covariates, 258
logistic regression, 116, 119
Common shocks assumption, 187
Comparative effectiveness research, 370-372, 371 (table)
Competing risk, 83
Complete case analysis, 90, 91, 93, 157
Composite end points, 81-87
competing risk, 83
coronary artery calcification (CAC) testing, 82, 86
how were composite end points used in this instance?, 85-86
interpretation of study's findings, 85-86
LIFE trial, 83
limitations, 83-85
major adverse cardiovascular event (MACE), 82, 83
weights reflecting component's utility, 85
why are composite end points used?, 82-83
Compound symmetry correlation structure, 108
Confirmatory studies, 143
Confounding, 223-229
caveats, 228-229
confounding by indication, 224, 227-229
confounding by severity, 225
E-value analysis, 216, 217
how to evaluate confounding by indication?, 229
identifying a confounding variable, 224
interpretation of study's findings, 227-229
mediation analysis, 235
National Cancer Database (NCDB), 411-412

Confounding (*continued*)
propensity score methods, 227, 228, 271
residual, 227, 228
statistical procedures, 226, 227
study design procedures, 226
Tricare data, 380
unmeasured, 227, 235
Confounding by indication, 224, 227-229, 271
Confounding by severity, 225
Congenital Heart Surgery Database (CHSD), 434, 437
Consensus methods (Delphi approach), 51, 52
Consortium paradigm, 204
Contamination, 28
Control, 194
Convolution, 328
Convolutional neural network (CNN), 326, 327 (video), 328-329
Coronary artery calcification (CAC) testing, 82, 86
Correlation structures, 108
Cost-effectiveness analysis, 309-316
comparing ICER to threshold value, 312
cost containment vs level of investment, 315
defined, 310, 311
description of the method, 311-312
how was cost-effectiveness analysis performed in this study?, 313-314
impact inventory, 313
incremental cost-effectiveness ratio (ICER), 311, 312
interpretation of study's findings, 314-315
limitations, 312-313
quality-adjusted life-years (QALYs), 311
quality-of life-related weights, 314
Second Panel recommendations, 313, 315, 320
time horizon. *See* Time horizon in cost-effectiveness analysis
Covariate adjusting. *See* **Adjusting for covariates**
Cox proportional hazards model, 76-79, 365
Cross-sectional study, 418

D

Data sets. *See* **Surgical database research**
DCA. *See* **Decision curve analysis (DCA)**
Deciles of risk, 124
Decision curve analysis (DCA), 125, 175-181
caveats, 181
defined, 176
expected benefit/expected harm, 177
graphic representation of DCA, 177-178
how was DCA used in this study?, 179
interpretation of study's findings, 179
limitations, 178-179
net benefit (benefit score), 177, 180 (figure)
probability threshold, 177, 180 (figure)
weighting factor, 177
why is DCA used?, 176-178
Deep learning, 325-331
convolution, 328
defined, 326
feature map, 328
filters, 326-327

hierarchical representation, 328-329
how convolutional neural network (CNN) works, 327 (video), 328-329
limitations, 329
motifs, 326
sharing strength, 329
Delphi approach (Consensus methods), 51, 52
DerSimonian-Laird method, 290
Difference-in-differences analysis, 183-189
caveats, 188-189
common shocks assumption, 187
conceptual illustration, 185, 186 (figure)
interpretation of study's findings, 188
limitations, 187
parallel trends assumption, 187
pre-post vs exposed-unexposed variables, 185
regression modeling, 185
spillover, 188-189
why is difference-in-differences analysis used?, 184-185
why was difference-in-differences analysis used in this instance?, 187-188
Direct care, 377, 379
Directed acyclic graph, 336 (box), 337, 344
Discrimination, 122-123, 123-124, 302
Discrimination score, 306
Distribution-based methods, 52, 53
Dose-finding trials, 9-15
caveats, 14
defined, 10
E_{max} model, 12
interpretation of study's findings, 14
limitations, 13
normal dynamic linear models, 13

SOCRATES-REDUCED trial, 11-13
why are dose-response models used?, 11-13
why use dose-response modeling in this instance?, 13
Dunnett method, 147

E

E_{max} **model,** 12
E-value analysis, 215-221
alternative approach to sensitivity analysis, 218
appealing features, 218-219
caveats, 220-221
confounding, 216, 217
interpretation of study's findings, 220
limitations, 219
why is E-value used?, 217-219
why was E-value used in this instance?, 219-220
Early stopping, 161-167
bias, 165
caveats, 166
interpretation of study's findings, 165-166
limitations, 164-165
O'Brien-Fleming method, 164
robustness analysis, 166
why is early stopping used?, 163
why was early stopping used in this study?, 165
Elixhauser comorbidities, 357
Emerging Risk Factors Collaboration (ERFC), 211 (figure)
Enthusiastic prior, 173
Epidemiological links, 319
Equipoise, 65-71
criticisms of, 69-70
fulfillment of three ethical obligations, 68

Equipoise (*continued*)
    how is equipoise applied in this instance?, 70
    interpretation of study's findings, 70-71
    principle of equipoise, defined, 66
Equivalence trial, 5
ERFC. *See* **Emerging Risk Factors Collaboration (ERFC)**
EXACT trial, 106, 110
Explanatory trials, 19, 20
Exploratory studies, 143
External validity, 18, 21-22

F

False discovery rate (FDR), 143
False-positive error rate, 149
False-positive inference, 138, 140
False-positive rate (FPR), 280, 281
Family-wise error rate (FWER), 139, 143
FDR. *See* **False discovery rate (FDR)**
Feature map, 328
FINER (Feasible, Interesting, Novel, Ethical, Relevant), 335, 336 (box)
Fixed-effect meta-analysis, 287, 288, 290
Fixed effects, 107
FPR. *See* **False-positive rate (FPR)**
Free-response receiver operating characteristic (FROC) curve analysis, 277-283
    CAMELYON16 competition, 279 (figure), 282
    caveats, 282
    false-positive rate (FPR), 280, 281
    HMS-MIT II team, 279 (figure), 282
    how are FROC curves constructed?, 280-281
    interpretation of study's findings, 281-282
    limitations, 281
    proximity criterion, 281
    ROC curve analysis, compared, 278, 281
    true-positive fraction (TPF), 280, 281
    universal acceptance of numerical indices?, 282
    why are FROC curves used?, 278-280
FROC curve. *See* **Free-response receiver operating characteristic (FROC) curve analysis**
FWER. *See* **Family-wise error rate (FWER)**

G

Gatekeeping strategies, 145-151
    Bonferroni procedure, 147
    CLEAN-TAVI study, 146, 147, 150, 151
    criteria for statistical significance, 148 (figure)
    description of the method, 147-149
    Dunnett method, 147
    false-positive error rate, 149
    how was gatekeeping used in this case?, 150
    interpretation of study's findings, 151
    limitations, 150
    steps in serial gatekeeping, 148-149
    transparency, 150
    why is serial gatekeeping used?, 147

General Thoracic Surgery Database (GTSD), 434, 437
Generalized estimating equations, 28-29
Genetic variants, 208
Glasgow Outcome Scale (GOS), 98, 99
GOS. *See* Glasgow Outcome Scale (GOS)
Graphical data summaries, 111
GTSD. *See* General Thoracic Surgery Database (GTSD)

Healthcare Cost and Utilization Project (HCUP), 350. *See also* HCUP data sets
Heterogeneity
  Bayesian hierarchical model (BHM), 297
  random-effects meta-analysis, 290, 291
Hierarchical models, 29
Hochberg sequential procedure, 140, 141 (table)
HOME trial, 322
Hosmer-Lemeshow statistic, 125

H

Hazard function, 74-75, 77
Hazard ratio, 76, 78
HCUP. *See* Healthcare Cost and Utilization Project (HCUP)
HCUP data sets, 349-358
  administrative data sets, 350-351
  downloadable statistical programming codes, 357
  KID, 351 (table)
  limitations, 354-355
  list of databases, 351-353 (table)
  NEDS, 352 (table)
  NIS. *See* National Inpatient Sample (NIS)
  NRD, 352 (table)
  P value, 355
  SASD, 353 (table)
  SEDD, 353 (table)
  SID, 352 (table)
  statistical significance, 355-356
  support features, 357
  surveillance bias, 355
  variable that track an individual over time, 357
Health policy evaluation, 371 (table), 372

I

I^2, 288, 291
ICC. *See* Intracluster correlation coefficient (ICC)
ICER. *See* Incremental cost-effectiveness ratio (ICER)
IER. *See* Individual error rate (IER)
Ignorability assumption, 234
Impact inventory, 313
Imputation methods
  mean value imputation, 91, 93
  MI. *See* Multiple imputation (MI)
  random number imputation, 91, 93
  single imputation methods, 154-155, 157
Incremental cost-effectiveness ratio (ICER), 311, 312
Incremental effect, 249. *See also* Marginal effects
Independence of test data, 127
Individual error rate (IER), 138
Information bias, 420
Informed consent, 38
Injury severity score, 355
Intention-to-treat (ITT), 97-103
  basic concepts, 98

Intention-to-treat (ITT) (*continued*)
  bias, 101
  caveats, 101-102
  Glasgow Outcome Scale (GOS), 98, 99
  limitations, 101
  modified intent-to-treat (MITT), 100, 102
  noninferiority trial, 7, 100-101
  per-protocol analysis, 100, 102
  superiority trial, 7
  why is ITT analysis used?, 99-101
Interim analysis. *See* **Early stopping**
Internal validity, 19, 22
Intracluster correlation coefficient (ICC), 29, 31
Inverse probability of treatment weighting, 273
ITT. *See* **Intention-to-treat (ITT)**

J

Joinpoint regression, 364

K

Kaplan-Meier curve, 75-76
Kids' Inpatient Database (KID), 351 (table)

L

Large data sets. *See* **Surgical database research**
Last observation carried forward (LOCF), 90, 93, 94

LIFE trial, 83
Lifetime horizon, 318
Likelihood ratio test, 108
Linear regression methods, 106
LOCF. *See* **Last observation carried forward (LOCF)**
Log odds, 241
Logistic regression, 113-119. *See also* **Logistic regression diagnostics**
  adjustment for confounding factors, 116
  caveats, 118-119
  collinearity, 116, 119
  constant magnitude of association, 116-117
  description of the method, 115-116
  goodness-of-fit tests, 172
  interpretation of study's findings, 117-118
  limitations, 116-117, 241
  marginal effects. *See* Marginal effects
  odds, 115
  odds ratio (OR), 115, 118. *See also* Odds ratio (OR)
  quick Sequential [Sepsis-related] Organ Failure Assessment (qSOFA), 117, 118
  risk ratio (RR), 118
  terminology (predictors/outcome), 115
  value of one predictor altering effect of another (interactions), 119
  why is logistic regression used?, 114-115
  why was logistic regression used in this instance?, 117
Logistic regression diagnostics, 121-128. *See also* **Logistic regression**
  area under the ROC curve (AUROC), 123

C statistic, 123
calibration, 123, 124-125
calibration plot, 125
caveats, 127
deciles of risk, 124
decision curve analysis, 125
description of the method, 123-125
discrimination, 122-123, 123-124
Hosmer-Lemeshow statistic, 125
independence of test data, 127
interpretation of study's findings, 126-127
pseudo-R^2, 125
receiver operating characteristic (ROC) curve, 123
sample size, 125-126
why is regression diagnostics used?, 122-123
why is regression diagnostics used in this instance?, 126
Longitudinal studies, 106. *See also* **Repeated measurements and mixed models**

M

MACE. *See* **Major adverse cardiovascular event (MACE)**
Machine learning, 327 (video). *See also* **Deep learning**
Major adverse cardiovascular event (MACE), 82, 83
Major Trauma Outcomes Study, 416
MAR. *See* **Missing at random (MAR)**
Marginal effects, 247-253
case-control studies, 251
interpretation of study's findings, 252
limitations, 251
odds ratio (OR), 248, 251
risk ratio, 248-249
statistical software, 251
what are marginal effects?, 249-251
why are marginal effects used?, 248-249
MC procedures. *See* **Multiple comparison procedures**
MCAR. *See* **Missing completely at random (MCAR)**
MCID. *See* **Minimal clinically important difference (MCID)**
MDD. *See* **Minimum detectable difference (MDD)**
MDR. *See* **Military Health System Data Repository (MDR)**
Mean value imputation, 91, 93
Mediation analysis, 231-237
bias, 235
caveats, 236
confounding, 235
description of the method, 232-234
limitations, 234-235
no confounding (ignorability) assumption, 234
objective, 234
overview, 233 (figure)
statistical, 232-234
why is mediation analysis used?, 232
why was mediation analysis used in this instance?, 235-236
Medicaid Analytic eXtract data set, 270
Medicare Advantage data, 369
Medicare claims data, 367-374
attributes, 368 (box)
comparative effectiveness research, 370-372, 371 (table)
health policy evaluation, 371 (table), 372

Medicare claims data (*continued*)
limitations, 370
Medicare Advantage data, 369
outcome variations, 371 (table), 372-373
usefulness as research tool, 369
where to find more information, 373
Medication exposure misclassification, 379
Mendelian randomization, 207-213
assumptions, 209
bias, 210
caveats, 212
genetic variants, 208
how was mendelian randomization used in this instance?, 210-212
limitations, 209-210
pleiotropy, 209, 212
statistical power, 210, 212
when is mendelian randomization used?, 209
Meta-analysis, 199-205
bias, 200
consortium paradigm, 204
fixed-effect design, 287, 288, 290
improvements, 202-204
mental health trials, 201, 203
preregistration, 203
PRISMA/PRISMA-P, 203
random-effects. *See* Random-effects meta-analysis
safeguards regarding conflicts of interest, 204
therapeutics research, 201, 204
update/ongoing analysis, 204
Metabolic and Bariatric Surgery Accreditation and Quality Improvement Program (MBSAQIP), 399-406
advantages, 404-405
attributes of MBSAQIP data, 401 (box)
data sets, 403 (table)
deidentification of patients, facilities, and clinicians, 402
limitations, 405
missing data, 404
outcomes, 403-404
participant use file (PUF), 401, 401 (box), 402-403
statistical considerations, 404
MI. *See* **Multiple imputation (MI)**
Military Health System Data Repository (MDR), 377, 378
Military health system Tricare encounter data, 375-382. *See also Tricare data*
Minimal clinically important difference (MCID), 49-55
anchor-based methods, 51, 52
caveats, 54
consensus methods, 51, 52
defined, 50
distribution-based methods, 52, 53
interpretation of study's findings, 53-54
limitations, 52-53
potential improvements vs costs and complications, 54
responder analysis, 54
statistical significance yet effect of intervention smaller than MCID, 54
why is MCID used?, 50-52
why was MCID used in this instance?, 53
WOMAC score, 50, 51
Minimization, 61
Minimum detectable difference (MDD), 44, 45
Missing at random (MAR), 92, 93, 109, 154
Missing completely at random (MCAR), 92, 109, 154
Missing data, 89-95, 110-111
baseline observation carried forward, 90-91
bias, 93
caveats, 94-95
censoring, 92

complete case analysis, 90, 91, 93
factors to consider when selecting method for handling missing values, 91
interpretation of study's findings, 94
last observation carried forward (LOCF), 90, 93, 94
limitations, 93
longitudinal studies. *See* Repeated measurements and mixed models
MBSAQIP, 404
mean value imputation, 91, 93
missing at random (MAR), 92, 93
missing completely at random (MCAR), 92
missing not at random (MNAR), 92
multiple imputation, 91, 94, 95. *See also* Multiple imputation (MI)
National Cancer Database (NCDB), 412
National Trauma Data Bank (NTDB), 420
random number imputation, 91, 93
reasons for "missingness," 90
SEER database, 365
surgical database research, 336 (box), 338, 344
Tricare data, 380
Vascular Quality Initiative (VQI), 427-428
VASQIP, 388-389
Missing not at random (MNAR), 92, 154
MITT. *See* **Modified intent-to-treat (MITT)**
Mixed linear models, 29
MNAR. *See* **Missing not at random (MNAR)**

Modified intent-to-treat (MITT), 100, 102
MOTIV, 138. *See also* **Multiple comparison procedures**
Multicenter clinical trials. *See* **Treatment effects in multicenter trials**
Multiple comparison procedures, 137-144
to adjust or not, 142-143
bias, 144
Bonferroni procedure, 139, 140, 141 (table)
caveats, 142-144
confirmatory vs exploratory studies, 143
definition of family, 144
false discovery rate (FDR), 143
family-wise error rate (FWER), 139, 143
Hochberg sequential procedure, 140, 141 (table)
individual error rate (IER), 138
interpretation of study's findings, 142
limitations, 140
why are MC procedures used?, 138-140
why were MC procedures used in this instance?, 142
Multiple imputation (MI), 91, 94, 95, 153-159
"auxiliary variables," 158
caveats, 158
interpretation of study's findings, 158
limitations, 157
single imputation, distinguished, 156
stages of, 155-156
why is multiple imputation used?, 155-156
why was multiple imputation used in this instance?, 157

N

National Cancer Database (NCDB), 407-413
  analytic and statistical considerations, 411
  best practices, 408 (box)
  bias, 411-412
  confounding, 411-412
  defined, 408
  hospital variables, 409-410
  missing data, 412
  outcomes, 411
  participant use file (PUF), 409
  readmission, 411
  statistical noise, 412
  survival analysis, 411
  "time from diagnosis to treatment" variables, 410
  treatment variables, 410
  tumor characteristics, 410
National Inpatient Sample (NIS), 354
  best practices, 356 (box)
  limitations, 355
  overview, 351 (table)
National Surgical Quality Improvement Program (NSQIP), 391-398
  access and logistics, 393-384
  best practices, 393 (box)
  complication data, 394
  composite morbidity outcomes, 394
  cost effectiveness, 396
  intraoperative factors, 395-396
  limitations, 396
  observed-to-expected event ratios, 395
  participant use file (PUF), 393-394, 397
  pediatric NSQIP (NSQIP-P), 392
  preoperative comorbidities, 394
  statistical methodology, 395
  variables and outcomes, 394
National Trauma Data Bank (NTDB), 415-422
  ACS TQIP, 417-418
  attributes of NTDB data, 417 (box)
  data compilation and structure, 416-418
  data quality, 417-418
  incident-based record, 416-417
  information bias, 420
  limitations, 419-420
  methods, 418-419
  missing data, 420
  mortality, 419
  NTDB Data Manual, 421
  recommendations for further reading, 421
  selection bias, 420
  validation rules, 417
Nationwide Emergency Department Sample (NEDS), 352 (table)
Nationwide Readmissions Database (NRD), 352 (table)
NCDB. *See* **National Cancer Database (NCDB)**
NEDS. *See* **Nationwide Emergency Department Sample (NEDS)**
Negative predictive value (NPV), 303
Nested case-control study, 194, 195. *See also* **Case-control study**
Neural networks, 326
Neutral prior, 170, 173. *See also* **Prior information**
NIS. *See* **National Inpatient Sample (NIS)**
NNT. *See* **Number to treat (NNT)**
No confounding (ignorability) assumption, 234
Noninferiority trials, 1-8
  caveats, 6-7
  determinants of noninferiority margin, 3
  equivalence trial, compared, 5
  how is noninferiority demonstrated?, 5
  intention-to-treat (ITT), 7, 100-101

interpretation of study's findings, 6
known effective treatments as controls, 3
limitations, 5
objective, 3, 5
sample size, 3-4
subjectivity of selection of noninferiority margin, 6
superiority trial, compared, 2-3, 7
why use noninferiority trial in this case?, 5-6
Normal dynamic linear models, 13
NPV. *See* **Negative predictive value (NPV)**
NRD. *See* **Nationwide Readmissions Database (NRD)**
NSQIP. *See* **National Surgical Quality Improvement Program (NSQIP)**
NTDB. *See* **National Trauma Data Bank (NTDB)**
Number needed to save one life, 134
Number to treat (NNT), 129-136
defined, 130
how was NNT applied in this study?, 134-135
interpretation of study's findings, 135
limitations, 132-134
number needed to save one life, 134
what is NNT?, 130-131
why is NNT important?, 131-132

O

O'Brien-Fleming method, 164
Observational data, 192
Observational studies

adjusting for baseline differences, 273
causal language, 336 (box)
confounding, 226, 271
directed acyclic graph, 337, 344
P value, 345
STROBE reporting guidelines, 343
uses, 184, 270
Odds, 115, 240
Odds ratio (OR), 239-245
arbitrary scaling factor, 242, 244
case-control study, 194-196
caveats, 244-245
how were odds ratios used in this instance?, 243-244
interpretation of study's findings, 244
limitations, 242-243
log odds, 241
logistic regression, 115, 118, 239-245
marginal effects, 248, 251
95% confidence intervals, 241, 254
probability/odds, compared, 240
relative risk ratio, 240, 242
uses, 240
Optimistic prior, 170. *See also* **Prior information**
OR. *See* **Odds ratio (OR)**

P

P **value,** 345, 355
Parallel trends assumption, 187
Participant use file (PUF)
MBSAQIP, 401, 401 (box), 402-403
National Cancer Database (NCDB), 409
NSQIP, 393-394, 397
STS National Database, 435-436

Pediatric NSQIP (NSQIP-P), 392
Per-protocol analysis, 100, 102
Permuted blocks and stratified randomization, 57-64
  advantages/benefits, 59-60
  alternatives to stratification, 61
  bias, 60-61
  how were these approaches used?, 61-63
  interpretation of study's findings, 63
  limitations, 60-61
  minimization, 61
  permuted blocks randomization, described, 59
  restricted randomization, 58, 63
  standard error of the treatment effect, 60
  stratified randomization, described, 59
Phase 2 dose-finding studies. *See* **Dose-finding trials**
PICO (Patient, Population, or Problem; Intervention, Prognostic Factor, or Exposure; Comparison or Intervention; Outcome), 335, 336 (box)
Pleiotropy, 209, 212
Positive predictive value (PPV), 303
Power analysis, 41-47
  baseline rate, 43
  caveats, 46
  interpretation of study's findings, 45-46
  limitations, 45
  minimum detectable difference (MDD), 44, 45
  power, defined, 43
  sample size, 45
  why was power analysis used in this instance?, 45
PPV. *See* **Positive predictive value (PPV)**

Practical guides to data sets, 349-438. *See also* **Surgical database research**
Pragmatic-Explanatory Continuum Indicator Summary (PRECIS), 22
Pragmatic trials, 17-23
  blinding, 21
  characteristics features, 19-20
  explanatory trials, 19, 20
  external validity concerns, 21-22
  internal validity concerns, 22
  interpretation of study's findings, 21-23
  limitations, 20-21
  why are pragmatic trials conducted?, 18-19
  why was pragmatic trial used in this instance?, 21
PRECIS. *See* **Pragmatic-Explanatory Continuum Indicator Summary (PRECIS)**
Preferred Reporting Items for Systematic Reviews and Meta-analyses (PRISMA), 203
Preferred Reporting Items for Systematic Reviews and Meta-analyses Protocols (PRISMA-P), 203
Prior information, 169-174
  Bayesian hierarchical model (BHM), 295
  enthusiastic prior, 173
  how was prior information used?, 172-173
  interpretation of study's findings, 173-174
  limitations, 172
  neutral prior, 173
  skeptical prior, 173
  what is it?, 170-171
  why is prior information important?, 171-172

PRISMA. *See* **Preferred Reporting Items for Systematic Reviews and Meta-analyses (PRISMA)**
PRISMA-P. *See* **Preferred Reporting Items for Systematic Reviews and Meta-analyses Protocols (PRISMA-P)**
Propensity score, 227, 271
Propensity score matching, 272, 273, 275
Propensity score methods, 269-276
  caveats, 275
  confounding, 227, 228, 271
  covariate adjustment, 272
  interpretation of study's findings, 274
  inverse probability of treatment weighting, 273
  limitations, 273-274
  methods of using propensity scores, 272-273
  propensity methods often used when randomized trials not feasible, 274
  propensity score, defined, 271
  propensity score matching, 272, 273, 275
  propensity score stratification, 272, 275
  why are propensity methods used?, 270-273
  why were propensity methods used in this instance?, 274
Propensity score stratification, 272, 275
PROSPERO, 203
Proximity criterion, 281
Pseudo-R^2, 125
PUF. *See* **Participant use file (PUF)**
Purchased care, 377, 379

Q

QALYs. *See* **Quality-adjusted life-years (QALYs)**
qSOFA. *See* **Quick Sequential [Sepsis-related] Organ Failure Assessment (qSOFA)**
Quality-adjusted life-years (QALYs), 311-312
Quality-of life-related weights, 314
Quick Sequential [Sepsis-related] Organ Failure Assessment (qSOFA), 117, 118
QUIK trial, 37-38

R

R, 251
Random effects, 107
Random-effects meta-analysis, 285-292
  caveats, 290-291
  DerSimonian-Laird method, 290
  description of the method, 288-289
  fixed-effect design, compared, 287, 288, 290
  heterogeneity, 290, 291
  interpretation of study's findings, 291
  why is random-effects design used?, 286-287
  why was random-effects design used in this instance?, 289-290
Random number imputation, 91, 93
Randomized clinical trial (RCT)
  case-control study, compared, 196

Randomized clinical trial (RCT) (*continued*)
cluster randomized trial, compared, 26. *See also* Clinical trial
confounding, 226
RCT. *See* **Randomized clinical trial (RCT)**
Receiver operating characteristic (ROC) curve, 123, 303
Receiver operating characteristic (ROC) curve analysis, 278, 281. *See also* **Area under the ROC curve (AUROC)**
Regression adjustment, 235
Relative risk ratio, 240, 242
Relative risk (RR), 196
Relative survival, 364, 365
Repeated measurements and mixed models, 105-111
caveats, 110-111
correlation structures, 108
EXACT trial, 106, 110
limitations, 109-110
missing at random (MAR), 109
missing completely at random (MCAR), 109
repeated measures ANOVA, 107, 109
why are mixed models used?, 107-109
why were mixed models used in this instance, 110
Repeated measures ANOVA, 107, 109
Residual confounding, 227, 228
Responder analysis, 54
RESTORE trial, 27-30
Restricted randomization, 58, 63
Risk ratio (RR), 118, 248-249
Robustness analysis, 166
ROC curve. *See* **Receiver operating characteristic (ROC) curve; Receiver operating characteristic (ROC) curve analysis**
RR. *See* **Relative risk (RR); Risk ratio (RR)**

S

Sample size
big data, 342-344
calculation of, for hypothesis test. *See* Power analysis
complete case analysis, 93
logistic regression diagnostics, 125-126
noninferiority trials, 3-4
power analysis, 45
stepped-wedge clinical trial, 35, 36
Vascular Quality Initiative (VQI), 427
SASD. *See* **State Ambulatory Surgery and Services Databases (SASD)**
SEDD. *See* **State Emergency Department Databases (SEDD)**
SEER. *See* **Surveillance, epidemiology, and end results (SEER) database**
Selection bias, 420, 425-426
Self-reporting bias, 437
Sensitivity analysis, 217, 235, 380
Serial gatekeeping, 147. *See also* **Gatekeeping strategies**
Shrinkage estimation, 297
SID. *See* **State Inpatient Database (SID)**
Single imputation methods, 154-155, 157
Skeptical prior, 170, 173. *See also* **Prior information**
Society for Vascular Surgery Vascular Quality Initiative (SVS VQI), 423-429
best practices, 424 (box)
data entry, 425
dedicated data analysts, 426
flow diagram, 427
limitations of data set, 425-426
missing data, 427-428
retrospective analysis, 426

INDEX **483**

sample size, 427
selection bias, 425-426
statistical considerations, 426-428
Vascular Study Group of Greater New York, 426
Society of Thoracic Surgeons (STS) National Database, 431-438
Adult Cardiac Surgery Database (ACSD), 432-434, 437
confounding, 436
Congenital Heart Surgery Database (CHSD), 434, 437
data collection, 434
details of STS National Database, 433 (box)
General Thoracic Surgery Database (GTSD), 434, 437
limitations, 436-437
outcomes and other key measures, 435
participant use file (PUF), 435-436
self-reporting bias, 437
speciality-specific variables, 435
statistical considerations, 436
type 2 errors, 436
SOCRATES-REDUCED trial, 11-13
Spaghetti plots, 111
Spillover, 188-189
Standard error of the treatment effect, 60
Standardized net benefit, 304
State Ambulatory Surgery and Services Databases (SASD), 353 (table)
State Emergency Department Databases (SEDD), 353 (table)
State Inpatient Database (SID), 352 (table)
Statistical mediation analysis, 232-234
Statistical power, 210, 212

Stepped-wedge clinical trial, 33-39
bias, 35
factors to consider in designing stepped-wedge trial, 35
informed consent, 38
interpretation of study's findings, 38
limitations, 36-37
main use, 38
QUIK trial, 37-38
sample size, 35, 36
time dependency concerns, 37
why is stepped-wedge design used?, 34-39
Stopping early. *See* **Early stopping**
Stratified randomization, 59. *See also* **Permuted blocks and stratified randomization**
Strengthening the Reporting of Observational Studies in Epidemiology (STROBE) reporting guidelines, 343
String plots, 111
STROBE. *See* **Strengthening the Reporting of Observational Studies in Epidemiology (STROBE) reporting guidelines**
STS National Database. *See* **Society of Thoracic Surgeons (STS) National Database**
Superiority trial, 2-3, 7
Surgical database research, 333-438
ACS NSQIP, 391-398
bias, 336 (box), 337
causal language, 336 (box), 337
competing risks, 336 (box), 338
data use agreements, 336 (box), 337
directed acyclic graph, 336 (box), 337
early preparation, 336 (box), 337
FINER criteria/PICO format, 335, 336 (box)

Surgical database research (*continued*)
  HCUP databases, 349-358
  inclusion criteria, exclusion criteria, outcome variables, 336 (box), 337
  institutional review board, 336 (box), 337
  list of databases covered, 335 (box)
  literature review, 336 (box), 337
  MBSAQIP, 399-406
  Medicare claims data, 367-374
  military health system Tricare encounter data, 375-382
  missing data, 336 (box), 338, 344
  National Cancer Database (NCDB), 407-413
  National Inpatient Sample (NIS), 349-358
  National Trauma Data Bank (NTDB), 415-422
  SEER data, 359-366
  solid research question and clear hypothesis, 335-337
  statistical tips, 341-347. *See also* Tips for analyzing large data sets
  STS National Database, 431-438
  take-home message, 336 (box), 338
  10-item checklist, 334-338, 336 (box)
  updates or significant changes over time, 336 (box), 337-338
  Vascular Quality Initiative (VQI), 423-429
  VASQIP, 383-390
Surveillance, epidemiology, and end results (SEER) database, 359-366
  cancer data, 362-363
  cancer-specific survival, 365
  Cox proportional hazard model, 365
  data sources, 360, 362
  details of SEER data, 363 (box)
  joinpoint regression, 364
  missing data, 365
  overview, 361-362 (table)
  relative survival, 364, 365
  SEER*Stat software, 364
  survival statistics, 364-365
  time trend data, 362
  treatment data, 364
  trend analysis, 364
  uses, 365
Surveillance bias, 355
Survival analysis, 74. *See also* **Time-to-event analysis**
SVS VQI. *See* **Society for Vascular Surgery Vascular Quality Initiative (SVS VQI)**

T

Thoracic surgery. *See* **Society of Thoracic Surgeons (STS) National Database**
Time horizon in cost-effectiveness analysis, 317-323
  effect of time horizon on interpretation of study, 322
  how was time horizon used in this study?, 321
  lifetime horizon, 318
  limitations, 318-320
  long time horizons, 320-321
  perspective (eg, patient, private or public payer, society), 320
  time horizon, defined, 317
  within-trial horizon, 318
Time-to-event analysis, 73-80
  bias, 75
  caveats, 78-79
  censoring, 75, 77, 78

Cox proportional hazards model, 76-79
hazard function, 74-75, 77
hazard ratio, 76, 78
interpretation of study's findings, 77-78
Kaplan-Meier curve, 75-76
limitations, 77
proportionality assumption, 78, 79 (figure)
why is time-to-event analysis used?, 74-76

Tips for analyzing large data sets, 341-347. *See also* **Surgical database research**
analytic and statistical considerations, 345-346
balancing between amount of information provided and journal space limits, 346
bar graphs, 344
data elements and presentation, 344-345
directed acyclic graph, 344
medical record abstraction, 345
methodological and sample size considerations, 342-344
methods of correction (Bonferroni correction, etc.), 344
missing data, 344
multivariate modeling, 345-346
pie charts, 344
power analysis, 343
predictor variables, 345-346
statistical significance, 343
STROBE reporting guidelines, 343
study population, 342

TPF. *See* **True-positive fraction (TPF)**

TQIP. *See* **Trauma Quality Improvement Program (TQIP)**

Trauma. *See* **National Trauma Data Bank (NTDB)**

Trauma Quality Improvement Program (TQIP), 417-418

Treatment effects in multicenter trials, 261-268
assumptions, 266
considering centers as fixed effects, 265
country-to-country variability, 267
external validity, 266
how were multicenter data analyzed in this study?, 266-267
interpretation of study's findings, 267
limitations, 265-266
uncertainty/independent repetition, 264
why are differences between centers considered?, 263-265

Tricare data, 375-382. *See also* **Veterans Affairs Surgical Quality Improvement Program (VASQIP)**
attributes, 376 (box)
Charlson comorbidity indices, 378
confounding, 380
direct care, 377, 379
how are data compiled?, 377-378
limitations, 379
medication exposure misclassification, 379
Military Health System Data Repository (MDR), 377, 378
missing data, 380
patient race/ethnicity, 380
purchased care, 377, 379
salient and unique features, 377
statistical considerations, 379-380
what common outcomes can be studied?, 378-379

True-positive fraction (TPF), 280, 281

Type 2 errors, 436

U

Unmeasured confounding, 227, 235
Unstructured correlation, 108

V

Vascular Quality Initiative (VQI). *See* **Society for Vascular Surgery Vascular Quality Initiative (SVS VQI)**
Vascular Study Group of Greater New York, 426
VASQIP. *See* **Veterans Affairs Surgical Quality Improvement Program (VASQIP)**
Veterans Affairs Surgical Quality Improvement Program (VASQIP), 383-390
  best practices (box), 385
  data considerations, 384-387
  hospital, 386
  missing data, 388-389
  outcomes, 387
  patients, 386
  procedure, 386
  statistical considerations, 388-389
  unique features, 387
VQI. *See* **Society for Vascular Surgery Vascular Quality Initiative (SVS VQI)**

W

Western Ontario and McMaster Universities Osteoarthritis Index (WOMAC score), 50, 51
Wilcoxon rank sum test, 75
Within-trial horizon, 318-319
WOMAC score. *See* **Western Ontario and McMaster Universities Osteoarthritis Index (WOMAC score)**

www.ingramcontent.com/pod-product-compliance
Lightning Source LLC
Chambersburg PA
CBHW060817170526
45158CB00001B/8